T0331005

China and the Globalization of Biomedicine

Rochester Studies in Medical History

Series Editor: Christopher Crenner
Robert Hudson and Ralph Major Professor and Chair
Department of History and Philosophy of Medicine
University of Kansas School of Medicine

Additional Titles of Interest

A complete list of titles in the Rochester Studies in Medical History series
may be found on our website, www.urpress.com.

China and
the Globalization
of Biomedicine

EDITED BY DAVID LUESINK,
WILLIAM H. SCHNEIDER, AND ZHANG DAQING

UNIVERSITY OF ROCHESTER PRESS

First published 2019

University of Rochester Press
668 Mt. Hope Avenue, Rochester, NY 14620, USA
www.urpress.com
and Boydell & Brewer Limited
PO Box 9, Woodbridge, Suffolk IP12 3DF, UK
www.boydellandbrewer.com

ISBN-13: 978-1-58046-942-5
ISSN: 1526-2715

Library of Congress Cataloging-in-Publication Data

Names: Luesink, David, 1974– editor. | Schneider, William H. (William Howard), 1945– editor. | Zhang, Daqing, 1959– editor.
Title: China and the globalization of biomedicine / edited by David Luesink, William H. Schneider, and Zhang Daqing.
Description: Rochester, NY : University of Rochester Press, 2019. | Series: Rochester studies in medical history, ISSN 1526-2715 ; vol. 45 | Includes bibliographical references and index.
Identifiers: LCCN 2019003201 | ISBN 9781580469425 (hardcover : alk. paper)
Subjects: LCSH: Medicine—China—History—19th century. | Medicine—China—History—20th century. | Medicine—Research—China—History. | Medical policy—China—History. | World health—History.
Classification: LCC R602 | DDC 610.951—dc23 LC record available at https://lccn.loc.gov/2019003201

This publication is printed on acid-free paper.
Printed in the United States of America.

This book is dedicated to all of those who built a system of health care in China—both foreign and Chinese, both health care workers and patients, both politicians and NGOs.

Contents

Part One. Hygiene and Disease Construction in Late Qing China

Part Two. The Indigenization of Biomedicine in Republican China

Illustrations

Figures

Tables

Preface

On a summer day at twilight in 2009, I sat with William Schneider at a coffee shop in Budapest during the Twenty-third International Congress of History of Science, Technology, and Medicine discussing the state of historical research on the global spread and exchange of modern medical technology. We agreed that there remains much work to do researching the history of medicine in modern China, and especially that there are many primary sources, hospital reports, and medical journals that have not been fully explored and utilized. Beginning in the mid-nineteenth century, medical missionaries practiced Western medicine in China and became important disseminators and practitioners. In the process, they left behind plentiful historical documentary sources—correspondence, diaries, and official reports—scattered in the libraries and archives of, among others, Chinese, American, British, and Canadian churches, universities, and hospitals. All of these, we agreed, should be systematically organized and completely researched, so we proposed collaborating to apply for a research grant that would address these lacunae.

On the strength of Bill Schneider's great efforts, the grant proposal gained the active support of the Luce Foundation, which first agreed to support preliminary research in order to prepare for the formal beginning of the project. On October 28–29, 2010, Peking University Medical History Center and Indiana University Philanthropy Center held an academic discussion conference called "Western Medicine and Philanthropy in China: History and Archive." Schneider and I each introduced a tentative overall plan and important research content for the project, while Martha Smalley introduced archival documents from Yale University Divinity School's library and archives collections about the missionary medical schools and universities in China; Xu Jinhua introduced the collections at the Shanghai Xujiahui Library that included documents on foreign medicine; Dang Yuewu introduced an outline of the complete collections of West China Union University Medical School, located at Sichuan University Archives; Zhang Xia and an American representative of the Chinese Medical Board introduced Peking Union Medical College and its associated records at the Rockefeller Archive Center; and Peng Jianping presented on the condition of collections at Sun Yat-sen University Medical School's Historical Archives. In addition, conference attendees presented reports on Suzhou's Boxi Hospital, Beihai's

Pokhai (Puren) Hospital, Guilin's Daosheng Hospital, and the early history and archives of several other Christian hospitals. Participants agreed to participate in the research project on the history of Western medicine in China and discussed what the next steps would be to make it happen. Suzhou University's Wang Guoping's passionate support ensured that the meeting organization proceeded smoothly, and he also organized a visit for all participants to the former site of Boxi Hospital, and its affiliated hospital and missionary graveyard. After the meeting concluded, participants also proceeded to Shanghai to tour the rich collection of documents on Western medicine collected at the Xujiahui Library, all of which left a deep impression.

When the Luce project officially began in 2011, participating Chinese archivists and historians came from Peking University Health's Science Center, Sichuan University's West China Medical Center, Sun Yat-sen Medical School, South Central University Hsiang-Ya Medical School, Peking Union Medical College, Fudan University, and others. North American archivists and scholars were affiliated with the Burke Library (Columbia University Libraries) at Union Theological Seminary, New York City; Harvard University; Presbyterian Historical Society; Rockefeller Archive Center; United Church of Canada Archives, Toronto; and United Methodist Archives, Yale University. This project's most important mission was to establish an open-access Internet database collecting information about the dissemination and development of Western medicine in China, both to make research access for historians more convenient and to promote accessibility of archives to a larger community in China and abroad. Important historical documents for the use of researchers include those chronicling the activities of medical missionaries and the Rockefeller Foundation, Chinese modern public health records, government documents, and hospital and medical school organizational archives. This website and database have been active for several years, hosted by the University Library of Indiana University–Purdue University Indianapolis at the following URL: http://ulib.iupui.edu/wmicproject/.

The project's other mission was to hold two conferences on the theme of Western medicine in China up to 1949, the first in June 2012 at IUPUI and the second in June 2013 at Peking University's Health Science Center. Participants at the conferences included archivists and historians from China, the United States, United Kingdom, Canada, Russia, Australia, Spain, and Singapore, as well as from Hong Kong and Taiwan. Participants presented historical studies on modern Chinese public health enterprises, analysis of the world of foreign medical workers in China, the origins and development of Chinese modern medical education, the perspective of female medical workers, Western medicine's early approach to the physician-patient relationship, the conflict between Chinese and Western medicine, the development of modern psychiatry in China, and other subjects.

This book is therefore a compilation of papers from the conferences that authors have spent significant time revising afterward.

The book moves scholarship forward by not presenting the transfer of Western medical knowledge to China as unidirectional, but instead emphasizing important instances from the nineteenth and twentieth centuries where knowledge created in semicolonial China influenced medicine in the universities and medical schools of Europe and America. I hope the publication of this book will entice more scholars to pay attention to historical research on the dissemination and development of Western medicine in China.

Zhang Daqing, 2018

Acknowledgments

This book has been many years in the making and so we, the editors, have amassed a long list of people without whom we would not have been able to complete it. Most importantly, the editors thank the authors for their patience and enthusiasm throughout the process. We would like to thank all members of the Program of the Medical Humanities at IUPUI and Peking University's Health Science Center Medical Humanities Research Center for logistical and moral support. We would also like to thank all of those, too many to mention here, who participated in the 2012 Indianapolis Workshop and the 2013 Peking Conference—altogether well over 50 presenters and many more support staff who made these conversations between Anglophone and Sinophone scholars a reality. Finally, the project and book would not have been possible without major financial support from the Henry Luce Foundation (especially Mary Brown Bullock and Helena Kolenda), the Rockefeller Archive Center, Indiana University's New Frontiers in the Arts and Humanities funding program, and the Office of the Vice Chancellor for Research and the School of Liberal Arts at Indiana University Purdue University Indianapolis.

Abbreviations

ABMAC	American Bureau for Medical Aid to China
CCP	Chinese Communist Party
CHC	County Health Center
CMA	Chinese Medical Association (1932–present)
CMMJ	*China Medical Missionary Journal*
CMPA	China Medical and Pharmaceutical Association
GMD	Guomindang (Nationalist Party)
NEPB	National Epidemic Prevention Bureau
NHA	National Health Association
NMAC	National Medical Association of China (1915–32)
NMC	National Medical College
PRC	People's Republic of China
PUMC	Peking Union Medical College (1927–45); *also* Peiping Union Medical College
SPHA	Sichuan Provincial Health Administration
TABC	combined cholera-typhoid vaccine
WHO	World Health Organization

Introduction

China and the Globalization of Biomedicine

DAVID LUESINK

This volume studies China-based biomedical work and its contribution to the common knowledge and practice of global biomedicine before the 1949 Communist Revolution. The basic contention of this book is that China was not merely a destination for biomedical knowledge and practice from elsewhere but was a fundamental site in the creation of biomedicine. In 1939, the prominent American pathologist Eugene L. Opie wrote the introduction for a special issue of the *Chinese Medical Journal* arguing that medical science produced in China and published in the issue demonstrated that Chinese physicians trained in the methods of Western medical science were addressing both "conditions particular to China" and also "fundamental problems of pathology and clinical medicine."[1] This book takes a much wider scope to examine the impact biomedicine had on Chinese society and the impact Chinese society had on biomedicine. It demonstrates that Chinese and foreign physicians based in China pursued research and practiced medicine relevant to China's particularities and also basic to experimental and clinical medicine around the world. China was unique because of the enormous scale of the problems of disease and medical delivery encountered by those who sought to establish a medical system as part of a modern state.

By the 1930s and 1940s, China's attempts to provide preventive and curative medical care for its citizens became an issue of international interest and a key policy problem for Chinese medical reformers like Robert K. Lim (Lin Kecheng) and C. C. Chen (Chen Zhiqian), encouraged by international observers who suggested that China might be a model for the world if it could bring health care to its people at a cost that could be borne through modest per capita government expenditures. As Henry S. Houghton of the Rockefeller Foundation put it, "If the Chinese Government can solve the problem of adjusting competent medical and nursing care to a sum total so that society can afford to pay, it will earn the grateful praise of a troubled world."[2] Certainly China took advantage of medical ideas and practices produced elsewhere, but it was also a laboratory for a new kind of state-based social medicine established to serve the people and not just the interests of physicians.

China's long "century of humiliation" from 1839 to 1949 covered in this volume coincides with the high point of capitalist imperialism in Asia, from the Opium Wars and treaty ports to Japanese occupation of the northeast and much of coastal China. Medicine was a tool of empire, even if China itself was never fully colonized by Britain, Russia, France, or Japan. Medicine helped soldiers survive who were sent to fight for imperial interests, and it cured merchants and missionaries bearing the messages of free trade and Christianity, thus playing an important part in the propaganda of Europe's "civilizing mission" to the world. In response, the Qing and Republican state used the new medicine as a tool to maintain and regain sovereignty. The power of Euro-American medicine was sometimes benign and sometimes malignant in the conflicting and often aligned goals of individuals and communities, or of imperialists and modern state-builders.

This volume originated in two international conferences held in Indianapolis in 2012 and Beijing in 2013 where many papers provided evidence of the power and complex ecology of biomedicine and public health in China between 1800 and 1949. The eight chapters of new research that follow in this volume demonstrate how this power was played out in tensions between the following sets of interests: those of governing regimes seeking health sovereignty versus those of individuals; biomedical versus traditional Chinese conceptions of disease; the use of medical knowledge and institutions to establish Chinese sovereignty vis-à-vis foreign encroachments; competition between physicians trained in the Anglo-American versus German-Japanese style; male versus female physicians; state ambition to establish health care for all Chinese versus the limitations of personnel and budget; and finally, efforts to spread the discipline, technology, and organization of modern medicine and public health to southwest China during the war even as conditions seemed most inhospitable for so doing. The question of biomedicine being part of imperialism and state power is the first major interpretive issue this volume addresses.

A second major interpretive issue addressed is the view that medical science was created in Europe and America, and then transferred more or less successfully to China. The contributions here add to a substantial literature that challenges and revises the technology-transfer model that valorizes medical progress in Germany, France, Great Britain, or the United States and then glosses over the colonial and semicolonial uses of modern medical science. This volume builds on other scholarly treatments that show how the knowledge and practice of medicine—as well as medical institutions themselves—were *remade* in the encounter with realities on the ground out-side the medical metropole.[3] There are numerous examples in the chapters below of how local Chinese conditions forced selective adaptation and accommodation (the easier argument to make), yet also of how medical realities encountered and addressed in China had an impact around the world and helped shape medicine in London, Paris, Berlin, and New York. As such this is a project critical of implicit Eurocentrism in studies of modern medicine. We reject the notion, explicit or not, that biomedicine was (and is) created in the laboratories of Euro-American centers and merely transferred to imperial peripheries, or that colonial medical science was "derivative, instrumentalist, and exploitative, with colonial scientists seen as mere fact gatherers, making few theoretical contributions in their own right."[4] Toward this end, we ask two questions: What role did medical work conducted in China actively play in the construction of global biomedicine? At the same time, how did this form of medicine, emanating at once from institutions both outside of and within China, reshape the polity of late Qing and Republican China, and the bodies and experiences of Chinese people themselves?

The contributions here provide evidence that biomedicine was not merely produced elsewhere to be consumed in China, but rather that medicine and even diseases themselves were coproduced at multiple sites partly despite, and partly because of, the unequal power relations between them. This introductory essay examines the historical context in which biomedicine came to exist in China. Key to that context is European, American, and Japanese imperialism, which is a historical precursor of neoliberal globalization today. It then asks what this rapidly changing medicine had to offer Chinese patients and nation-builders. The argument is built on a survey of the growing literature on this topic in English and Chinese, in order to situate the contributions of the essays that follow. Finally, each of the chapters is introduced and then an argument is made for the contributions of the volume as a whole.

Evaluating Europe and America
as Sources of Biomedicine

If you ask most Chinese about the source of biomedicine in China, they will usually say that it came from Euro-America (*ou-mei*).[5] If you ask in Chinese, the very words you will be using will indicate that this is *Western* medicine (*xiyi*) as opposed to Chinese medicine (*zhongyi*). In fact, this commonplace understanding is not so different from the assumption of contemporary health providers and even some historians of Euro-American medicine. A crude statement of that assumption is this: biomedicine was and continues to be largely created in Europe and America, and is then transferred around the world as a result of globalization.[6] A more nuanced argument for the technology-transfer thesis would acknowledge the give and take of local negotiations as biomedicine has grown around the world,[7] but that the United States and Europe were, and continue to be, the location of the most prestigious hospitals and medical schools that attract students and residents from around the world, and so are also the origin of most published research and scientific discoveries. The result is that studies of biomedicine in Europe and America are taken to be of both local and worldwide importance, while those outside of these areas are merely of local interest. Historians of medicine have questioned the idea that biomedicine is an untarnished benefit of civilization as it was transferred in colonial settings, but the history of the role of the "non-West" in the development of biomedicine has tended to be omitted or slighted.[8]

There are good reasons for the Eurocentric perspective. These are rooted in an analysis of the wealth and power of Euro-American medical institutions for the past two hundred years. When researchers and practitioners in Western Europe and North America accumulated enough knowledge of anatomy, physiology, chemistry, and physics, they were able to understand the workings of the human body and its illnesses in a fundamentally new and effective way. They also developed increasingly sophisticated statistical analyses of human populations that produced the field of public health, which was always at the service of state and empire. These rapidly changing disciplines at once increased the gaze of medicine inwardly, reductively to the microscopic and molecular level, as well as outwardly, simultaneously aggregating beyond the individual patient to the macro level of the city and nation. These changes were based in impressive institutions that included hospitals, medical schools, pharmaceutical companies, and government and nongovernmental public health organizations. In the nineteenth and twentieth centuries the growing complexity and power of the biomedical professions and the institutions they controlled, combined with increasing links between public health and the nation-state and a belief in the endless progress and capacity of industrial civilization, gave Euro-American physicians in China and around the world confidence about the superiority of their form of medicine. But we must not take their word for it.

The miracles of twenty-first-century medicine are largely based in the development of antibiotics during and after World War II.[9] True, Western surgery had made great advances by the mid-nineteenth century in emergencies and removal of external tumors, thanks to detailed anatomical knowledge. The discovery of anesthesia and antisepsis by the end of the century, also allowed many more surgical cases to survive. Yet histories of Western medicine have had a tendency to project backward to the prewar period this overwhelming curative power of biomedicine against infectious diseases.

Lewis Thomas, prominent physician and mid-twentieth century author, reminds us that this is a false assumption that is fundamentally ahistorical. In his memoirs, Thomas describes in great detail the limits of a medicine previously devoted primarily to diagnosis before World War II: "it gradually dawned on us that we didn't know much that was really useful, that we could do nothing to change the course of the great majority of the diseases we were so busy analyzing, that medicine, for all its façade as a learned profession, was in real life a profoundly ignorant occupation."[10] Thomas McKeown, also arguing from inside the medical establishment in the postwar period, provided much research to back up the anecdotes of Thomas and argued that the population growth in Britain since the late eighteenth century had little or nothing to do with medical interventions and much to do with improved nutrition.[11] If we accept these limits on what Western medicine had to offer until the mid-twentieth century, why would this "profoundly ignorant" profession spread so inexorably around the world in the nineteenth and early twentieth centuries before antibiotics? If it was not obvious curative power, there must have been power of another kind, and diagnostic power can be only part of the answer. Roy Porter sees the ongoing spread around the world of this form of medicine since the nineteenth century as largely due to "western political and economic domination." Although it had become effective in diagnosing disease, this power grew "largely independent of its efficacy as a rational social approach to good health."[12] This medicine—with all its strengths and weaknesses for identifying disease and improving the health of people—spread around the world, and to China, along with European, American, and Japanese imperialism. Its spread was then indigenized as part of China's attempt to regain sovereignty over its territory and population from those very forces of imperialism.

Western medicine, from 1800 to 1945, developed in conjunction with, and sometimes in opposition to, the military, cultural, and economic violence of imperialism. Imperialist wars and subsequent "free" trade ensured the rapid transfer of disease from one port to another, what Emanuel Le Roy Ladurie has called "the unification of the globe by disease," and Alfred Crosby has called Europe's "ecological imperialism."[13] Meanwhile, dislocation of traditional economies saw the movement of colonized and semicolonized people to towns and urban centers where in the aggregate—statistical thinking about the population became essential to the new medicine—they were seen to be a reservoir of disease.[14] The phrase "tropical medicine" was coined in one of these new cities, Hong Kong, by Patrick Manson, who served as the imperial customs medical officer. The plague bacillus was codiscovered, also in Hong Kong, by Alexandre Yersin and Shibasaburo Kitasato. Major advances in understanding the pneumonic form of plague resulted from two epidemics and a Chinese state antiplague organization, the Manchurian Plague Prevention Service, led by Wu Lien-teh. If Manson and Yersin were representatives of Europeans pursuing scientific goals, Kitasato and Wu deserve a place for Japan and China at the international table of globalizing imperial medicine.[15] All of these medical discoveries were made in colonial and semicolonial enclaves of China.

Equally important is to recognize how the pharmacology of modern biomedicine was formed by colonial practices of botanical collecting since the eighteenth century, a process now often referred to as bioprospecting. Long before the eighteenth century, in medieval monasteries and university towns, Europeans established thousands of botanical gardens and gradually developed a standardized nomenclature to identify these plants. In a second phase, following Lavoisier's chemical revolution, they began to identify and standardize the chemically active agents, such as in the case of cinchona extracted as quinine, that gave birth to the modern pharmaceutical industry.[16] Fa-Ti Fan has described in great detail how British naturalists in nineteenth-century China created a translated pharmacological knowledge in conjunction with a large network of Chinese collectors, informants, and interlocutors.[17] Sean Hsiang-lin Lei has described the process of how Chinese pharmaceuticals, like the antimalarial *changshan*, could be renetworked into biomedical pharmaceutical networks.[18] So we can say that China contributed to the making of biomedicine through this unequal exchange of botanical and pharmaceutical knowledge.

Some of the best work in the history of medicine today examines just how much the context of imperialism and colonialism shaped medicine at home in Europe and America, just as nonmedical work is demonstrating how much British, French, German, or American history in the nineteenth and twentieth centuries was shaped by their colonial and neocolonial projects.[19] There is no doubt that the Euro-American metropole shaped the periphery, but it is now becoming clear how much the periphery shaped the imperial centers as well. The situation only becomes more complex when we begin to consider the role of Japan as a late-coming imperial medical power in East Asia.[20]

Yet a history of medicine as merely cultural imperialism ignores the degree to which Western medical therapies and forms of knowledge were desired by Chinese actors for their own purposes. The reality of medical and public health imperialism in China must be examined along with a perspective that allows us to see how successive Chinese government bodies and elites like their Western counterparts pursued strategies to employ medicine for state and other goals. Furthermore, the conditions of imperialism in China initiated immense dislocation and misery, which were compounded by longstanding patterns of human-made and natural disaster.[21] Organized medical interventions could bring temporary and long-term relief, as well as prevention, to millions of Chinese individuals. It is difficult to untangle the acquisition of biomedicine by the Chinese from its imposition on them, but recent analysis that examines both offers the most productive path forward. The next section offers a brief, if incomplete, narrative of the relationship between medicine and politics in China during the long century of imperialist influence that is useful for understanding the interpretation of the historical literature and the intervention of the authors of the chapters to follow.

A Political History of the Development of Biomedicine in China

Before and during the rapid expansion of Euro-American medicine, between the 1830s and 1949, a number of physicians trained in Euro-American institutions established medical practices in China. Qing China (1644–1912) had expelled most foreign missionaries after the Rites Controversy of the early eighteenth century, and merchants and missionaries were restricted to Portuguese-controlled Macao and a tiny island outside the city walls of Guangzhou. In 1793, a British diplomatic mission unsuccessfully attempted to persuade the Qianlong emperor to dissolve the Chinese-dominated embassy system and join the European system of international relations. With much of the world's silver still flowing into China in exchange for silk, porcelain, and tea, Europe had no choice but to accept the limits of the Chinese system.[22] Between the 1790s and 1830s, however, opium produced in British India reversed the flow of silver. Dutch and English traders laced tobacco with opium to produce *madak*—a remarkably potent substance. By the nineteenth century this drug—with such great medical potential as a pain reliever—became widely used, recreationally, at all levels of Chinese society, but it was also disastrously addictive. Official corruption and a series of civil wars in the very heartland of the Qing Empire led to despair among the poor and cynicism among the elite—perfect conditions for a new culture of drug dependency.[23] When the Qing government decided to exercise its sovereign prerogative to enforce a law prohibiting opium by destroying twenty thousand chests of illegal opium, the British responded with war. Brand-new, industrially produced military technology led to Chinese defeat and the first of many unequal treaties and massive indemnities, which, among other things, gave Western medicine a foothold in China.[24]

After the occupation of the Qing capital of Beijing in the climax of the Second Opium War of 1856–60, the British forced the establishment of a Chinese Imperial Customs Service to ensure regular repayment of the new indemnities. This Customs Service also produced regular medical reports.[25] The increasingly onerous unequal treaties also had clauses written into them that allowed foreigners to open hospitals and similar institutions.[26] If philanthropic supporters of this work in the United States or Britain thought it benign, anti-imperialist Chinese nationalists did not: "The strength of imperialism is to anaesthetize the Chinese people's spirit and not let go, this is their method of cultural aggression," Mao Zedong later said, "[s]preading their religion, establishing hospitals, establishing schools, establishing newspapers and attracting students to study abroad, this was their policy of aggression in action."[27] Sympathetic Western scholars have generally agreed. Christian missionaries first sought to use medicine to advance evangelism, but eventually medical care became its own end as part of a larger "civilizing mission" of Euro-American culture that sought to remake China in its own image.[28] Historians have argued that these medical missionaries who set out to change China were driven by arrogance in their belief that they carried a superior religion, culture, and form of medicine. Jonathan Spence has argued that the medical missionaries "were sure that their own civilization, whatever its shortcomings, had given them something valid to offer, something that China lacked . . . and [f]or the Chinese to protest against this made no sense, since it was self-evident."[29] As late as the 1920s, missionaries grossly overestimated the curative power of medicine in the West while underestimating that of Chinese medicine. The medical missionary Edward Merrins wrote in 1924, for example, that China's "medicine has always been very backward," while in the West "medicine has been much more fortunate from the very earliest times."[30]

Yet the historical record is clear that the limited accomplishments of medical missions were made through adaptation to local conditions, cooperation with local elites, and free service to the poor. As Bridie Andrews has argued, for missionaries attempting to practice medicine before the Republic of China, "medicine turned out to be not so much a marker of cultural difference as a tool for reducing the perception of alterity."[31] Peter Parker, the first American medical missionary working before the revolutionary developments of biomedicine described above, realized that his medicine was only an advance on Chinese medicine in two skills: eye surgery and external surgical removal of tumors. This led to the popular Chinese view that Western medicine was good for external medicine, while Chinese medicine was better for internal medicine. Even the hospital—that most basic institution of medical power of the nineteenth and twentieth centuries—had to be adapted to Chinese realities.[32] In the immediate decades after the opening of hospitals in the nineteenth century, rumors of missionaries conducting black magic in their medical spaces demonstrated the degree to which missionaries showed both too much and too little of their strange spaces to Chinese.[33] Among more than eight hundred antimissionary cases recorded in nineteenth-century China, many resulted from rumors related to medical practice.[34] The violence against missionaries, in turn, led to a structural reaction embedded in treaty terms that eroded Qing sovereignty, the power of local elites, and the economic viability of existing tradespeople and laborers.[35]

At this same time, a few Chinese began medical training in Europe and the United States, the first being Wong Fun (Huang Kuan), who graduated from Edinburgh University around 1853. He came back to China as a missionary under the auspices of the London Missionary Society and then moved to a series of positions in government and private practice, followed by a teaching position at the Canton Hospital, where missionary John Kerr praised Wong's competent and independent leadership of the Chinese staff of surgeons who together conducted a record number of surgical operations.[36] Later, in 1896, two women, Kang Cheng (Ida Kahn) and Shi Meiyu (Mary Stone), opened a small clinic for women and children that inspired generations of Chinese women to enter the medical profession.[37] But most Chinese trained by missionaries until the first decade of the twentieth century were trained merely to become assistants. A major problem was that medicine as a full-time profession was not respected in China. Few elite Chinese men would enter the field of medicine to support themselves, and most practitioners were either of low status or practiced as an avocation for their friends.[38]

There were notable but limited exceptions. The Self-Strengthening movement among Chinese elites in the 1860s–1890s led to the adaptation of military and scientific technology and some acceptance of medical ideas through new government-sponsored translation bureaus in Shanghai and Fuzhou. There was also some elite interest in the Chinese-language anatomical works of Benjamin Hobson (1850) and John Dudgeon (1885).[39] But by 1895 this movement seemed a complete failure to a new generation of gentry elite who were in Beijing for the triennial examinations when the Treaty of Shimonoseki forced the Qing Empire to accept humiliating terms from tiny Japan. The longstanding elite preference for neo-Confucian orthodoxy withered, and the shift was institutionalized when the imperial examination system was abolished in 1905, thus leaving a vacuum in the production of officials. This vacuum was gradually filled by students returning from overseas study who adapted and transplanted the educational systems of Germany, Japan (which was based on the German system), and the United States. Some of these elites studied medicine and began to challenge foreign leadership in the medical arena, even while they were divided into Anglo-American and German-Japanese camps based on the languages and institutional priorities of their training. What most of the new elite physicians did agree on, however, was that medicine, once a tool of imperialism, must now become a tool of state building. Even private philanthropic and missionary medicine needed to increasingly fall in line with the goals of state health programs.

The last years of the Qing dynasty and early years of the Republic were decisive in establishing systems for major health interventions in China. In the British colony of Hong Kong in the 1890s, the appearance of plague led to an end of the British laissez-faire approach to quarantine and the onset of invasive and even violent enforcement, while also launching the international careers of several scientists, such as Shibasaburo Kitasato, who became Japan's leading bacteriologist.[40] War with Japan in 1894–95 led to the province of Taiwan becoming a colony of Japan, while the Russo-Japanese War of 1904–5 over influence in Korea and its hinterland of Manchuria, led directly to the plague epidemic there in 1910–11. Both the Russians who controlled the city of Harbin in the north of Manchuria and the Japanese who controlled railway lines farther south where the plague was spreading, increasingly functioned like modern colonial rulers, and Western-trained politicians in Beijing saw that the Qing government's assertion of its ability to control the plague was directly tied to sovereignty. Cambridge-educated bacteriologist Wu Lien-teh's leadership of the medical and political situation stopped the spread of the epidemic through repressive police measures and mass incineration of plague corpses.[41] Cremation was a radical change for China, as Wu would later write to a friend, "for the first time in our history, I have obtained permission in getting the Imperial Consent of the burning of bodies and post-mortems. In other words, history is being made, and a proper independent medical profession will be a mere matter of time."[42] Wu held an international plague conference in Harbin to demonstrate Chinese mastery of the outbreak, then he established the Manchurian Plague Prevention Service in Harbin as the beachhead for further government public health and medical research institutes.

Despite the internationally recognized success of these measures, other countries now firmly associated plague and disease with China. Long the cultural and economic envy of the world, China was now carved up into zones of imperialist influence and called "the Sick Man of East Asia." This phrase, in both English and Chinese, then became a metaphor applied to the health of China's people.[43] Even as the writer Yan Fu translated the social Darwinian writings of Herbert Spencer, and as European powers scrambled to control every square mile of the globe that could not defend itself against their Maxim guns, Chinese intellectuals saw Confucian China as unable to meet the challenges of industrial capitalist imperialism. Japan had quickly learned the essence of political power from the West, within a few decades throwing off its own unequal treaties with the Western powers. So despite its own military aggression toward Qing China, Japan became a model and a haven for reformers like Liang Qichao and revolutionaries like the medically trained Sun Yat-sen. A growing number of young elites, many sponsored by the Qing government, flocked to Japan to study and learn the lessons of how to marry science, technology, medicine, and industry to give birth to a powerful state and army, or *fukoku kyōhei*. Physicians like Gotō Shinpei played key political roles in Japan's twin processes of modernization and colonization, in his case in Taiwan, Manchuria, and Tokyo.[44] Many Chinese medical students in Japan, such as Tang Erhe, became involved in anti-Qing movements and participated directly in the 1911 Revolution and postrevolutionary attempts to set up a constitutional government.[45] Yet when Qing military strongman Yuan Shikai took up the presidency and disbanded the legislature and finally rejected Republicanism by declaring himself emperor, despair about China's weakness became even more widespread. After Yuan's death in 1916, the Beijing government was controlled by a revolving set of warlords, while many provinces were run as independent fiefdoms. Attempts to bring Japanese-style medical reforms under these conditions were mostly unsuccessful.

The late Qing and early Republic saw new roles for women in society, and this included medicine. If missionaries (both American and Chinese) created new spaces for women and women's work in their institutions, elite women and elite men argued that China could never be strong if women's feet were bound and if women did not receive education and have equal rights to marry and divorce as men, or have careers outside the home.[46] Urban institutions of higher learning and the new professions allowed some space for women, although in health this was often limited to gendered roles like nursing, midwifery, and obstetrics and gynecology.[47] Yet even enlightened males tended to think they had a right to speak for women, and while women did have an increased role in the public sphere, they tended to be subordinated to men in modern institutions. For example, the new profession of nursing that in China had begun exclusively male soon became gendered as female.

Cultural changes more favorable to biomedicine intensified as a result of political changes. When, in 1919, diplomatic promises to return German holdings in Shandong to Chinese sovereignty were betrayed in favor of giving these to Japan at the Versailles Peace Conference, students in China began protesting against the Beijing government's acceptance of the treaty. The beginning of active student movements and nationalism built on a larger "New Culture" movement that rejected Confucianism and Chinese medical and scientific ideas completely while embracing science from the West. In the radical journal *Xin Qingnian* (*New Youth*), Communist Party cofounder Chen Duxiu argued that "if the old and rotten elements fill society, then it will cease to exist," while the writer Lu Xun memorably described Confucian society as cannibalistic, and the physician-politician Tang Erhe castigated practitioners of Chinese medicine as superstitious and ignorant.[48] Debates ensued about whether European science and technology—having just obliterated millions of young men in the mud of France—were actually a force for progress in the world. Could science successfully create a new Chinese spirit or would it just destroy the old one? But elites increasingly accepted the materialist terms of scientific and industrial society. The old Chinese medicine appeared weak, disorganized, and apolitical, while the

new scientific medicine revealed itself as dynamic and expedient for building state power and (re)establishing sovereignty.

All of these changes played out in a growing public sphere thanks to an
explosion of print media that included daily newspapers, weeklies, radical
periodicals, and professional journals in which health and medicine issues
were increasingly prominent. Journals for women and youth often had regular columns devoted to medical advice. Advertisements for patent medicines jostled with advertisements for cosmetics or famous physicians. Some
medical titles were tied to professional associations, like the *National Medical
Journal* of the National Medical Association, or the *Journal of the Republic of
China Medico-Pharmaceutical Association.* Others tried to mix Chinese and
Western medicine, or sought to organize Chinese medicine along increasingly professional lines in response to pressures from professionalizing physicians of Western medicine.[49]

The end of the Qing dynasty also saw the birth of the first Western-style
medical schools in China. Nineteenth-century efforts at medical education
"on a humble scale" included the training of assistants in Guangzhou and
a more rigorous program in Tianjin after 1881 and in Hong Kong after
1887.[50] Attempting to raise standards, Protestant missionaries formed union
medical colleges by pooling resources and staff. An influx of Rockefeller
Foundation grants by the 1910s accompanied a second round of consolidation in key centers like Guangzhou, Jinan, and Chengdu, while the
Rockefeller Foundation set up its own world-class medical school after purchasing the missionary union medical school in Beijing.[51] Government medical schools also sprang up, although after the opening of the Peking Union
Medical College (PUMC) in Beijing in 1921, they all tended to fall under its
enormous shadow.[52] These government schools were part of a larger expansion of modern education to replace the imperial examination system. Yet,
for all the expense of a medical education, physicians could only make a
desirable income in major cities. In the Republican period, up to half of
all modern-trained Chinese physicians practiced in Shanghai, where wealthy
Chinese and foreign patients could support a bourgeois professional lifestyle. Few rural areas could support even basic food and housing for a full-
time physician and family, and only missionaries or Chinese supported by
income from abroad could afford to work in the vast countryside where
most Chinese lived. The "rural problem" thus became key to the goal of
health sovereignty.

But medical policies did begin to address rural health in the 1920s and
1930s in a fast-shifting political environment that can be understood as a tale
of two political parties.[53] Providing health for ordinary people became part
of the governing logic of both the Nationalist and the Communist regimes.
In the 1920s a new revolutionary movement led by Dr. Sun Yat-sen and the
Nationalist Party established itself in Guangzhou, and after his death in 1925,

the movement was taken over by Chiang Kai-shek, head of a disciplined and loyal military. A Moscow-brokered alliance between the Chinese Communist Party (CCP) and the Nationalists in Guangzhou became uneasy after Sun's death.[54] Yet CCP mobilizations of peasants and workers in a vast swath of southeastern China between Guangzhou and Shanghai, combined with the military strength of Chiang Kai-shek's army, saw a Northern Expedition succeed that unified much of East China. In April 1927, Chiang and his allies in Shanghai betrayed the Communists and began massacring them along with labor unionists and peasants who appeared to threaten the economic interests of his landlord and capitalist allies. Survivors fled to mountainous regions and under CCP leadership set up independent soviets, like that in Jiangxi, where they gave up urban revolution and began experimenting with new social forms that included a basic health system for peasants.[55] Years of encirclement campaigns finally drove the CCP out of Jiangxi, and Chiang Kai-shek's Nationalist government attempted to appease brutalized peasants by supplying some basic health care to these regions as a way of establishing governing legitimacy. In a few regions close to the cities with medical schools, experimental rural health centers were set up that generated some new ideas for addressing the newly identified needs of rural health.[56] Meanwhile, a small group of CCP members survived the Long March by regrouping in remote Yan'an and there had some success reestablishing some basic medical services, one plank in a larger program of winning local people over to their program.[57]

In 1928, with help from the League of Nations Health Organization, the Nationalists set up a Ministry of Health—the first in Chinese history—in their new capital of Nanjing.[58] Yet only 0.11 percent of the total national budget in 1929 and 0.7 percent in 1936 went to health work, with 44 percent going to support the civil war against the Communists, and 35 percent to service indemnities and new debts to the Western powers and Japan.[59] Imperialism continued to hinder China's capacity to develop comprehensive state health programs. Nevertheless, the ministry attempted a series of programs to consolidate and register all health work in areas controlled by the Nationalists. This in turn led to conflict with missionary medical schools unwilling to accept government supervision and give up foreign control.[60] Meanwhile, modernizers from Japan, led by Yu Yunxiu, attempted to use the ministry to abolish traditional medicine, following the Japanese model.[61] This attempt failed, but nonetheless both forms of medicine became increasingly organized and disciplined under state leadership and the forces of professionalization. In the end, the modernizers overplayed their hand, and the Ministry of Health was demoted and placed under the Ministry of the Interior. And by 1934 the League of Nations Health Organization had retreated from China.[62] It appeared that state medicine in China had suffered a major blow.

It was in this context of expansive ambition limited by resources and politics that the beginning of total war with Japan in 1937 led to new opportunities for the growth of biomedicine in China. In March 1937, on the eve of the war, Robert Lim and C. C. Chen argued that the goal of state medicine could be accomplished through new types of social mobilization and management of the economy. Lim and Chen saw state medicine, as a policy, "defined as the rendering available for every member of the community, irrespective of any necessary relationship to the conditions of individual payment, of all the potentialities of preventive and curative medicine." This would be achieved through the "personnel discipline of a military machine" and the "economic management of an industrial enterprise."[63] While wartime medicine faced many of the same problems of scarcity as prewar medicine, desperate times nonetheless led to extraordinary achievements.[64] Soldiers were mobilized, refugees were vaccinated, and nursing was expanded. This increased wartime mobilization in Nationalist-controlled southwest China, CCP-controlled northwest China, and even in Japanese-controlled coastal areas, and set the stage for an increased expectation and capacity for subsequent Chinese regimes to penetrate rural society with medicine and public health.

Disappointments nonetheless abounded as official corruption, incompetence, and the White Terror of Chiang Kai-shek's secret police eroded public support for the Nationalists. American financial, military, and medical support was maintained after victory over Japan in 1945; however, and despite almost unanimous cries from the US State Department to work with the CCP, the victorious United States supported Chiang in the subsequent resumption of civil war. The United States then established Chiang in the United Nations as a puppet ally with one of five Security Council seats, which Chiang's regime maintained even after 1949 when he had de facto ceded all of mainland China to the People's Liberation Army by retreating to Taiwan. American medical aid in the McCarthy era, exemplified in the American Bureau for Medical Aid to China, shifted to military medical support and disease eradication programs in Taiwan.[65] The People's Republic of China (PRC) ejected missionaries and nationalized all private institutions while welcoming Soviet Russian medical experts.

Two Chinas now existed: the Republic of China on Taiwan and the PRC, centered in Beijing. Both Chinas used the politics of health to increase their legitimacy. Both sides of the Taiwan Straits developed modern health care for their populations, but followed divergent reactions to the legacy of colonialism and imperatives of state building. In Taiwan, aid from the United States and many existing medical leaders clashed with a large group of physicians trained before 1945 in Japan or Taipei.[66] In the PRC, attempts to bring medicine to the people accelerated through the clash between the ongoing technocratic methods of the Ministry of Health, staffed by pre-1949 leaders who had not moved to Taiwan, and the radical approach of Mao and the

Communist Party that sought to equalize medical care by dispersing person-nel and resources from the cities to the countryside. While the technocrats in the Ministry of Health dominated through much of the first fifteen years of the PRC and failed to deliver government health care to most of China's people living in rural areas, the radical approach of the Cultural Revolution resulted in the Barefoot Doctor movement (1966–1980s), which brought basic paramedic care and antibiotics to everyone in China, but these devel-opments are beyond the scope of the present volume.[67]

Historiography of a Hybrid Field

In China today there are two state-sponsored forms of medicine, often in the same hospital: traditional Chinese medicine and biomedicine. Like the contemporary Chinese hospital, the historiography of medicine in China cannot be understood apart from the relationship between the two forms of medicine. The most significant developments in medicine in China between 1835 and 1949 studied in the secondary literature are (1) the sinification of Euro-American medicine, (2) the scientization of Chinese medicine, and (3) the resulting convergence and conflict of the two. These issues have not yet been definitively resolved in contemporary health care, and one could argue that it is the dual nature of official medicine in China in the twentieth and twenty-first centuries that has led to a hybrid field of historiography.

This hybrid literature can be traced back as far as the beginning of mod-ern historical writing about medicine in China, to the late 1910s when Chen Bangxian began serially publishing his history of medicine in China in popular journals.[68] Like K. Chi-min Wong and Wu Lien-teh, who pub-lished two editions of their English-language tome in the 1930s, Chen, in his Chinese-language work, aimed to tell the history of medicine in China as a single story with multiple origins. Wong and Wu argued, "Chinese medicine, to be understood, and its significance appreciated, must be studied as one whole."[69] During the Maoist period (1949–76) until the early 1980s, Chinese scholars were highly critical of missionary and philanthropic medicine dur-ing the semicolonial modern period (*jindai*) from 1800 to 1949, seeing medicine as the cultural arm of imperialism. The institutionalization and scientization (*kexue hua*) of Chinese medicine was supported by the state out of pragmatic necessity of fulfilling the goals of state medicine and for pur-poses of cultural nationalism.[70]

In the West, the student protest movement of 1968 was partly inspired by Maoism, and Maoist policies also influenced young scholars of medicine in China. In that year, Ralph Crozier wrote, "The fact is that Western medicine was an integral part of Western cultural aggression and ultimately of Chinese cultural revolution."[71] Crozier's critical interpretation of biomedicine is

significant in that his main argument was that the survival of Chinese medicine was based on the political expediency of the Maoist period. A generation later, E. Richard Brown argued that the Rockefeller Foundation used its
influence in China to produce "modernization," a process that made poor
countries dependent on, and profitable for, Western interests. American
directors of the PUMC insisted on training a small number of medical
elites, not the large number of medical workers state medicine required.
Thus, Brown argued, the extensive Rockefeller medical project in China did
not target Chinese health problems, but rather aimed to create a system of
medicine "ideologically and culturally conducive" to China's development
as a dependent partner in the industrialized, capitalist economic system.[72]
The Cold War also saw the beginning of the work of Joseph Needham and
his many collaborators who sought to ask why China had failed to generate a scientific revolution despite being economically and technologically
ahead of Europe for centuries. Nathan Sivin and Paul Unschuld have also
played a role in mediating the historiographies of Chinese medicine and
biomedicine, with Sivin arguing that Needham's question is less interesting
than asking what *did* happen in China, while Unschuld's impressive corpus of scholarship and translations of ancient texts have greatly advanced
understanding of the social and political context of earlier medical
developments.[73]

With the death of Mao and the end of the Cold War, both Washington
and Beijing embraced neoliberal policies, and most scholars in the West and
in China have adopted a vocabulary emphasizing "modernization" (*jindai-
hua*) in Chinese-language literature and "modernity" in English-language
literature.[74] Terms such as "cultural aggression" have disappeared. With
many new primary sources available, two new patterns are discernible in the
Chinese-language literature. The first is an empirical approach that shies
away from explicit analysis and has a biographical or institutional focus.
Although this trend appears to avoid ideology, it tends to valorize anything
leading to medical modernization as unimpeachable progress. The best
among these studies offer careful exposition of new archives without challenging the reigning modernization orthodoxy. A second trend might be
broadly described as a "postcolonial" approach, which accepts some of the
Marxist and Maoist criticisms of medical imperialism but without relying
on wooden formulations of these criticisms, while also taking note of the
complexities of negotiation, collaboration, and accommodation. This new
approach sees Chinese people as active in receiving, adapting, and rejecting
aspects of Western medical policy.

In 1989, Zhao Hongjun's *History of the Modern Controversies over Chinese vs.
Western Medicine* appeared as an empirical work that put the (historical and
ongoing) controversies between Chinese and Western medicine at the center of analysis.[75] Zhao's was the first book-length treatment of the subject

since Ralph Crozier's in 1967, and Nathan Sivin published an English summary translation. While Crozier privileged the inevitable progress of China in adopting Western medicine at the expense of Chinese medicine, the new literature demonstrated in a symmetrical manner not only that traditional Chinese medicine was formed by the encounter with biomedicine, but that the reverse was also true.[76] Both medicines must be understood to have formed the other in the twentieth-century encounter. This point is now taken for granted in the English-language literature.

The most important work in this vein is Ruth Rogaski's *Hygienic Modernity*. Eleven years after its publication in English, and eight years after its popular translation in Chinese, *Hygienic Modernity* has made studies of health, hygiene, medicine, and healing a central part of the study of modern Chinese history.[77] Like a Warwick Anderson or David Arnold, Rogaski does not shrink from describing the Janus-faced nature of public health and biomedicine: at once it is a power to protect health and restrain bodies, ensuring the long life of the many at the expense of personal liberty.[78] A more recent volume edited by Angela Leung and Charlotte Furth, *Health and Hygiene in Chinese East Asia*, picks up where Rogaski left off by looking at case studies beyond the borders of China proper.[79] That book demonstrates the leading role of Taiwan-based scholars in the literature in this field.[80]

Another approach to the hybrid field has been through the study of the evolution of a particular disease nosology over time. This approach has the advantage of naturally focusing on the diagnostic conflicts between Chinese medicine and biomedicine while also emphasizing the indigenization of biomedicine. The work has tended to maintain a strong focus on the modern development of historical nosologies, as exemplified by Angela Leung on *li/lai*/leprosy and by Marta Hanson on the Chinese concept of warm diseases (*wenbing*), which now includes SARS, and to a lesser degree by Carol Benedict's earlier book on plague.[81] Leung's book well illustrates an increasing trend toward medical confinement and even violence, with the modernizing Chinese state demonstrating public health sovereignty through wholesale extermination of lepers.[82] An edited volume by Ka-che Yip compares colonial biomedical attempts to fight malaria in China, Hong Kong, Okinawa, and Taiwan since the nineteenth century but does not take seriously earlier nosologies.[83]

In China the social history of disease has also become an important field of inquiry, with Yu Xinzhong using a wide variety of sources to study "warm diseases" in the culturally central *Jiangnan* region around Suzhou, Hangzhou, and Shanghai in the late Qing period, while Zhang Daqing's more general account of disease in China discusses the various developments of attempts to control disease in prewar Republican China.[84] The key to such social history approaches has been to escape from the elite medical perspectives of most sources by also examining patient perspectives. Yu

Xinzhong has pursued this kind of social history of public health by examining how the lucrative and ubiquitous business of night soil became a public health issue.[85]

Perhaps the most influential Chinese-language work on the experience of patients encountering medicine is Yang Nianqun's *Remaking Patients*.[86] Directly addressing the issue of the indigenization of biomedicine, Yang approaches the issue of power subtly through a series of well-selected anecdotes that demonstrate both the exercise of power by missionary and state physicians and their need to take indigenous concerns seriously. While some historians have questioned the broad arguments of Yang's work, it nonetheless opens up new questions for further empirically *and* theoretically driven studies and shifts the field away from the ongoing influence of modernization theory.[87]

A response to that call is Hu Cheng's recent book, whose title aligns it with the themes of the current volume: *Medicine, Hygiene and China in the World*.[88] Hu is also interested in going beyond elite accounts to the experiences of patients living under the increasingly interventionist health regimes in China. Hu argues that it is in the ordinary experiences of Chinese common people dealing with health and illness that world history is made. He covers many of the topics addressed in the present narrative, from the indigenization of biomedicine in the work of missionaries and their assistants, to the spread of epidemics through economic expansion, to the politicization of public health during the plague epidemic in Manchuria. One can hope that scholars in China and abroad will continue to search for the elusive sources that might expand our knowledge beyond top-down policies and explore the lived experience of patients and physicians.

China and the Globalization of Biomedicine

This book does not address the full range of topics in the burgeoning field outlined above but rather makes its intervention in three major categories that are both thematic and divided by era: the first section contains two chapters examining aspects of nineteenth-century hygiene and disease construction; the second explores the indigenization of biomedicine in the Republican era to the Japanese invasion in 1937; and the third section explores how war remade medicine in China. Medicine, which appeared to be only a promise in the nineteenth century and the frustrated ambition of modernizing elites in the early Republic, ironically became most deeply entrenched during the destruction of war.[89]

In part 1, two sides of global biomedicine in the nineteenth century are explored. Yu Xinzhong builds on his large corpus of empirical scholarship to argue that hygienic modernity cannot be accepted uncritically. Yu observes many of his fellow Chinese historians of medicine who portray all developments in modern medicine as progress, no matter the cost to individual liberty. Although the bulldozer of modernity may have made a clear and hygienic space appealing to colonial elites (whether foreign or Chinese), those subject to involuntary displacement and the constricting disciplines of hospitals saw massive disruptions to their lives. This is a well-established research project in the English-language social history of medicine, but Yu is one of few scholars writing in Chinese who dares to be openly critical of modernization at a time when modernization is still the official policy of the People's Republic. If Yu's argument is that the globalization of biomedicine was sometimes coercive for Chinese, his purpose is to further integrate Chinese medical historiography into norms that recognize the role of historians to speak not only to the power of physicians and institutions, but also for the weakness of patients and subjects in the history of medical exchange.

Xi takes a very different approach by examining an institution that can be said to have conducted significant two-way exchanges of medical knowledge via its regular medical reports—the Chinese Imperial Customs Service. Building on her book about John Dudgeon, Gao sees a lacuna in studies of Western medicine in nineteenth-century China that have focused exclusively on missionary medicine.[90] More important than the tiny medical clinics established by missionaries in terms of the development of the institutions of state and public health that came later in the Republic and PRC was the Chinese Imperial Customs, which was established on behalf of the Chinese government by the British after the Second Opium War and Treaty of Tianjin in 1860. The customs medical officers organized a nationwide network of informants to gather information on a variety of subjects including diseases and fed a steady stream of knowledge to the institutions of global medicine through its widely circulated and reviewed reports. Patrick Manson, the founder of tropical medicine, got his start and inspiration as a medical officer in China. But the "discovery" of new diseases in China, including the Hong Kong plague epidemic of 1893 and the Manchurian plague of 1910–11 had a fundamental impact on global biomedical knowledge, and the customs reports played a key role in mediating knowledge of these diseases.

In part 2, four chapters explore diverse aspects of the key question of how biomedicine became Chinese. Arguably, the process of indigenization was facilitated by the transition to state and elite interest in medicine. A chapter by Daniel Asen and David Luesink on the early history of the National Medical School in Beijing demonstrates the importance of the Chinese government and Japanese medicine (derived from Germany) in the early Republic. This influence was institutionalized in the National Medical School in Beijing. Never as well funded as the richest missionary medical schools or the lavishly endowed Peking Union Medical College, the National

Medical School, these authors argue, was nonetheless modestly successful in accomplishing its stated goals of providing a large number of competent medical graduates. Following the Japanese model, rather than immediately attempting to build a world-class medical school, state medicine sought to establish a basic quorum of biomedical physicians at a level of training feasible under semicolonial conditions. The best of these physicians were then sent to Japan, Germany, or even the United States for further training to become medical teachers and researchers in a growing network of government medical schools, resulting in a kind of "sliding scale" model of medical education.

The present volume does not have a chapter devoted to the Rockefeller Foundation and its PUMC, but the influence of the PUMC, more or less allied with Wu Lien-teh and the Anglo-American school of biomedicine, is in the background of several chapters. This is most notable in the chapter by Shi Yan that describes the little-known attempt to amalgamate the German-Japanese and Anglo-American styles of medicine into one organization. The Chinese Medical Association (itself a merger of the National Medical Association and the Medical Missionary Association) and the German-Japanese-oriented China Medical and Pharmaceutical Association attempted, unsuccessfully, to merge in 1934. Several factors had seemed to point toward a successful merger of all professional associations of Western-style physicians, including funding from the Rockefeller Foundation and a successful 1932 merger of two Anglo-American associations, the National Medical Association (founded by Wu Lien-teh and others in 1915) and the China Medical Association (founded as the China Medical Missionary Association in 1886). Shi reveals that it was Lee Tao, a single faculty member of PUMC and chief editor of the CMA publication, who derailed the merger. In the *Chinese Medical Journal*, Lee wrote editorials dismissive of the German-Japanese group, thus making union impossible. By 1928, Anglo-Americans dominated China's first Ministry of Health and other state organizations and used their power to favor the priorities of Anglo-American medicine over other possible goals. The key issue between the Anglo-American group and the German-Japanese group was said to be different standards of education, but Shi's analysis points to a more structural reason for the inability of the two groups to merge rooted firmly in China's semicolonial condition. The key takeaway, however, is even more basic and important to emphasize: that China's Western-style practitioners were divided among themselves and so failed either to form a union or to find agreement on many issues that might have improved medicine in Republican China.

He Xiaolian takes us even further toward understanding the cleavages in the field of biomedicine.[91] For He, it is no longer the politics of national preference between Anglo-American and German-Japanese groups, but gender politics that form the center of analysis. He Xiaolian's research demonstrates a strong patriarchal dominance in the biomedical field in Shanghai in the Republican period. The sole exception was the field of obstetrics and gynecology in which female practitioners predominated. Yet He demonstrates that a kind of class system based on the origin of training further divided female practitioners: those with a foreign medical degree formed a wealthy elite that charged exorbitant fees for child delivery and could afford luxuries such as cars and houses staffed with drivers, chefs, and nurses. But even these elite female physicians could not compare to the upper-class wealth of elite male physicians. Graduates of elite Chinese medical programs in Shanghai or a handful of other medical centers were the second strata of female physicians, but there was a much larger group, possibly up to one thousand, of non-MD practitioners (most of them approved midwives but some merely former hospital workers) who claimed that they were female physicians who could deliver babies. Unlike men, female physicians who got married were expected to give up their career; therefore, many remained unmarried. He Xiaolian's chapter describes not only the earlier Republican period but also life under Japanese occupation. Most remarkable, of course, is the fact that it is completely an urban story of women making a space for themselves in the medical marketplace in a period when up to 50 percent of all biomedical practitioners in China practiced in the city of Shanghai.

A global conception of state medicine and public health motivated the League of Nations Health Organization and the Chinese Ministry of Health in the 1920s and 1930s to find a way to enable biomedicine to reach rural China. The health of the rural poor was increasingly conceived of as a "problem" for intervention not only for reasons of international humanitarianism and national strength but also because the poor might be seen as reservoirs of disease threatening cosmopolitan urban populations through intensifying trade networks. Yet spreading the power and benefits of biomedicine to the countryside met with numerous obstacles. The reach of state medicine was only beginning to penetrate rural areas by the end of the Nanjing Decade in 1937 when the Nationalist government was forced to retreat up the Yangzi River to Wuhan and Chongqing to escape the advance of the Japanese forces.

Part 3 demonstrates that the Second Sino-Japanese War (1937–45) has, until recently, been overlooked in the history of biomedicine in China. Also called the War of Resistance against Japan, it was, in fact, a major turning point for biomedicine, not least because this is also the period of dramatic discoveries in biomedicine, such as antibiotics, vaccinations, and other public health measures. In addition, it was a period when the state began to utilize its increasing capacity to intervene medically in the lives of individuals. The war in China called for a level of social mobilization that penetrated deep into local society in ways unthinkable and impossible only a few years prior. If one may forgive the metaphor, the cause of state medicine and public health in China received a major shot in the arm under wartime conditions.

A dramatic example of the social disruption of the period was the massive migration of biomedical workers from Japanese-occupied eastern cities to interior regions where Western medicine had hardly been practiced before. The migration of millions of people was a major contributing factor to the spread of diseases. But at the same time, wartime medical workers were able to stem the spread of epidemics among the population in the southwest, thanks to significant funding and supplies from the United States. What is clear in all three of these chapters is that with medical and public health infrastructure almost nonexistent, even by Chinese standards of the time, the government in wartime mobilization mode was nonetheless able to build infrastructure from the ground up with limited resources.

Li Shenglan argues that nurses have been overlooked in the history of medicine in China generally and that the wartime was a period of particular metamorphosis for the nursing profession. Diverging from most existing literature on missionary nurses, Li takes an inside-out view of the profession with the direct translation of *hushi* as the "warriors in white uniforms" playing a key part of state medicine.[92] While giving information on the growth of the profession as a whole, Li focuses her study on the Hunan-Yale Nursing School in Changsha, which later moved to Yuanling in western Hunan, and then to Guiyang. Although the private institution maintained independence throughout the war, it increasingly took on state goals such as midwifery and public health training. Significantly, gender played an important part in nursing roles and the experience of nurses themselves. While there was a positive sisterhood that developed among nursing students, Li finds, the hierarchy of nurses was subordinated to physicians, thus increasing the gender divide. Early nurses in China had been male, but by the war period, nursing became almost exclusively a female profession. Yet Li finds that whereas white nursing uniforms for American nurses clearly distinguished gender roles for American wartime nurses in Vietnam, in wartime China white nursing uniforms were gender-neutral, as evidenced in a theatrical revival of the traditional cross-dressing tale of Mulan in 1939.

Mary Augusta Brazelton describes technological and organizational work of vaccinators and immunologists who developed, produced, and distributed vaccines throughout southwest China under the threat of daily bombardment by Japanese aircraft. This work was one of the keys to the globalization of biomedicine in China. The movement of millions of troops and refugees in wartime inevitably led to an increased threat from diseases such as smallpox, cholera, plague, typhus, tuberculosis, and diphtheria. Chinese medical and public health personnel had increased interaction with their overseas counterparts, even as they worked to make Nationalist China independent from expensive shipments of vaccines and sera from foreign sources.

Brazelton describes how the National Epidemic Prevention Bureau (NEPB), founded in Beijing in 1919, was transformed first by the expanding state health infrastructure of the Nationalist government in Nanjing after 1927, and secondly after its wartime migration to Kunming. Despite wartime inflation, the NEPB did its best to maintain affordable prices for the dozens of vaccines and sera it produced. Brazelton, even more than other contributors in this volume, addresses the trend of globally relevant Chinese biomedical research pointed out by Eugene Opie. International networks of funding and research included the American Bureau for Medical Aid to China (ABMAC) and the National Health Administration (NHA) in the wartime Nationalist capital of Chongqing, which had clinical research sites in Yunnan Province. Many Chinese medical scientists who had never previously worked in bacteriology, immunology, or public health now turned their considerable combined talents to this collective effort, which was of relevance not only in "Free China" but also throughout the Allied wartime areas. While such efforts were successful in preventing disease, as Yu Xinzhong points out in his chapter, they also led to an increase in state and collective rights over individuals. For example, Brazelton also describes how, in 1942, proof of inoculation for cholera became necessary to enter or exit Yunnan Province, and without such proof, vaccination was mandatory.

Nicole Barnes describes how Chen Zhiqian (C. C. Chen), a trainee of "medical Bolshevik" John B. Grant at PUMC and leader of the model rural health facility of Dingxian in Hebei before 1937, developed the Sichuan Provincial Health Administration (SPHA) between 1939 and 1945. Before 1937, rural health programs remained only token experimental projects in a handful of counties near large cities in eastern China, but Barnes shows how under wartime emergency mobilization conditions Chen was able to establish county health centers (CHCs) in 131 of 139 counties, the immediate legacy of his experimental work in faraway Dingxian, Hebei Province. Not only did most of these previously remote counties get public health and medical services in this manner, but the expansion of state services also played the political role of incorporating this previously independent province into the nation, echoing themes throughout this volume about the twin roles of state-building and expanding health services. Barnes argues that from the beginning of his medical training, Chen sought to find a way to bring modern health to rural people, unlike many of his classmates from PUMC who built their careers through research accolades or lucrative private practice. For Chen, the key was focusing on the more mundane practice of disease prevention, which was made possible by the vaccines produced in Yunnan, even if ongoing transportation and shortages provided significant obstacles to distribution. Barnes does careful work in comparing four CHCs to reveal exactly what was accomplished, rather than relying merely on general reports. These mini–case studies reveal that more centrally located health centers were also better staffed and equipped, but that for this very reason, they also experienced more epidemic outbreaks than did more isolated areas. Health outcomes thus diverged widely. Ultimately, however, Barnes' account provides a narrative of how wartime conditions and the technologies of public health allowed the state to incorporate rural Sichuanese into "the disciplined body of the nation."

The volume ends with an afterward by William Schneider that puts the themes of the volume in conversation with issues of global health today. Schneider's perspective is that of a comparative historian of medicine in Europe and Africa. Schneider offers us a review of the problems of this field by surveying the work of theorists and historians of global health. While acknowledging many differences between warlord-era China and contemporary Africa, Schneider sees at least one similarity. This is the tendency for the balkanization of medical efforts by governments "less able to resist and more likely to take advantage of multiple outside offers of assistance." As discussed above, due to the unequal treaties, the Chinese government during much of this period was simply unable to stop foreign interests from developing hospitals and medical schools. While international health assistance, whether by missionaries or philanthropic organizations, appeared (and appears) to the average donor to be an uncomplicated benefit that relieved apparent misery, Schneider uses the comparative framework of China a century ago and Africa both then and now to challenge neoconservative and neoliberal orthodoxy. He points out that weak governments and strong international organizations of health, working together, do not necessarily, *or even typically*, result in better health outcomes. In fact, the evidence points to the opposite conclusion. Moreover, weakened states that allow extensive foreign involvement in health, like those of late Qing and especially Republican China, or those of sub-Saharan Africa today, are perceived as being corrupt and ineffective. The question is thus raised (if not answered) as to whether, and to what degree, overseas health care assistance is implicated in the weakening of central states and of overall health outcomes. Schneider does not suggest it, but the case of medical development seems parallel with Andre Gunder Frank's concept that so-called economic development actually leads to underdevelopment.[93] If we applied the concept rigorously to biomedicine in China, would we find that all of the foreign aid described in this book served to underdevelop health care, and that only indigenous medical service advances were significant in the long term?

The chapters herein all point to the increasing ambition of the Chinese government to take control of the health of its citizens. Remarkably, only fifteen years after the Rockefeller Foundation established its private, elite-focused medical school and hospital in Beijing in 1917, the PUMC had shifted its position to support state medicine. This about-face was led by faculty member John B. Grant, who called for a full Marxist analysis of capitalist medicine and heralded a worldwide trend toward socially organized medicine and away from individualistic practice. Such ideas also increasingly appealed to liberals like Henry S. Houghton, who thought that state control was "the only way" to spread the benefits of medical science to all of China's people.[94] Moreover, even for Houghton, the key to making this successful depended on supporting "the power and authority of the National Government."[95] Although we should recognize the concessions made by PUMC faculty and Rockefeller Foundation staff to the realities of medicine in China, the pivot from emphasizing elite medicine to health for the masses was limited and driven more by Chinese nationalism and the growth of a stronger state than by the good intentions of American physicians and philanthropic officers.[96]

We have already encountered the ideas of two of the most important leaders of Chinese state medicine, Robert K. S. Lim and C. C. Chen. Writing on the eve of war with Japan in 1937, they stressed the need to reevaluate all private and government medical activities and redirect them as needed. They argued that a military level of discipline must envelop medical workers, while the economic management of an industrial enterprise must take over the financial outlay of medical services. All roles of medical workers from doctors, to nurses, to midwives, to pharmacists, as well as all "spaces" of medicine, must be "scrutinized, and if they do not fit adequately in the new scheme, they must be altered," they wrote.[97] Presaging the Barefoot Doctor movement that began with the Cultural Revolution, the direction had been set before 1949 of state-directed attempts to reevaluate and redirect all medical resources according to collective and not individual aims. And, as Houghton prophesied in 1935, Chinese allocation of limited medical resources for the collective benefit of the nation would come to be seen as a model for global health care when limited local means have so often not matched the ambition and technical capacity of biomedicine.

Globalization in nineteenth- and twentieth-century China led to economic inequality beginning with the perverted role played by a medical substance—opium. It also led to the spread of pandemic diseases to and from China. But globalized problems could also lead to globally relevant solutions—none more pressing in 1949 or today than that of equal access to affordable health care. The tensions of the globalization of biomedical research in China are evident in the words of Eugene Opie above. Capitalist medicine, as developed in the United States and exported to China in the Peking Union Medical College, succeeded very well in producing original research on "fundamental problems of pathology and clinical medicine," whether addressed to the "pressing questions concerning the welfare of the Chinese people" or not. But this model of elite medicine was increasingly critiqued even by PUMC faculty like Lim, Chen, Grant, and Houghton. By 1935, G. Canby Robinson, who had as much influence as any other doctor in establishing this elite research model in the United States, acknowledged that the time of private medicine appeared to be over, and that "China may point the way to the world for the solution of some of the vexing questions now involved in the establishment of an adequate governmental health service for all the people."[98]

Eighty years later, that tension still exists in China's current round of medical reforms. Today we see the robust medical delivery system developed since the 1930s alternately dismantled or patched up, in a series of reforms attempting to allow full engagement with, and production of, the latest expensive medical interventions and biomedical research, while also providing equal access to such care. We watch carefully, for in the twenty-first century, the medical problems and solutions of China are surely aligned with those of the whole world.

Notes

1. Eugene L. Opie, "Introduction," *Chinese Medical Journal*, Supplemental Volume, 1938–39, n.p.

2. Henry S. Houghton, "Trends in Medical Education," *Chinese Medical Journal* 49 (1935): 941.

3. For more on the conferences and multiyear Luce-funded project, see IUPUI University Library, "History of Western Medicine in China," The History of Western Medicine in China, Beijing Workshop, June 22–23, 2013, http://ulib.iupui.edu/wmicproject/conference.

4. Mark Harrison, "Science and the British Empire," *Isis* 96 (2005): 56.

5. The Chinese term for biomedicine is *shengwu yiyao*, but it is more commonly used as the adjectival "biomedical" to describe biomedical engineering (*shengwu gongcheng xue*) or biomedical technologies (*shengwu yixue jishu*). The *Oxford English Dictionary* defines biomedicine conservatively as "the branch of medicine concerned with the application of the principles of biology, biochemistry, etc., to medical research or practice" and observes its first published occurrence in 1922 in the *Pennsylvania Medical Journal* to reference the problem of the exponential growth of biomedical knowledge, such that an internist would find it impossible to absorb the advances relevant to internal medicine. I submit that there is no single accurate term to represent the form of medicine and public health described here: "allopathic medicine" is a term used by homeopathic physicians to emphasize how biomedicine uses pharmacological agents to treat symptoms; "Western medicine" ignores how this medicine was formed as much in colonies as in Europe and America; "scientific medicine" is closer to what we are trying to describe here in that by the late nineteenth century medicine became increasingly tied to the laboratories of physiology, chemistry, and biology, but it tends to be viewed as prejudicial toward other forms of medicine.

6. The classic statement of the technology-transfer model is George Basalla, "The Spread of Western Science," *Science*, n.s., vol. 156, no. 3775 (1967): 611–22.

7. See, for example, Peter Buck, *American Science and Modern China, 1876–1936* (Cambridge, MA: Harvard University Press, 1980).

8. See Roy Porter, *The Greatest Benefit to Mankind: A Medical History of Humanity from Antiquity to the Present* (New York: Norton, 1997). Despite adding significant chapters to summarize the history of medicine in China, Porter's magisterial survey nonetheless presents Chinese developments as merely a sideline to those in Europe and America. It is worth comparing early twentieth-century histories of medicine by Fielding H. Garrison and by K. Chi-min Wong and Wu Lien-teh. For analysis of this historiography, see David Luesink, "*History of Chinese Medicine*: Empires, Transnationalism and Medicine in China, 1908–1937," in Iris Borowy, ed., *Uneasy Encounters: The Politics of Medicine and Health in China, 1900–1937* (Frankfurt: Peter Lang, 2009): 149–76.

9. Much of modern medicine is currently at risk due to the development of antibiotic-resistant diseases and a sharp decline in the manufacture of new antibiotics. See "Antibiotic/Antimicrobial Resistance (AR/AMR)," Center for Disease Control and Prevention, accessed September 1, 2018, http://www.cdc.gov/drugresistance/.

10. Lewis Thomas, *The Youngest Science: Notes of a Medicine-Watcher* (New York: Viking, 1983), 29.

11. For an entry point to McKeown, see Bill Bynum, "The McKeown Thesis," *Lancet* 371 (February 23, 2008): 644–45.

12. Porter, *Greatest Benefit to Mankind*, 6–8.

13. Emanuel Le Roy Ladurie, "A Concept: The Unification of the Globe by Disease," in *The Mind and Method of the Historian* (Chicago: University of Chicago Press, 1984), 28–91; Alfred Crosby, *Ecological Imperialism: The Biological Expansion of Europe, 900–1900* (Cambridge: Cambridge University Press, 1986).

14. Robert Peckham and David M. Pomfret, *Imperial Contagions: Medicine, Hygiene, and Cultures of Planning in Asia* (Hong Kong: Hong Kong University Press, 2013).

15. On Manson, see Douglas M. Haynes, *Imperial Medicine: Patrick Manson and the Conquest of Tropical Disease* (Philadelphia: University of Pennsylvania Press, 2001). On Yersin's preeminence in the Yersin-Kitasato controversy, see Thomas Butler, *Plague and Other Yersina Infections* (New York: Plenum Medical Book Company, 1983), 22–24. The best account of Wu's politics is Sean Hsiang-lin Lei, "Sovereignty and the Microscope: Constituting Notifiable Infectious Disease and Containing the Manchurian Plague (1910–1911)," in Angela Ki Che Leung and Charlotte Furth, eds., *Health and Hygiene in Chinese East Asia: Policies and Publics in the long twentieth century* (Durham, NC: Duke University Press, 2010), 73–106.

16. Pratik Chakrabarti, *Medicine and Empire* (London: Palgrave Macmillan, 2014), 20–39.

17. Fa-ti Fan, *British Naturalists in Qing China: Science, Empire and Cultural Encounter* (Cambridge, MA: Harvard University Press, 2004).

18. Sean Hsiang-lin Lei, "From Changshan to a New Anti-Malarial Drug: Re-Networking Chinese Drugs and Excluding Chinese Doctors," *Social Studies of Science* 29, no. 3 (1999): 323–58.

19. For a synthesis of the literature on imperialism and medicine, see Chakrabarti, *Medicine and Empire*. For the case of imperialism and medicine in China, see the contributions in Borowy, *Uneasy Encounters*.

20. Michael Shiyung Liu, "The Ripples of Rivalry: The Spread of Modern Medicine from Japan to Its Colonies," *East Asian Science, Technology and Society* 2 (2008): 47–71.

21. Kenneth Pomeranz, *The Making of a Hinterland: State, Society, and Economy in Inland North China, 1853–1937* (Berkeley: University of California Press, 1993); Kathryn Edgerton-Tarplay, *Tears from Iron: Cultural Responses to Famine in Nineteenth-Century China* (Berkeley: University of California Press, 2008).

22. Joanna Waley-Cohen, "China and Western Technology in the Late Eighteenth Century," *American Historical Review* 98, no. 5 (1993): 1525–44.

23. Timothy Brook and Bob Wakabayashi, "Introduction: Opium's History in China," in *Opium Regimes: China, Britain and Japan, 1839–1952* (Berkeley: University of California Press, 2000).

24. Li Chuanbin, *Tiaoyue tequan zhidu xia de yiliao shiye: Jidujiao zai hua yiliao shiye yanjiu (1835–1937)* [Healing activities under the unequal treaties: Research on Christian healing activities in China, 1835–1937] (Changsha: Hunan Renmin Chubanshe, 2010).

25. On the Customs Service see Gao Xi's contribution to this volume; Donna Brunero, *Britain's Imperial Cornerstone in China: The Chinese Maritime Customs Service, 1854–1949* (New York: Routledge, 2006); and Robert Bickers, "'Good Work for China in Every Possible Direction': The Foreign Inspectorate of the Chinese Maritime Customs, 1854–1950," in Bryna Goodman and David Goodman, eds., *Twentieth-Century Colonialism and China: Localities, the Everyday, and the World* (New York: Routledge, 2012), 25–36. On the significance of the 1860 occupation, see James Hevia, *English Lessons: The Pedagogy of Imperialism in Nineteenth-Century China* (Durham, NC: Duke University Press, 2003).

26. K. Chimin Wong and Wu Lien-teh, *History of Chinese Medicine* (Shanghai: National Quarantine Service, 1936), 367.

27. Mao Zedong, *The Chinese Revolution and the Chinese Communist Party*, as quoted in Gong Chun, "Woguo jinbainian lai de yixue jiaoyu" [The last hundred years of Western medical education in China], *Zhonghua yishi zazhi* 12, no. 4 (1982): 209.

28. Yuet-Wah Cheung, *Missionary Medicine in China* (Lanham, MD: University Press of America, 1988); Theron Kue-Hing Young, "A Conflict of Professions: The Medical Missionary in China, 1835–1890," *Bulletin of the History of Medicine* 47 (1973): 250–72.

29. Jonathan D. Spence, *To Change China* (New York: Penguin, 1980), 292. Catholic medical missions could be radically different from Protestant, as seen in a recent article, Henrietta Harrison, "Rethinking Missionaries and Medicine in China: The Miracles of Assunta Pallotta, 1905–2005," *Journal of Asian Studies* 71 (2012): 127–48.

30. Edward M. Merrins, "Medical Ethics in China," *China Medical Journal* 38, no. 8 (1924): 679–94.

31. Bridie Andrews, *The Making of Modern Chinese Medicine, 1850–1960* (Vancouver: University of British Columbia Press, 2014), 55.

32. Michelle Renshaw, *Accommodating the Chinese: The American Hospital in China, 1880–1920* (New York: Routledge, 2005).

33. Yang Nianqun, *Zaizao "Bingren": Zhongxi yi chongtu xia de kongjian zhengzhi* [Remaking "Patients": Spatial politics in the conflict between Chinese and Western medicine] (Beijing: China Renmin University Press, 2006).

34. Xiaoli Tian, "Rumor and Secret Space: Organ-Snatching Tales and Medical Missions in Nineteenth-Century China," *Modern China* (March 2014): 1–40.

35. Hevia, *English Lessons*; Lydia Liu, *The Clash of Empires: The Invention of China in Modern World Making* (Cambridge, MA: Harvard University Press, 2004).

36. Gerald H. Choa, *"Heal the Sick" Was Their Motto: The Protestant Medical Missionaries in China* (Hong Kong: Hong Kong University Press, 1990), 80–81.

37. Connie Shenmo, *The Chinese Medical Ministries of Kang Cheng and Shi Meiyu, 1872–1937* (Lehigh, PA: Lehigh University Press, 2011).

38. Angela Leung argues that the decline in status was due to an increase in the number of healers with only limited knowledge of the medical classics. See "Organized Medicine in Ming-Qing China: State and Private Medical Institutions in the Lower Yangzi Region," *Late Imperial China*, 8, no. 1 (1987): 134–66. See Andrews, *Making of Modern Chinese Medicine*, 25–50, for an excellent survey of the spectrum of practice in late Qing and Republican China.

39. Gao Xi, *Dezhen zhuan: Yige Yingguo chuanjiaoshi yu wan Qing yixue jindai hua* [A biography of John Dudgeon: An English missionary and the modernization of late Qing medicine] (Shanghai: Fudan University Press, 2009).

40. Carol Benedict, *Bubonic Plague in Nineteenth-Century China* (Stanford, CA: Stanford University Press, 1996).

41. Lei, "Sovereignty and the Microscope," 73–106; Mark Gamsa, "The Epidemic of Pneumonic Plague in Manchuria, 1910–1911," *Past and Present* 190 (2006): 147–83; see also William C. Summers, *The Great Manchurian Plague of 1910–1911: The Geopolitics of an Epidemic Disease* (New Haven, CT: Yale University Press, 2012).

42. Wu Lien-Teh to Elliot, March 25, 1911, courtesy of the Wu Lien-teh Society and the Penang Historical Trust.

43. Larissa Hinrich, *The Afterlife of Images: Translating the Pathological Body between China and the West* (Durham, NC: Duke University Press, 2008), 149–56; Liping Bu, "Social Darwinism, Public Health and Modernization in China," in Borowy, *Uneasy Encounters*, 93–124.

44. James Bartholemew, *The Formation of Science in Japan: Building a Research Tradition* (New Haven, CT: Yale University Press, 1993); Ruth Rogaski, *Hygienic Modernity: Meanings of Health and Disease in Treaty-Port China* (Berkeley: University of California Press, 2004), 136–64.

45. See the contribution by Daniel Asen and David Luesink in the present volume. On the general trend, see Douglas Reynolds, *China, 1898–1912: The Xinzheng Revolution and Japan* (Cambridge, MA: Council on East Asian Studies, Harvard University, 1993).

46. Dorothy Ko, *Cinderella's Sisters: A Revisionist History of Footbinding* (Berkeley: University of California Press, 2005); Susan Glosser, *Chinese Visions of Family and State, 1915–1953* (Berkeley: University of California Press, 2003).

47. Tina Phillips-Johnson, *Childbirth in Republican China: Delivering Modernity* (Lanham, MD: Lexington Books, 2011).

48. David Luesink, "State Power, Governmentality and the (Mis)remembrance of Chinese Medicine," in Howard Chiang, ed., *Historical Epistemology and the Making of Modern Chinese Medicine* (Manchester: University of Manchester Press, 2015).

49. See Wang Youpeng, "Humanist Analysis on Periodicals of Chinese Medicine from the Late Qing and Republican Periods," trans. David Luesink, *Twentieth-Century China* 40, no. 1 (2015): 69–78. On professionalization, see Xiaoqun Xu, *Chinese*

Professionals and the Republican State: The Rise of Professional Associations in Shanghai, 1912–1937 (Cambridge: Cambridge University Press, 2001).

50. Harold Balme, *China and Modern Medicine: A Study in Medical Missionary Development* (London: United Council for Missionary Education, 1921), 107–17.

51. Karen Minden, *Bamboo Stone: The Evolution of a Chinese Medical Elite* (Toronto: University of Toronto Press, 1994); Jessie Lutz, *China and the Christian Colleges, 1850–1950* (Ithaca, NY: Cornell University Press, 1971); Mary Brown Bullock, *An American Transplant: The Rockefeller Foundation and Peking Union Medical College* (Berkeley: University of California Press, 1980).

52. Mu Jingjiang, *Minguo xiyi gaodeng jiaoyu (1912–1949)* [Advanced medical education in Republican China, 1912–1949) (Hangzhou: Zhejiang Gongshang University Press, 2012), 120–41.

53. John Fitzgerald, *Awakening China: Politics, Culture, and Class in the Nationalist Revolution* (Stanford, CA: Stanford University Press, 1996).

54. Michael Murdock, *Disarming the Allies of Imperialism: Agitation, Manipulation, and the State during China's Nationalist Revolution, 1922–1929* (Ithaca, NY: Cornell University Press, 2006).

55. John R. Watt, *Saving Lives in Wartime China: How Medical Reformers Built Modern Healthcare Systems amid War and Epidemics, 1928–1945* (Leiden: Brill, 2014), 73–114.

56. The most prominent health center was in Ding Xian, near Beijing. See C. C. Chen, "Ting Hsien and the Public Health Movement in China," *Millbank Memorial Fund Quarterly* 15, no. 4 (1937): 380–90.

57. Watt, *Saving Lives in Wartime China*, 253–98.

58. AnElissa Lucas, *Chinese Medical Modernization: Comparative Policy Continuities, 1930–1980s* (Westport, CT: Praeger Publishers, 1982). It is worth noting that Britain's Ministry of Health was established only in 1919, and the Soviet People's Commissariat for Health only in 1923.

59. Ka-che Yip, *Health and National Reconstruction in Nationalist China: The Development of Modern Health Services, 1928–1937* (Ann Arbor, MI: Association for Asian Studies, 1995), 62–63.

60. Kai-yi Chen, *Seeds from the West: St. John's Medical School, Shanghai, 1880–1952* (Chicago: Imprint Publications, 2001).

61. Zhao Hongjun, *History of the Modern Controversies over Chinese vs. Western Medicine* (Hefei: Anhui kexu Jishu chubanshe, 1989); Andrews, *Making of Modern Chinese Medicine*; Sean Hsiang-lin Lei, *Neither Donkey nor Horse: Medicine in the Struggle over China's Modernity* (Chicago: University of Chicago Press, 2014).

62. Jürgen Osterhammel, "'Technical Co-operation' between the League of Nations and China," *Modern Asian Studies* 13, no. 4 (1979): 661–80.

63. R. K. S. Lim and C. C. Chen, "State Medicine," March 18, 1937, 4–5, 1937 General Correspondence, folder 1119, box 151, Record Group (RG) 2, Rockefeller Foundation Archives, Sleepy Hollow, New York [hereafter cited as RFA].

64. Watt, *Saving Lives in Wartime China*.

65. John R. Watt, *A Friend in Deed: ABMAC and the Republic of China, 1937–1987* (New York: American Bureau for Medical Aid in China, 1992), 10.

66. See, for examples, Michael Shiyung Liu, "From Japanese Colonial Medicine to American-Standard Medicine in Taiwan: A Case Study in the Medical Profession and Practices in East Asia," in Liping Bu and Darwin Stapleton, *Science, Public Health*

and the State in Modern Asia (New York: Routledge, 2012), 161–76; Ming-cheng M. Lo, Doctors within Borders: Profession, Ethnicity, and Modernity in Colonial Taiwan (Berkeley: University of California Press, 2002).

67. David M. Lampton, The Politics of Medicine in China: The Policy Process, 1949–1977 (Boulder, CO: Westview Press, 1977); Xiaoping Fang, Barefoot Doctors and Western Medicine in China (Rochester, NY: University of Rochester Press, 2012).

68. Chen Bangxian, Zhongguo yixue shi [Chinese medical history] (Beijing: Tuanjie Publishing, 2005).

69. Wong and Wu, History of Chinese Medicine, vii.

70. Kim Taylor, Chinese Medicine in Early Communist China, 1945–63: A Medicine of Revolution (London: Routledge Curzon, 2005); Volker Scheid, Currents of Tradition in Chinese Medicine: 1626–2006 (Seattle: Eastland Press, 2007).

71. Ralph Crozier, Traditional Medicine in Modern China: Science, Nationalism, and the Tensions of Cultural Change (Cambridge, MA: Harvard University Press, 1968), 37.

72. E. Richard Brown, "Rockefeller Medicine in China: Professionalism and Imperialism," in Philanthropy and Cultural Imperialism: The Foundations at Home and Abroad, ed. Robert F. Arnove (Boston: G. K. Hall and Co., 1980), 123–46, quotation at 136.

73. Nathan Sivin, ed., Traditional Medicine in Contemporary China (Ann Arbor: University of Michigan Center for Chinese Studies, 1987); Nathan Sivin, ed., Science and Technology in East Asia (New York: Science History Publications, 1977); Paul Unschuld, Medicine in China: A History of Ideas (1985; reprint, Berkeley: University of California Press, 2010), final chap.

74. See Arif Dirlik, "Reversals, Ironies, Hegemonies: Notes on the Contemporary Historiography of Modern China," Modern China 22, no. 3 (July 1996): 243–84.

75. Zhao's account should be contrasted with earlier ones still caught in the unreflexive modernization paradigm of the Cold War—for example, Crozier, Traditional Medicine in Modern China.

76. Symmetry refers to treating both "true" and "false" scientific theories the same way in scholarly accounts of science and was first put forward by David Bloor and extended by Bruno Latour.

77. Rogaski, Hygienic Modernity; Luo Fuyi, Ruth Rogaski, and Xiang Lei, trans., Weisheng de xiandai xing: Zhongguo tongshang kou'an weisheng yu jibing de hanyi (Nanjing: Jiangsu People's Press, 2007).

78. Warwick Anderson, Colonial Pathologies: American Tropical Medicine, Race and Hygiene in the Philippines (Durham, NC: Duke University Press, 2006); David Arnold, Colonizing the Body: State Medicine and Epidemic Disease in Nineteenth Century India (Berkeley: University of California Press, 1993).

79. Angela Ki Che Leung and Charlotte Furth, eds., Health and Hygiene in Chinese East Asia: Policies and Publics in the Long Twentieth Century (Durham, NC: Duke University Press, 2010).

80. See also Michael Shiyung Liu, Prescribing Colonialization: The Role of Medical Practices and Policies in Japan-Ruled Taiwan, 1895–1945 (Ann Arbor, MI: Association of Asian Studies, 2009). For Chinese-language literature from Taiwan, see the bibliography in Leung and Furth, Health and Hygiene; Yu Xinzhong, "Guanzhu shengming—Haixia liang an xinqqi jibing yiliao shehui shi yanjiu" [Saving lives—the rise of historical research into disease and medicine on both sides of the Taiwan Strait],

Zhongguo shehui jingji shi yanjiu [Journal of Chinese Social and Economic History] 3 (2002): 94–98.

81. Angela Ki Che Leung, *Leprosy in China: A History* (New York: Columbia University Press, 2009); Marta Hanson, *Speaking of Epidemics in Chinese Medicine: Disease and the Geographic Imagination in Late Imperial China* (New York: Routledge, 2011); Benedict, *Bubonic Plague in China.*

82. Leung, *Leprosy in China,* 142–43, 163; Leung is also known for an important article on organized medicine in late-imperial China, "Organized Medicine in Ming-Qing China," and an important statement on the field in Chinese, "Yiliao shi yu zhongguo xiandai xing wenti" [The history of medicine and the problem of modernity in contemporary China], in *Zhongguo shehui lishi pinglun* [Chinese Social History Review], ed. Chang Jianhua, vol. 8 (Tianjin: Tianjin guiji chubanshe, 2007).

83. Ka-che Yip, *Disease, Colonialism and the State: Malaria in Modern East Asian History* (Hong Kong: Hong Kong University Press, 2009).

84. Yu Xinzhong, *Qingdai jiangnan de wenyi yu shehui: Yi xiang yiliao shehui she de yanjiu* [Epidemics and society in Qing Jiangnan] (Beijing: Beijing Normal University, 2014); Zhang Daqing, *Zhongguo jindai jibing shehui shi* [A social history of diseases in modern China] (Jinan: Shandong Jiaoyu chubanshe, 2006).

85. Yu Xinzhong, "The Treatment of Night Soil and Waste in Modern China," in Leung and Furth, *Health and Hygiene,* 51–72.

86. Yang Nianqun, *Zaizao "Bingren."*

87. Yu Xingzhong, "Writing about a Different Kind of Medical History: A Critical Review of *Zaizao "Bingren"* by Yang Nianqun," trans. Li Yi, *Journal of Modern Chinese History* 1, no. 2 (2007): 239–48.

88. Hu Cheng, *Yiliao, weisheng yu shijie zhi zhongguo: Kua guohe kua wenhua shiyu zhi xia de lishi yanjiu* [Medicine, hygiene and China in the world: A transnational and transcultural history study] (Beijing: Kexue Publishing, 2013).

89. This book does not address post-1949 developments for a variety of reasons, the key one being that it focuses on the coherent period of foreign imperialism known as the "century of humiliation," from the First Opium War to the establishment of the People's Republic of China and end to all unequal treaties. Modern (*jindai*) historians in China do not research past the 1949 divide (a notable exception is Yang Nianqun's *Zaizai "Bingren."* When originally conceived by Zhang Daqing and William Schneider, the project retained these boundaries, as did the conference papers on which the following chapters are based. Some of the authors represented here are writing monographs that cross the 1949 divide, and we look forward to future collaborative projects that will do the same.

90. Gao, *Dezhen zhuan.*

91. Compare also He's previous published work: He Xiaolian, *Xiyi dongjian yu wenhua tiaoshi* [Western medicine's eastern advance and cultural accommodation] (Shanghai: Shanghai Guji Chubanshe, 2006).

92. Sonya Grypma, *Healing Henan: Canadian Nurses at the North China Mission, 1888–1947* (Vancouver: University of British Columbia Press, 2008); Kaiyi Chen, "Quality versus Quantity: The Rockefeller Foundation and Nurses' Training in China," *Journal of American–East Asian Relations* 5, no. 1 (2003): 77–104.

93. Andre Gunder Frank, *On Capitalist Underdevelopment* (Oxford: Oxford University Press, 1976); see also Andre Gunder Frank, Sing C. Chew, and Robert

Allen Denemark, *The Development of Underdevelopment: Essays in Honor of Andre Gunder Frank* (Armonk, NY: Sage Publications, 1999).

94. John B. Grant, "Relations between Public Health and Social and Economic Conditions in the Community," March 18, 1937, 1937 General Correspondence, folder 1119, box 151, series 1937-601, RG 2, RFA. See also Bullock, *American Transplant*, 134–61.

95. Houghton, "Trends in Medical Education," 939.

96. On the adaptability of the Rockefeller International Health Commission to local conditions, see Steven Palmer, *Launching Global Health: The Caribbean Odyssey of the Rockefeller Foundation* (Ann Arbor: University of Michigan Press, 2010).

97. R. K. S. Lim and C. C. Chen, "State Medicine," March 18, 1937, 1937 General Correspondence, folder 1119, box 151, RG 2, RFA.

98. Robinson helped establish Johns Hopkins–style research medical schools at the Rockefeller Institute (1910–13), Washington University (1913–20), Vanderbilt University (1920–23), and Cornell University Medical School (1923–34) and was visiting professor of medicine at PUMC at the time of his speech. G. Canby Robinson, "The Influence of the Past on the Present and Future of Medicine," *Chinese Medical Journal* 49, no. 9 (1935): 836.

Part One

Hygiene and Disease Construction in Late Qing China

Chapter One

Reflections on the Modernity of Sanitation Policies in the Late Qing Dynasty

YU XINZHONG

China's post-Mao embrace of market socialism has transformed its society over the past forty years, and modernization has become the prime directive in almost every realm of life. Yet in this headlong embrace of modernity, there is little space for a healthy critique of the processes and unintended consequences of modernization. Modernity has arguably offered increased wealth and comfort for millions in China, but the increased *convenience* of life has not necessarily led to an increased *quality* of life—we need only look to the dramatic health effects of pollution on *all* residents in cities like Beijing as an example. Interestingly, this headlong turn to praise modernization has led to a reevaluation of China's semicolonial past. While the twentieth century largely saw the historical disparagement of foreign missionaries and other foreign physicians as agents of imperialism, the turn toward modernization as the *goal* (rather than the *means* to an egalitarian socialist society) has resulted in most Chinese-language accounts today praising the contributions of medical missionaries and other foreign builders of public health systems. This, despite the complicated impact of such systems on the lives of Chinese people of all classes and their arrival under the unequal conditions of foreign imperialism. Yet our histories of public health must not merely be paeans of praise to the pioneers of public health; they must also recognize the sacrifices that these measures forced on ordinary people. Although something was gained by increased hygiene, much was also lost. This chapter is a reflection on the empirical findings in my recent book, *Qingdai weisheng fangyi jizhi jiqi jindai yanbian* (Qing-era hygienic prevention mechanisms and their modern transformation), where I elaborate on the issues of quarantine and the management of water and night soil in the rapidly growing urban centers at the end of the Qing dynasty. For all that was gained in disease management, whole economies and livelihoods were disrupted, while personal freedoms were severely restricted.[1]

In the late nineteenth and early twentieth centuries, Western conceptions of health and hygiene that were designed primarily to avoid the spread of epidemic disease by ship or train gradually began to infiltrate port cities of China where unequal treaties allowed foreigners to trade, reside, and establish local settler governments. European and American settlers in treaty ports like Shanghai and Tianjin had daily contact with a wide variety of Chinese people, especially people of lower status than themselves such as their servants and the destitute people they encountered on the street. From these encounters foreign observers drew broad generalizations about the hygiene or lack of hygiene of the Chinese people. In 1896, one of the most careful and sympathetic of these observers, William Alexander Parson Martin (1827–1916), wrote in his memoirs about the remarkable freedom the Chinese seemed to feel in conducting themselves in public:

> So far are the Chinese from presenting the aspect of an oppressed people, that no people in the world are more exempt from official interference. You might spend days in a Chinese town without seeing a policeman. Every man seems free to do what is right in his own eyes. He throws his garbage in the street, and no one calls him to account. He stops his cart in the street, and everybody turns out without complaining. In most places, though not in the capital, on the occurrence of a marriage or funeral, in both of which the festivities last for several days, he may enlarge his house by taking in a part or the whole of the street; and other people submit to the inconvenience, knowing that time and circumstance will bring their revenge.[2]

Martin was not completely clear about whether this trait among Chinese people was to be praised or condemned, and the reader may doubt whether such freedom existed, even in the late Qing era. Yet it is worth considering the possible implications. Today it is unlikely that many would interpret it as saying that formerly the Chinese were particularly liberated among the peoples of the world; most are likely to take the exact opposite position, that Chinese people were lacking in expressing the norms of civilization, and especially lacking notions and consciousness of public health that they could not understand. In this view, Chinese people of the late Qing era simply did not pay attention to hygiene. Yet these criticisms of late Qing Chinese hygienic practices are not new. For example, that giant of modern Chinese thought, Liang Qichao, contrasted Chinese hygienic practices with those of America after he visited the United States at the beginning of the twentieth century:

On the sidewalks on both sides of the streets in San Francisco (vehicles go in the middle of the street), spitting and littering are not allowed, and violators are fined five dollars. On New York trolleys, spitting is prohibited and violators are fined five hundred dollars. They value cleanliness so much as to interfere and restrict freedom. No wonder Chinese are despised, since they are such messy and filthy citizens.[3]

Although not a direct response to the words of Martin, Liang's conclusions about the lack of Chinese hygienic practices are perfectly clear; it is as if he took Martin's positive words that Chinese people are particularly free, but instead saw this as a defect. The resulting judgment is that Chinese behave as "messy and filthy citizens." Whether considered within its original late Qing context, or in the eyes of one of today's public figures—emotional flag-wavers supporting traditional Chinese culture—it is natural that Liang Qichao's very public criticism of Chinese people evokes a similar reaction. Clearly, there is good reason for Liang's criticism of Chinese culture. Precisely for this reason we can see that at that time the saying "Chinese people are unhygienic" (*bu jiang weisheng*) was already a widely accepted concept, and up to the present day it continues to have considerable purchase. But such judgments ignore the long Daoist and medical traditions of "guarding life," or *weisheng*, in China that emphasize moderation in both eating and the frequency of sexual intercourse, but also included larger-scale efforts to prevent epidemics.[4] Two examples stand out to illustrate this: Wu Youxing's Warm Disease school, and the spread of variolation to prevent smallpox. During the civil wars of the Ming-Qing transition, an epidemic was successfully treated through Wu Youxing's innovative thinking about the spread of disease, while smallpox variolation was used to prevent the disease in China for centuries before Jennerian vaccination arrived from Europe.[5]

Yet whatever antiepidemic mechanisms had been used previously, by the late nineteenth century it was the *lack* of Euro-American-style public health measures that came to characterize China, not the *existence* of other antiepidemic practices. Since the Opium War and China's experience of a series of failures and humiliations, China's pride and self-respect as the Celestial Empire of civilization gradually diminished as it was increasingly characterized by a condition of conservatism, arrogance, and stubbornness that made it unable to adapt to global trends. This historical process evoked two simultaneous and seemingly contradictory reactions. Chinese people came to feel lost, humiliated, and helpless, while at the same time a healthy sense of self-respect was transformed into self-abasement even among some of the most prominent intellectuals like Liang Qichao and Lu Xun. Lu Xun, China's greatest modern writer and critic of traditional culture, described China's loss of self-respect as a "misfortune that leads to sorrow and incontestable resentment." Lu Xun tended to describe the Chinese character as barbarous, citing cases of cannibalism, looting, murder, human trafficking, superstition, polygamy, and linking the wearing of the pigtail, opium use, and foot-binding as comparable to habits of aboriginal peoples whom he might have called "savages" if writing in English. Lu Xun was deeply influenced by paternalistic, Orientalist representations of the Chinese character by the missionary Arthur Smith in his widely influential *Chinese Characteristics.*[6] The idea that the Chinese were "unhygienic," another source of humiliation, also originated in the late Qing period. The narrative of the racial superiority of Europeans during the heyday of European imperialism and social Darwinism became foundational to Chinese modern history. Yet these simplistic caricatures of "the Chinese" by foreigners, which Chinese writers accepted, not only fostered a sense of national humiliation, summarized in phrases like "the Sick Man of East Asia," but also created a strong reaction among some that led to an imaginary national pride, wounded as it may be. Chinese, by the twentieth century, might at one moment feel the disgrace of national failure, and at the next, the smugness of being part of a great world civilization. So an appropriate question to ask is whether this phenomenon is a product of a kind of self-hating imagination, or does it reveal the historical reality of a specific Chinese character?

In the last forty years of reform and opening up, as China has made remarkable achievements on the road of modernization—great developments eulogized by international society—what in Chinese is called "civil quality" (*wenming sushi*) of Chinese people has nonetheless been generally criticized. Chinese people, are, on the one hand, proud of the advancement of material accumulation, while being worried and feeling repulsed by the backwardness of their national soft power and the low standard of civil quality, on the other.[7]

"Being hygienic" (*jiang weisheng*) has become an essential component of modern "civility"; therefore, "being not hygienic" undoubtedly reflects the lack—or at least low quality—of Chinese people's "civility." To this day, Chinese people still feel largely uncomfortable and insecure because of society's failure to fully establish a modern public health system. For a developing country eager to pursue modernization, China is still in pursuit of establishing a modern public hygiene system that first originated in the West. But does this insecurity about the current situation of public health in China mean that an idealized modern "hygiene" should only be a goal to strive for rather than an object to be pondered and reflected upon? I think that both hygienic accomplishments *and* reflection on those accomplishments are needed. As my research on the sanitization history of the Qing period has demonstrated, the modern system of Western hygiene and public health not only involves the beautiful cloak of being "modern," representing the evolution of civilization, but also has become an omnipresent power that penetrates people's daily life in sometimes unwelcome ways.[8]

One of China's classic novels from the Ming dynasty, known and loved by children and adults alike, tells the supernatural story of Sun Wukong, the irascible monkey king who accompanies the monk Xuanzang on a journey to India in pursuit of Buddhist scriptures. The mission of Xuanzang was historical, yet in this popular account the author was able to use supernatural beings to describe truths in a kind of parable that transcends and transgresses the historical record. The supernatural abilities of Sun Wukong, the monkey king, can be used here as a metaphor, particularly useful for Chinese readers, to describe the power of modern hygiene with its sometimes negative consequences. At one point in the story, Sun Wukong, who provides significant assistance to Xuanzang on his journey, causes enormous damage in heaven and on earth and is no longer trusted with his freedom. To gain rebirth, Sun is persuaded to wear a hooplike golden crown around his head, which can not be removed, and which the monk Xuanzang uses to control him if he becomes too independent minded. This crown gives the monkey a new life, yet he never comes to understand its true nature found in the incantation the monk Xuanzang recites to inflict pain to control him. The enormous popularity of the story for many centuries in China may be because the monkey king has both positive and negative qualities. He is mischievous and naughty, but also perceptive, brave, and intelligent. In contrast, Xuanzang, the monkey king's master, is boring and inflexible.[9] The crown relies on the restraint of freedom produced by this incantation, but also allows the monkey king to achieve reincarnation. Readers of the story tend to focus only on the restraint provided by the crown, not the enormous benefit.

Modern hygiene might be compared to this golden crown. Yet in considering modern hygiene in China, the situation is exactly the opposite. It is not the restraints but only the benefits of hygiene that are discussed. Maybe Chinese people are too eager to be modernized, so when they think about modern hygiene, they naturally see only the aura of "modernization" that hygiene presents and symbolizes, as well as the concrete benefits it has for Chinese society. But it seldom occurs to them that behind such a system is political and cultural power, which can interfere with and restrain a body that is naturally free in the manner described by W. A. P. Martin. If we can see this common feature of the monkey king's golden crown and the modern system of hygiene, can we not also observe other similarities between the two?

Such an analogy is not merely a literary device to draw the reader's attention. Nor is the intention to deny all the good brought by the modern system of hygiene to mankind generally and to Chinese society in particular. I only hope to remind people that besides providing order, tidiness, and a more comfortable environment with less chance to catch disease, hygiene also brings political and cultural hegemony and power, unfairness and injustice, and the monitoring and restraint of the human body. To recognize this, it is necessary to overcome the prevalent narrative of modernization found in histories of sanitization in the country, as well as the lack of reflection on modernity. Building on my own empirical research,[10] I can summarize this argument as follows:

First, through examining the founding of the modern inspection and quarantine system, it is obvious that the modern public sanitization system was not developed only out of the motive of defending public health; it also contained elements of racial or class bias. For example, when introducing the Western inspection and quarantine system to China, the imperial powers placed the highest priority on the safety of their citizens in concessions and other places. In the process they sacrificed the interests, and sometimes even the lives, of Chinese people. The introduction of this kind of blatant bias in the inspection and quarantine system was not only an invasion of China's sovereignty, but also a demonstration of colonial power and the superiority of civilization and race. Although modern sanitization had the effect of maintaining good health, the introduction and promotion of such a system was not driven only by this goal. It was also driven by the interests of imperial powers that promoted their own ideological discourse onto Chinese society in the name of science and the civilizing mission.[11]

Second, the introduction and implementation of the modern public health system contributed to the improvement of the urban environment, sanitization infrastructure, and lowering the rate of disease infection. From the perspective of the upper and middle classes in Chinese society, this was undoubtedly praiseworthy progress. However, the process of enforcement always exacted great costs but with little benefit for the much greater number of people of the lower classes. The reform of night soil manure processing, for example, not only meant new taxes upon ordinary people; it also raised the cost for farmers to acquire manure as fertilizer.[12]

In traditional times, night soil in the city was mainly taken care of by professional manure fertilizer organizations and handled through market mechanisms. The workers who dug out the night soil, according to a schedule for each neighborhood, would go up to each house to collect their night soil and other organic waste (usually for free) and then sell it to nearby farmers or professional managers. From the 1860s forward, beginning in Shanghai's foreign concessions, professional hygiene management organizations were established to take responsibility for managing night soil and garbage. They began by using existing urban networks, but then strengthened regulations, such as requiring that night soil buckets add lids, that night soil removal must happen at set times, and that night soil removal contractors pay a set fee. All of this added to the cost of removal and management. For those involved in the night soil business, such reforms aimed at the "improvement of the city environment" certainly did not seem necessary, and were at least not urgent. At the worst, such reforms might put these workers out of business or even lead to violence, as in 1907 when police patrolmen in Suzhou detained and tortured a night soil worker who they claimed they had caught breaking regulations.[13]

Meanwhile, the implementation of health inspection systems always infringed upon most people's practical benefits and freedom, often merely to please the aesthetic preferences of foreign residents and with few benefits for working people.[14] From the perspective of sanitization, many "advancements" brought by modernization were realized by the sacrifice of people from lower social classes. Mandatory cleaning, sterilization, and hygienic inspection brought Chinese society improved sovereignty, health, and progress, but also the infringement and deprivation of people's rights and freedom in the name of hygiene and civility.[15] Although it is inevitable that some people's interests and freedom would be sacrificed in order to promote modernization and national revival, during the process of enforcement, should we ignore the legitimate rights and appeals of ordinary people, or denounce their resistance as conservative, ignorant, and backward? Or should we give more thought as to whether the sacrifice they made was worth of it? I think the answer is obvious.

Third, at the beginning of the Qing period, the state seldom interfered with public hygiene and health, and had no corresponding systematic mechanism to do so. Thus the construction of the public health and sanitization system in the late Qing era turned the business of health and hygiene from individualized, self-initiated practices without specialized management to systemized and organized work under the official jurisdiction of the state. Yet, the interference of the state in public health and sanitization increased gradually; the establishment of state health responsibility was the result of a more specific state duty as well as the expansion of the state power. If the power discourse hidden within the health system cannot be recognized and society fails to establish a mechanism of corresponding checks and balances, then governmental power can, in the name of legitimacy, expand infinitely, while people's practical needs are overlooked.[16] In that case, the progress and achievements of "modernization" would merely be a mirage posing a significant cost to everyone in society.

One last observation is that the Western models of modern public health and sanitization that were introduced during the late Qing era in the name of importing science, civilization, and progress arrived in the context of a series of domestic and foreign-initiated crises. During this time, the pressures of the crisis of Chinese sovereignty had an indirect influence, but it was also the result of concrete and conscious choices over a one-hundred-year period by Chinese gentry elites who sought to modernize the nation and its citizens. Obviously, the gentry elites made such choices for a wide variety of reasons, yet during the internal and external crises, they considered such measures to be a panacea for Chinese society without much consideration about their practical necessity and specific suitability. In fact, there were not many opportunities or much time for them to think things through, and in the interest of expediency and convenience they could only simplify the complicated situation to basic issues such as defending sovereignty, pursuing civilization, and modernizing.[17]

Today, however, as time has passed and society has changed, it is no longer a luxury to carefully deliberate about the resources available to society. Reflecting on the past, we should not merely criticize the efforts and limits of that generation, but rather try to appreciate historical complexity in order to provide a chance for people to reconsider the process of Chinese modernization and reflect on the sources of and inspirations for modernity from an adequately sophisticated historical perspective.

If we reflect on the process of modernizing public health and sanitization in China, we might realize that history has repeated itself, even as society in general has ignored that history. Once again, Chinese society is uncritically embracing anything presented to it under the guise of "modernization." Is this because Chinese society is unwilling to examine its own history, or is there some kind of built-in tendency within modernizing Chinese society? Whatever one's perspective, historians should encourage society to recognize the role historical narratives play in legitimizing real-world actions.

Compared to that which came later in the second half of the twentieth century, the transformation of the late Qing public health system is no doubt a modest beginning that failed to fully transform society. Perhaps for this reason, in most scholarship concerning modern public health, the reforms of the late Qing era are mentioned merely in passing without much analysis. However, as the previous argument shows, the late Qing origins of public health were not insignificant. "Hygiene" became a signifier of social status and the pursuit of a new mainstream ethos, yet in addition the state made many substantial statutes and regulations regarding public health, especially those related to health inspection. But also, more importantly, the specific character of hygiene during the Chinese modernization process was already entrenched within the late Qing reforms, given their systematic nature.

During the twentieth century, diseases such as plague, smallpox, cholera, and tuberculosis declined as the major causes of death in China while many other diseases continued to be an important influence on Chinese society and people's health. Yet public health and hygiene measures paid special attention to those epidemic diseases most likely to produce social panic and disrupt international trade.[18] That is to say, although public hygiene measures were no doubt related to protecting health, at the same time they were a large part of the attention paid to establishing a stable social sphere. In fact, public health has always been primarily an exercise of political power to ensure economic ends.[19] This can be illustrated by some of the public health incidents at the turn of the twentieth century when, for example, the central and local governments established public health projects not necessarily for the sole purpose of disease treatment, but because of external political pressure. When plague struck Hong Kong in 1893–94, and again in Manchuria in 1910–11, the driving force behind public health measures such as quarantine and isolation were concerns for political sovereignty and the viability of trade routes by rail or by sea.[20] In the case of plague in Manchuria, the original reason for the government to commit fully to inspections was international pressure and to control the plague to avoid further encroachment on state sovereignty by Japan and Russia. This was why the incident was managed by the Ministry of Foreign Affairs and not another branch of government. The direct aim was to secure a hygienic cordon to stop the spread of plague, but the means by which the state managed this was to control the free movement of people suspected of plague with quarantine. In many cases, inspection was an opportunity for further state intervention in the lives of people, and many public health projects were initiated more because of ideological reasons, the power of public opinion, or the need of the ruling class to maintain its rule, rather than preserving people's health.

In this way diseases, including plague, were not merely pathological conditions that are scientifically measurable. They should be considered hybrid cultural constructions based on popular and scientific discourse; physician and patient experience; and the manipulation of existing religious, social, and medical concepts.[21] Viewed in this way, public health is not merely a medical and technical problem. It cannot be solely explained by means of science but must also be understood in the context of deep social, political, and cultural factors. If these points are obvious to Anglophone historians of medicine, they are not necessarily so to Sinophone historians.

The preceding is an example of the social determination of disease, a perspective that is generally appreciated by Western academics, but that has received little attention in China. It was only at the end of the twentieth century, with the appearance of AIDS—a disease with a growing impact and influence on Chinese society—that Chinese researchers and public health workers were compelled to pay more attention to nonmedical factors of disease and public health. Reflections prompted by this turn of events are no longer limited to social issues arising from inspection but also relate to issues of fair distribution of medical resources and social discrimination against AIDS patients. This disease also raised deep concern about the right of all to health and life, as well as issues of the overexpansion of political power over the bodies of patients.[22]

The result has been a turn among scholars and activists to reflect on the myths of health modernization since the beginning of the twentieth century. In examining the purpose of hygienic measures, the focus has been less on the growth of national and state power connected to economic gains, and more on the realization of individual rights. Meanwhile, the logic of the creeping expansion of state influence in the area of public health—with the concomitant expansion of political power—is no longer considered self-evident and above criticism. These new approaches seem to support a new view of public health in the twenty-first century. After a long century in which the bodies and health of Chinese people were increasingly subject to state control due to the construction of the public health system, there is now a demand to return rights over their bodies back to individuals.

Looking at the development of public health projects since the late Qing era, it is obvious that in the beginning of public health construction, with its emphasis on institutionalizing the public health system and hygiene, the focus was on the reform of the system of hygienic management. With the gradual introduction of modern public health science, as well as the founding of research institutes like the Central Inspection Bureau in the early twentieth century, the construction of public health relied more and more on the development of scientific power. At the end of the twentieth century, as the influence of AIDS kept growing, it led people to question the suitability of a model of a single biomedical science, a mechanism for understanding health issues that privileges the perspective of public health. People have started to think through social and cultural factors in addressing health issues by coordinating efforts from all of society, using multidisciplinary and more-comprehensive approaches.[23]

In twentieth-century China, one could say that the pursuit of hygiene has been a significant national goal of modernization aiming to reverse the humiliation of the late Qing dynasty. Achieving a fair and relatively complete system of national public health, even today, is still the goal, and there are ongoing efforts in that direction that benefit both the collective nation and individuals.

Without doubt, the construction of public health in twentieth-century China brought huge changes to Chinese society and people, although in many places to this day such developments remain at a preliminary stage. Thus far some readers may consider this essay to be merely a minor criticism of the public health system, which is actually beneficial to people's health and to national power. Here I reiterate that I have no intention to deny the significance and value of the construction of public health to Chinese society; however, this aspect is already acknowledged and discussed in most scholarship. But admitting its value and significance does not mean that there is no need to conduct criticism and reflection about its potential problems and oversights. By such reflection and criticism, I not only hope to challenge the mainstream modernization narrative of researchers about public health history in China, but also to provide historical context for contemporary public health practitioners in China. I further wish to suggest that in the long term, merely emphasizing development and prosperity while ignoring the guarantee of people's rights may not be ideal for the future development for China.

Notes

1. Yu Xinzhong, *Qingdai weisheng fangyi jizhi jiqi jindai yanbian* [Qing-era hygienic prevention mechanisms and their modern transformation] (Beijing: Beijing shifan daxue chubanshe, 2016).
2. Martin's memoirs were originally published as W. A. P. Martin, *A Cycle of Cathay; or, China, South and North; with Personal Reminiscences* (New York: F. H. Revell, 1896), 335–36. Author quotation was from Ding Weiliang et al., trans., *Huajia jiyi—yiwei Meiguo chuanjiaoshi yanzhong de wan Qing diguo* [Recollections from sixty years on: The late Qing Empire from the perspective of an American missionary] (1896; reprint, Guangxi: Normal University Press, 2004), 227.
3. Original from Liang Qichao, "Xin dalu youji ji qita: Lun Zhongguo ren zhi quedian" [Travels in the New World and other matters: On the defects of Chinese] (original 1903), in Zhong Shuhe, ed., *Toward the World Collectanea*, vol. 10, rev. ed. (Yuelu Bookstore, 2008), 561–62. Translation from R. David Arkush and Leo O. Lee, "Excerpts from 'Observations on a Trip to America' by Liang Qichao," in *Chinese Civilization: A Sourcebook* (New York: Patricia B. Ebrey, 1993), 335–40.
4. Yu, *Qingdai weisheng fangyi jizhi jiqi jindai yanbian*, 42–43; Ruth Rogaski, *Hygienic Modernity: Meanings of Health and Disease in Treaty-Port China* (Berkeley: University of California Press, 2004), 4–6.
5. Marta Hanson, *Speaking of Epidemics in Chinese Medicine: Disease and the Geographic Imagination in Late Imperial China* (New York: Routledge, 2011); Angela Ki Che Leung, "'Variolation' and Vaccination in Late Imperial China," *History of Vaccine Development*, S. A. Plotkin, ed. (Springer Science, 2011).
6. Lu Xun, "Mo luo shi li shuo" [On the function of poetry] (1890; reprint, Shanghai: North China Herald, 1907). For a critical discussion, see Lydia Liu, "Translating National Character: Lu Xun and Arthur Smith," in *Translingual Practice: Literature, National Culture, and Translated Modernity—China, 1900–1937* (Stanford, CA: Stanford University Press, 1995).
7. On the contradictions at the heart of contemporary Chinese nationalism, see William Callahan, *China: The Pessoptimist Nation* (Oxford: Oxford University Press, 2010).
8. See especially Yu Xinzhong, *Qingdai jiangnan de wenyi yu shehui: Yi xiang yiliao shehui she de yanjiu* [Epidemics and society in Qing Jiangnan] (Beijing: Beijing Normal University, 2014); and Yu Xinzhong, "The Treatment of Night Soil and Waste in Modern China," in Angela Ki Che Leung and Charlotte Furth, eds., *Health and Hygiene in Chinese East Asia: Policies and Publics in the Long Twentieth Century* (Durham, NC: Duke University Press, 2010), 51–72; see also Yu Xinzhong, ed., *Qing yilai de jibing, yiliao he weisheng* [Disease, medicine, and hygiene since the Qing] (Beijing: Sanlian Books, 2009); "Qingdai Jiangnan wenyi dui renkou zhi yingxiang chu tan" [A preliminary investigation into the influence of disease and population in Qing dynasty Jiangnan], *Chinese Population Science* 2 (2001); and "Qingdai Jiangnan de

weisheng guannian yu xingwei ji qi jindai bianqian chutan—yi huanjing he yongshui weisheng wei zhongxin" [A preliminary investigation into modern changes in ideas and activities of health and hygiene in Qing Jiangnan—placing environment and water use hygiene at the center], *Qing shi yanjiu* [Research in Qing History] 2 (2006).

9. The significance of this story to Chinese popular culture cannot be overestimated. There have been two big-budget Chinese films about this story released within twelve months while this manuscript was being prepared, and television adaptations are in almost continuous development.

10. Regarding the Chinese historiography of hygiene, see Yu Xinzhong, "Hewei weisheng: Zhongguo jinshi weisheng shi yanjiu chuyi" [What is hygiene? My humble opinion on the historiography of hygiene in China], *Research on the Theory of History*, no. 4 (2011): 133–41.

11. Yu Xinzhong, "Fuzhaxing yu xiandaixing: Wan Qing jianyi jizhi yinjian zhong de shehui fanying yanjiu" [Complexity and modernity: Research on social reaction created by late Qing quarantine mechanisms], *Jindai shi yanjiu* [Research in modern history] 2 (2012): 47–64.

12. Yu, "Treatment of Night Soil," 51–72.

13. Ibid., 66.

14. See ibid., 51–72; and Yu Xinzhong, "Fangyi, weisheng, shenti kongzhi—Wan Qing qingjie guannian he xingwei de yanbian" [Epidemic prevention, public health, and the domination of the body: The transformation of sanitary concepts and actions in the late Qing], in *Xin Shixue* [New History], ed. Huang Xingtao, vol. 3 (Beijing: Zhonghua shuju, 2009), 57–99.

15. See Yu, "Fangyi, weisheng, shenti kongzhi"; Yu Xinzhong, "Wan Qing de weisheng xingzheng yu jindai shenti de xingcheng—yi weisheng fangyi wei zhongxin" [Late Qing sanitary administration and the formation of the modern body—placing public health epidemic prevention at the center], *Research in Qing History* [Qing shi yanjiu] 4 (2011): 48–68; Yu Xinzhong, "Complexity and modernity"; 47–64.

16. Yu, "Qingdai Jiangnan de weisheng guannian yu xingwei ji qi jindai bianqian chutan," 12–26.

17. Yu Xinzhong, "Late Qing Sanitary Administration and the Formation of the Modern Body—Placing Public Health Epidemic Prevention at the Center" [Wan Qing de weisheng xingzheng yu jindai shenti de xingcheng—yi weisheng fangyi wei zhongxin], *Research in Qing History* [Qing shi yanjiu] 4 (2011): 48–68; Yu, "Complexity and modernity," 47–64.

18. Regarding causes of death of urban citizens from epidemic disease in modern China, see Jia Hongwei, *Ershi shiji sanshi niandai chengshi jumin de jibing yu siwang—yi Nanjing, Beiping, he Guangzhou weilie* [Disease and death among urban residents in the 1930s: The example of Nanjing, Beiping, and Guangzhou] (Shanxi University: Chinese Social History Association 14th Annual Meeting, 2012); and for acute infectious diseases as the target of public health since the late Qing, see Yu Xinzhong, "Epidemics and Public Health in Twentieth-Century China: Plague, Smallpox, and AIDS," in Bridie Andrews and Mary Brown Bullock, eds., *Medical Transitions in Twentieth-Century China* (Bloomington, IN: Indiana University Press, 2014), 91–105.

19. Yu, "Epidemics and Public Health," 91–105.

20. Sean Hsiang-lin Lei, "Sovereignty and the Microscope: Constituting Notifiable Infectious Disease and Containing the Manchurian Plague (1910–11)," in Leung

and Furth, *Health and Hygiene*, 73–106; Carol Benedict, *Bubonic Plague in Nineteenth-Century China* (Stanford, CA: Stanford University Press, 1996).

21. See Byron Good, *Medicine, Rationality and Experience: An Anthropological Perspective* (Cambridge: Cambridge University Press, 1994); Kai Bo-wen, *Kutong he jibing de shehui genyuan: Xiandai Zhongguo de yiyu, shenjing shuailuo he bingtong* [The social origin of pain and disease: Depression, neurasthenia, and illness in contemporary China] (Shanghai: Shanghai Sanlian Bookstore, 2008); and Kai, *Jitong de gushi: Kunnan zhiyu yu ren de jingkuang* [The story of pain: Financial difficulty, cure, and human circumstances] (Shanghai: Yiwen Press, 2010).

22. Yu, "Epidemics and Public Health," 91–105; Joan A. Kaufman, Arthur Kleinman, and A. Saich, eds., *AIDS and Social Policy in China* (Cambridge, MA: Harvard University Press, 2006).

23. Yu, "Epidemics and Public Health," 91–105.

Chapter Two

Discovering Diseases

Research on the Globalization of Medical Knowledge in Nineteenth-Century China

GAO XI

In 1869, Dr. Alexander R. Jamieson, a medical officer of Shanghai Customs Station, suggested to Sir Robert Hart (1834–1911), the inspector-general of Chinese Imperial Customs, that the customs establishment should take advantage of its unique position to collect information about the diseases of foreigners and natives in China. Hart then issued a circular on December 31, 1870, to the commissioners of customs at all treaty ports, in which he invited the medical officers and medical missionaries of the various ports to investigate the general health and disease prevalence at their ports for the observation of local peculiarities of diseases, especially those diseases that were rarely or never encountered anywhere outside of China.[1] Hart reasoned: "If carried out to the extent hoped for, the scheme may prove highly useful to the medical profession both in China and at home, and to the public generally."[2] On September 11, 1871, the first issue of the *Medical Reports* was published in Shanghai at Hart's order, which was the first of eighty volumes published over the next forty years with hundreds of reports from China, Hong Kong, and Korea as well as Japan.[3] They provided an abundance of data that offers historians a largely untapped resource for research on medicine and public health in nineteenth-century China and Asia. By presenting the scope of the *Medical Reports*, this chapter demonstrates that research activities related to the biomedical discovery of diseases began in nineteenth-century China and Asia and should be considered a significant episode in the narrative of the spread of Western medicine. In particular, it demonstrates the role of medical officers of the Maritime Customs Service and medical missionaries in promoting the globalization of scientific medical knowledge by establishing a standard of classification for investigating epidemic diseases not only in China and Asia more generally, but also in Europe and Africa.[4]

The present chapter will explore why the customs service was organized and why it issued medical reports, in addition to the relationship between these; and also how foreign medical officers and medical missionaries discovered and identified the diseases that they had never encountered anywhere else. Building on the resources of the *Medical Reports*, this study extends our understanding of the history of modern Chinese medicine, and the history of the globalization of medical knowledge, by focusing on the role that the Chinese Maritime Customs Service and its medical officers played in these historical processes.

The Chinese Imperial Maritime Customs and Its *Medical Reports*

The Imperial Maritime Customs Service in China was an international bureaucracy predominantly staffed by British officials at senior levels that was under the control of successive Chinese central governments from its founding in 1854 to the resignation of the last foreign inspector-general in January 1950. The inspector-general of customs gradually established a standardized British-style statistical and trade report system beginning in 1860.[5] In the aggregate, the system created a huge database of information on modern Chinese economic development, including international trade between China and the world. More than one thousand volumes of reports and publications were issued by the inspector-general of customs from 1859 through 1949. Scholars in China and around the world have recognized this collection as a remarkable database for modern Chinese history in general, and they have taken full advantage of this resource in studies of Chinese economic history in particular.[6] In addition to the trade reports, the inspector-general of customs also published a series of special reports on topics that included medicine, skills, opium, tea, and drugs. Most of these are one- or two-volume special editions and differ in format from the eighty volumes of regularly published medical reports. However, the customs reports have rarely been referenced in the history of medicine and public health, except in K. Chi-min Wong and Wu Lien-teh's *History of Chinese Medicine* published in 1932 (and revised in 1936).[7] This leads to two questions. First, why did an imperial revenue and trade institution take responsibility for medical reports? And second, what do these eighty volumes of medical reports indicate about the development of Chinese modern medicine and epidemic diseases in the nineteenth century?

To answer the first question, it is necessary to make a brief review of the relationship between the main practitioners of Western medicine—medical missionaries—and the Customs Service. The earliest Western physicians who came to China were employed by the British East India Company to serve their staff as well as other foreigners who lived and worked in Guangzhou (hereafter Canton) and Macao, then after 1842 in Hong Kong.[8] Dr. Alexander Pearson (1780–1874) of the East India Company, considered to be the first Western physician in modern China, introduced the practice of vaccination to the inhabitants of Canton and Macao beginning in 1805, only seven years after Edward Jenner published the results of his research.[9] In the next thirty years, there were at least five surgeons from the East India Company who cared for foreign and Chinese patients in Canton until 1835, when Peter Parker (1804–88), the first medical missionary, arrived.[10] In 1838, the Medical Missionary Society was established by Parker and others who followed him at Canton. After that, medical missionaries played an important role in the spread of Western medicine in China, although they were not the only group to contribute to the introduction of medical science in nineteenth-century China. The historical record shows that private, secular physicians and the surgeons of the British military also introduced Western medicine to the Chinese people.[11]

With the signing of the Treaty of Tianjin (Tientsin) in 1860, more Westerners and missionaries settled in the treaty cities, where they found an increase in demand for medical services.[12] Due to limited resources, medical missionaries and private physicians often collaborated to carry out medical practice. For example, private physicians sometimes assisted in running mission hospitals while the medical missionaries were sometimes employed by official foreign institutions. John Dudgeon (1837–1901), a doctor with the London Missionary Society, was in charge of the mission hospital in Beijing while he was simultaneously employed as a medical attendant to the British and American consulates and served as the medical officer of the Imperial Maritime Customs Service.[13] Inspector-General Hart was clearly aware of the extent of medical missionary activity when he decided to publish the *Medical Reports*.[14] Evidence of this can be found in the fact that ten medical missionaries were among the twenty medical officers on the first list of physicians published by Hart.[15] In fact, examples of medical missionaries holding concurrent posts as customs medical officers in the *Medical Reports* can be found well into the twentieth century. Some of them were famous nineteenth-century missionaries, such as Dr. H. N. Allen (1858–1932) of the Board of Foreign Missions of the Presbyterian Church in Seoul; Dr. W. W. Myers of the London Missionary Society in Wenzhou (Wenchow); and Dr. Edward H. Hume (1876–1957) of the Yale-in-China Mission in Changsha, who was the last medical officer to submit a report in the final volume.

In nineteenth-century China, before the Chinese government considered medicine or public health as part of its responsibility, it was difficult for foreigners to find information about basic environmental information or local health conditions as they had come to expect in Europe. Because no health inspection system or health law yet existed in China, there were no national health administration institutes to issue regular health reports on morbidity and mortality statistics and also no medical officers to inspect urban health or monitor epidemic diseases. The Imperial Maritime Customs Service was established as an agency of the Chinese government under the management of a Western system. The service had a number of stations served by a group of medical officers who had received a medical education in the West and then practiced in China. Their training gave them the tools and ambition to investigate epidemic disease and explore the local disease ecology.

Jamieson was the sole force behind the development and publication of the *Medical Reports*. Hart commissioned him to take charge of the publication in 1870.[16] Jamieson had been the chief commentator of the *North China Herald* and the *North China Daily* from 1862 to 1866, but he resigned in 1866 to go back to Ireland to study medicine. In 1869, when he returned to Shanghai as a physician at St. Luke's Hospital, he was employed as a medical officer in the Customs Service. Despite this change in his professional career, Jamieson's experience as a journalist served him well in managing the *Medical Reports* since he had experience providing instructions to contributors, preparing and formulating reports, and in the actual tasks of publication. He was the most prolific among the contributors to the *Reports*, authoring forty-five contributions from 1871 until he left the Customs Service in 1894. Of the 126 medical men (there were no women), some had received an Anglo-American medical education, some had training in German laboratory medicine, and some had been trained in clinical practice by French doctors. Contributors also included the medical missionaries stationed in customs ports of Japan and Korea. All therefore had some training in modern experimental science and a background in researching epidemiology. Because of their common cross-cultural experience, they all shared an interest in what would now be called medical geography and medical anthropology. The longest-serving contributor was a Dr. Ring, who served first at Canton (Guangzhou) and then moved to Amoy (Xiamen), eventually returning to Canton, for a total of twenty-eight years in China from 1874 through 1902. As mentioned above, the last contributor was Edward Hume, one of the most important figures in modern medical education during the Republican era of China. Dr. Wong Foon (Huang Kuan; 1828–78) was the only Chinese physician commissioned by Hart. He was considered one of the best surgeons east of the Cape of Good Hope, and in addition to private practice, he worked in the Canton Hospital in cooperation with John Kerr, who had succeeded Peter Parker.[17] Wong contributed seven reports on the health of Canton and one monograph on leprosy.

The reports were published semiannually—on March 31, with accounts from the winter season; and on September 30, for the summer season.[18] There were a total of 540 reports and fifty-nine monographs. Two examples of the monographs include one by Patrick Manson about the parasite now known as paragonimiasis, but which he named distoma ringer, that led to chronic hemoptysis (coughing up blood) if unboiled water was consumed[19] and one comparing the etiology of cholera in Japan by D. B. Simmons that included a map demonstrating the spread of cholera epidemics throughout East Asia.[20] Altogether, there were six reports from Japan and six reports from Korea. The *Medical Reports* reprinted six outside articles: three from the prestigious European pathology journal *Virchows Archiv*, one from the International Medical Congress of 1881, one from a Dutch journal, and one from the *China Medical Missionary Journal* (*CMMJ*). In turn, the *CMMJ* reprinted several articles of the *Medical Reports* beginning in 1890 and continuing until 1921, well after the *Medical Reports* ceased publication in 1910. [21] Dr. J. L. Maxwell offered an index of the printed *Medical Reports* in the *CMMJ*.[22]

The *Medical Reports* initially covered seventeen treaty ports from the most northern city of Niuzhuang (Newchwang, now called Yinkou) through the most southern, Huangpu (Whampoa), and included one inland city, Hankou (Hankow). During the half century of the publication history, reports came from thirty-two cities and regions, which included the capital Beijing and the important coastal port cities of Tianjin, Shanghai, Ningbo, and Guangdong, and Taiwan's key ports of Dansui and Tainan, as well as Yangzi River port cities such as Hankou, Nanjing, and Chongqing. But reports were also regularly included from Korea (Corea, also called Chemulp) and Yokohama in Japan. Thus the network of medical reporting extended throughout East Asia from Chongqing in the west to Yokohama in the east, and from Guangzhou and Tainan in the south to Tianjin in the north.[23]

This network of epidemic monitoring and ecological investigation, which was gradually built up by the medical officers and medical missionaries, extended throughout East Asia and created a huge medical database, comprising hundreds of reports. The *Medical Reports* were published by the Customs Service, as a public periodical rather than an internal report, and the issues were distributed around the world.[24]

Average circulation each year was 500, ranging from 488 in 1882 to 578 in 1890. Each issue was distributed to the 170 custom stations throughout the country, including Hong Kong, but also to Korea, Japan, and the Chinese Imperial Maritime Customs office in London. More than 130 foreign envoys, consulates, and commercial counselors as well as navy officers

Table 2.1. *Customs Medical Reports* circulation, 1882 and 1890

Region	Recipient	1882	1890
Total Asia		364	399
	Imperial Customs headquarters, stations, etc.	175	168
	Envoys, consulates, naval officers	139	131
	Hong Kong viceroy; Indian Ministry of Health	4	29
	Imperial college, libraries, societies	13	21
	Media in Shanghai, Hong Kong, Yokohama	7	14
	Physicians in Hong Kong, Fuzhou, Shanghai	26	36
Total Europe and United States		124	181
	Chinese offices overseas: Chinese Embassy, Imperial Customs in London	20	25
	Great Britain: libraries of medical schools, museums, royal societies, media, and individuals	60	68
	France: government, public affairs, media, publishers	20	24
	Germany and Austria: government, public affairs, media, publishers	6	30
	Russia: Ministry of Foreign Affairs	1	1
	Italy: Ministry of Foreign Affairs	—	1
	Sweden and Norway: governments	—	3
	United States: libraries and publishers	17	29

Source: China Imperial Maritime Customs, Customs Publications: Free List (Shanghai: Statistics Department of the Inspectorate General, 1882, 1890).

in China received each issue. The libraries of medical schools and public libraries and museums in Britain were the largest foreign subscribers, but the *Reports* also were received in France, Germany, the United States, Russia, and India. In addition to the customs medical officers, subscribers included diplomats, individual physicians, and media outlets. Its total circulation was not large, but the *Medical Reports* reached a truly global audience.

Although the medical officers and medical missionaries at the various ports were responsible for the content of the volumes, Hart formulated the structure of the *Medical Reports* according to six general categories:

1. The general health; the death rate among foreigners; and, as far as possible, a classification of the causes of death;
2. Disease prevalence;

3. General types of disease; peculiarities and complications encountered; special treatment demanded;
4. Relation of disease to season, alteration in local conditions—such as drainage;
5. Peculiar disease; especially leprosy;
6. Epidemics: absence or presence, causes, course and treatment, fatality.[25]

Generally, the main structure of each report was divided into three parts. First, brief six-month health reports were given for cities of foreign residence, including a description of the location, monthly meteorological observations, the sanitary situation, hospital reports, and statistics regarding foreigners arrived, born, and dead. Further attention was paid to urban public health facilities, basic health-related infrastructure such as housing construction materials, ventilation, indoor spatial distribution, food, water supply, drainage systems, and so on, with reference to the foreign residents' housing and their state of health. The second part of each report recorded epidemics, mapping their geographical spread while researching their history, pathology, treatment, and statistics. Attention was also given to exploring the different terms and names for diseases and contrasting varying diagnoses and treatments between the West and the East. Third, some items of information were provided by medical officers regarding Chinese medical knowledge, including theories of medicine and materia medica. Some scholars in the 1880s observed that "the remarkable divergence between some of those theories and those which are current among Western nations is no less striking than the approach which in other instances is manifest between them."[26]

The Classification of Disease

Historical nomenclatures differ radically from those in use today, and some current scholars even question whether it is possible to adequately capture the meanings contained in historical medical terminology using today's terms.[27] Analysis of the *Medical Reports* data, therefore, can help shed some light on this issue. Dr. Peter Parker published the first hospital report in modern China in February 1836—the first medical report that described Chinese patients' diseases using Western medical concepts.[28] His account described three diagnoses he had made in China: amaurosis of the eye (amaurosis fugax), abscess of the ear, and abscess of the parotid gland.[29] Later (1840–41) in Macao, Dr. Benjamin Hobson reported a range of conditions, from ophthalmic diseases, to cutaneous diseases, abdominal diseases, urinary diseases, uterine diseases, as well as wounds and contusions.[30] Both reports indicated that most patients attended their clinics with diseases of the eye. Among a great amount of missionary hospital reports available in mission archives and newspapers published before the 1870s, many registers of disease were relied on as furnishing accurate information on the statistics of disease in the cities where the medical missionaries opened dispensaries to care for Chinese patients.[31] The register of cases in Dr. W. Lockhart's report of Zhoushan (Chusan) demonstrates that most of his patients suffered from fevers rather than eye conditions, so his classification of disease was different from those of Drs. Parker and Hobson.[32] But they noted that they were unable to classify some general and local diseases.[33]

The initial *Customs Medical Reports* submitted from each port were based on the regular hospital reports of physicians like Parker. But the reports also extended to the regional ecological environment and general health conditions. However, as the contributors came from a variety of Western countries, missionaries with different educational backgrounds had no idea how to define or classify the new diseases they encountered in various regions of China. At first, there were no principles or patterns to follow in listing these diseases in English. Some disease nomenclatures listed diseases in alphabetical order, but in other reports diseases were listed in random order. For example, a total of eleven categories of disease were used in the second issue of the report from Amoy in 1871 by Drs. Müller and Patrick Manson. Their list demonstrates both the scale of diseases encountered and the prebacteriological or genetic terminology of miasmatic, enthetic (introduced from without), or diathetic (constitutional) diseases, followed by more familiar ones such as diseases of the digestive organs, diseases of circulatory and respiratory organs and generative organs, or diseases of the integuments (includes dermis, epidermis, hair, nails, sebaceous and mammary glands, and subcutaneous tissue). These were followed by eye diseases and parasitic diseases, but in between these categories Müller and Manson listed "accidents," which would not appear to be a disease category at all, followed by the catchall "other disease" that included cynanche tonsillaris (inflammatory sore throat leading to an abscess), epilepsy, alcoholism, debility (loss of strength), and adenitis (inflammation of a gland).[34] But at least the Müller and Manson report attempted organization: some early reports did not even attempt to classify diseases, but only recorded the method of treatment and the number of patients.

Later in 1871, when the second volume of the *Medical Report* was issued, Dr. Scott of Shantou (Swatow) made clear that his purpose was to use Victorian epidemiologist William Farr's classification system of diseases to "classify the diseases which have come under his notice among foreigners . . . indicating the number of cases seen under each head in each month of the half year."[35] Table 2.2, which is taken directly from that issue, gives a sense of how much Scott was influenced by Farr's classifications.

Table 2.2. Jamieson's classification of Chinese diseases, 1871–72

Disease name	Disease description	Total cases, October 1871– March 1872
fenghan	seems to include bronchitis and pneumonia	7
shengchan	childbirth	10
laobing	a convenient term covering every disease at the end of which the patient dies exhausted, including tuberculosis and the syphilitic and cancerous cachexiae	69
jibing	or "violent disease," another beautifully convenient and comprehensive term	35
shanghan	seems to be characterized by intense heat of skin, including probably typhus, pneumonia, and acute tuberculosis	17
tuxie	haemoptysis [haematemesis]	5
kesou	or cough; chronic bronchitis no doubt, often supplemented by asthma	1
fasha	which I am told, includes every state of insensibility	8
guzhang	or "drum dropsy," Ascites	2
fuji	choloraic diarrhea	2
xunsi	suicide	7
tongfeng	acute rheumatism [gout]	2
tianhua	smallpox	1
—	accidental burning	1

Source: "Dr. Alexander Jamieson's Report on the Health of Shanghai for the Half-year Ended 31st March 1872," *Medical Reports*, no. 13 (January–March 1872): 82.

Nor was Scott alone. In the previous thirty years, William Farr (1807–83) had developed the first British national vital statistics system as a public health surveillance instrument as well as a system for conducting epidemiological studies.[36] Farr's endeavors to craft a disease nosology usable by vital statisticians and epidemiologists eventually led to the creation of the International Classification of Diseases (ICD), derived from a proposal made in 1860.[37] This, in turn, was based on the first annual report of the registrar-general for Great Britain that he submitted in 1839, which included the following principles that should govern a uniform classification of disease:

> The advantages of a uniform statistical nomenclature, however imperfect, are so obvious, that it is surprising no attention has been paid to its enforcement in Bills of Mortality. Each disease has, in many instances, been denoted by

three or four terms, and each term has been applied to as many different diseases: vague, inconvenient names have been employed, or complications have been registered instead of primary diseases. The nomenclature is of as much importance in this department of inquiry as weights and measures in the physical sciences, and should be settled without delay.[38]

The utility of a uniform classification of the causes of death was so positively recognized at the first International Statistical Congress, held in Brussels in 1853, that the congress requested that William Farr and Marc d'Espine of Geneva prepare an internationally applicable uniform classification of the causes of death. At the next congress, in Paris in 1855, Farr and d'Espine submitted two separate lists that were based on very different principles. Farr's classification was arranged under five categories: (A) epidemic diseases; (B) constitutional (general) diseases; (C) local diseases arranged according to anatomical sites; (D) developmental diseases; (E) diseases that are the direct result of violence. D'Espine classified diseases according to their nature (gouty, herpetic, haematic, etc.). The congress adopted a compromise list of 139 rubrics.[39] This decision was most significant because it recognized the importance of uniformity in analyzing and comparing illnesses across the world. The specific categories were less important because of the ongoing debate on etiology. For example, Farr classed epidemic, endemic, and contagious diseases as "zymotic,"[40] which was similar to Müller and Manson's unfamiliar terminology of the mid-nineteenth century.[41] Of course, after acceptance of the germ theory of diseases, the categories changed dramatically.

In China, the first person to adopt Farr's nosology was not Dr. Scott, but Dr. Robert Meadow of Ningpo.[42] Although Meadow did not specify the reference for his classification of diseases, we can speculate that he used Farr's nosology. He divided his diseases into five classes: (I) Zymotic, (II) Constitutional, (III) Local, (IV) Developmental, (V) Accidental—almost identical to Farr's divisions.

Farr and the statistical congresses were not the only ones proposing a uniform disease classification system. Dr. Somerville of Fuzhou (Foochow) explained in his report that "in the classification of disease I adopt the form issued by the Admiralty for the use of Naval Surgeons:—Nomenclature of Disease, London 1868." These were:

I. General Diseases-Schedule A;
II. General Diseases-Schedule B;
III. Diseases of the Nervous System and Organs of the Special Senses;
IV. Diseases of the Circulatory System;
V&VI. Diseases of the Absorbent System;
VII. Diseases of the Respiratory System;
VIII. Diseases of the Digestive System;

IX. Diseases of the Urinary and Generative Systems;
X. Diseases of the Cellular Tissue and Cutaneous System; Unclassed
   Debility and Delirium Tremens and Wounds and Injuries.[43]

Somerville used this system of classification in his nine medical reports.[44] The lords commissioners of the Admiralty ordered the compilation of Statistical Reports of the Health of the Royal Navy in order to collect disease data by medical officers on board Her Majesty's naval ships for reports back to London. These reports included statistics of disease from stations in Great Britain, the Mediterranean, North America and the West Indies, South America, the Pacific, China, the East Indies, Australia, the west coast of Africa, and the Cape of Good Hope. Different from Farr's nosology, which focused on examining secular change in mortality, specific causes of death, and deaths by area, by occupation, and by marital state,[45] the naval surgeon's formulation made use of a symptom-based nosology, in which diseases were classified according to the symptoms they exhibited.[46]

The contrast between Farr's system and that of the Royal Navy was obvious. In editing the second *Medical Reports* issue, Jamieson was aware that uniformity of terminology and classification of diseases was needed. He noted:

> I take this opportunity of suggesting through you to Surgeons to the Customs at the various ports, that for purposes of comparison it is advisable for all to adopt some one recognised classification of disease. *The Nomenclature of Disease* (London, 1869), drawn up by a Committee appointed by the Royal College of Physicians of London, though doubtless not the best possible, is in the hands of nearly every member of profession, and adherence to it would for this reason, if for no other facilitate the collection of statistics from the tables supplied by the Surgeons.[47]

The 1869 edition of *The Nomenclature of Disease* was quite different from that of 1868. The new edition was divided into three categories of diseases: General Diseases (A), which included smallpox, measles, typhus, cholera, yellow fever, and plague; General Diseases (B), which included various forms of rheumatism, syphilis, gout, cancer, and diabetes; and Local Diseases, which covered those ailments particular to a specific part of the body. Jamieson was looking forward to receiving and comparing opinions on this question. He stated that if such expressions of opinion were forwarded to him, he would inform each surgeon as soon as possible what direction the majority were inclined to take. But his desire for uniformity of terminology was not realized. In later reports, a variety of classifications of diseases continued to be employed, with Farr's nosology and the *Nomenclature of Disease* becoming the main standards. Jamieson, along with Dudgeon of Peking (Beijing), used death certificates from hospitals for their reports. Dr. Wong did not use any kind of classification but listed the names of diseases with the numbers of patients. Dr. Reid of Hankow gave the statistics of diseases according to corresponding anatomical systems (which corresponded to "Local Diseases" in the *Nomenclature* of 1869), while Dr. Allen of the Port of Korea listed diseases in alphabetical order.[48] While each system had an internal logic, there was little or no overlap between them, making comparisons difficult.

In 1864, the international classification of the causes of death was revised in Paris on the basis of Farr's model and was subsequently further revised in 1874, 1880, and 1886. Although this classification was never universally accepted, the general arrangement proposed by Farr, including the principle of classifying diseases by anatomical sites, survived as the basis for the International List of Causes of Death.[49] The statistics provided by the customs medical officers not only covered the treaty ports, but also expanded inland to the rest of the country as the Chinese increasingly accepted treatment at mission hospitals. But the Imperial Maritime Customs Service was an economic institution of tax management and customs inspection; it did not have the authority to formulate uniform terminology and academic standards for classification of diseases. The *Medical Reports* merely built up a communication platform to collect the disease information for research conducted by the medical officers and the medical missionaries. Before this classification was uniformly agreed upon in the Western world, doctors working in China had limited input to the diseases being made by doctors in Europe regarding the classification of diseases. In his "*Epitome*" of the *Medical Reports*, Charles Gordon wrote:

> [Details in the reports] do not support theories which for the time being occupy a good deal of professional attention in England in regard to the etiology of what are called "zymotic diseases"—on the contrary, they are in direct opposition to some at least of those theories. This is a point of view the importance of which is manifest alike in its bearing on the causation of the very large class of diseases so designated, and, most important of all, in the treatment of persons suffering from those diseases.[50]

From a global perspective, information on nosologies from the *Medical Reports* challenged prevailing European theories of disease transmission, and thus contributed to opening up space for newer theories that took into account the East Asian diseases. Their investigation and classification of diseases could be regarded as part of the formation process of defining disease patterns in the West. The contributors were practitioners of these modes and applied Western classifications of disease to an Asian environment very different from that of Europe. Their description and understanding of the diseases they encountered in China and other parts of Asia therefore constitute an important dimension for research on the modern history of disease.

However, they ran into other problems when they tried to standardize diseases according to the *Nomenclature of Disease*. For example, a number of

Table 2.3 William Farr's classification of diseases, 1871

Class	Order
I. Zymotic	Miasmatic
	Enthetic
	Dietic
	Parasitic
II. Constitutional	Diathetic
	Tubercular
III. Local	Nervous system
	Organs of circulation
	Respiratory organs
	Urinary organs
	Generative organs
	Locomotive organs
	Integumentary system
	Disease of eye
IV. Developmental	—
V. Contusions	Contusions

Source: "Dr. Scott's Report on the Health of Swatow for the Half-year Ended September 30," *Medical Reports*, no. 11 (July–September 1871): 7.

Chinese diseases were beyond the descriptive categories in the *Nomenclature*. When they reported the native mortality in the British and American settlements of Shanghai, Dr. Jamieson chose to give the table of causes of death compiled from Chinese sources.[51] Jamieson acknowledged that, as a classification, the *Nomenclature of Diseases* was utterly worthless for China. Nonetheless, one or two important facts might be extracted from the descriptions.

For example, *jibing* was "violent diseases," a beautifully convenient and comprehensive term; *shanghan*, which seemed to be characterized by intense heat of skin, including probably typhus, pneumonia, and acute tuberculosis; *laobing* was a convenient term covering every disease at the end of which the patient died exhausted. Tuberculosis and the cachexia caused by syphilis and cancer found their places under this category. A variety of diseases were combined under one name, such as *fenghan*, which included bronchitis and pneumonia. On the one hand, Western doctors tried to define the disease found in China according to the *Nomenclature of Disease*; on the other hand, they tried to understand the background of Chinese interpretation of diseases in order to trace the metaphor of language, culture, and religion.

For example, using English, Irish, and continental European statistics, Dr. Jamieson reported that childbirth mortality was 1.21 percent in European lying-in hospitals, where complicated cases were frequently received, whereas doctors in China were surprised by the excessive puerperal mortality among Chinese women. They found a relevant term to describe this condition: "Blood lake," which was one of the layers of Buddhist hells originating from a Buddhist motet, *xue peng jing*. Dr. D. B. McCarter, who for many years resided in Ningbo (Ningpo), had an intimate knowledge of Chinese language. He visited a temple there in order to try to explore the meanings and influence of "Blood lake" among pregnant women and their families who suffered from puerperal fever.[52]

In terms of using the Chinese culture, lifestyle, habits, behavior, morality, and religion to discuss the meanings of Chinese disease terminology, Dudgeon's report in 1872 was a high point of academic rigor among all of the *Medical Reports*. For example, he found that diphtheria was called *nao sangzi, houdan, houyong*—all signifying more or less a malignant sore throat, or a narrowing of the air passages to suffocation.[53] Dudgeon found that the Chinese classified diseases according to three categories: the cancerous, malignant, and other sores. Several varieties are mentioned and named according their locality on the body. Ague (malaria) was the most common affliction in Beijing during the summer, Dudgeon reported:

> The popular name here for ague is yau-tze [*yaozi*]. The character is not found in Morrison's Dictionary, although it is in Kanghi's [Kangxi's]. The book name is nio-chi [*nüeji*], so called, according to a medical writer of this dynasty, from its resemblance in its treatment of people to a harsh and cruel man. Several kinds of ague are specified in Chinese medical works. The principal are the following ranged according to their causes, wind *feng*, cold *han*, heat *ri*, damp *shi*, phlegm *tan*, food *shi*; excessive exertion of body or mind *lao*, spirits (devils) *guixie*, epidemic *yi*, pestilential vapours issuing from deep valleys, and old age. The latter is caused by phlegm, water and bad blood getting coagulated into one lump, which is buried in the body, and which becomes enlarged and painful.[54]

Discovering Disease

As a record of the ecological environment of disease, the epidemiological situation, physical geography, weather reports, public health response measures, and the charity activities in most areas of China, the *Medical Reports* also explored the history of Chinese medicine, natural history, and materia medica during the last half century of the Qing dynasty. This information is of great value in recounting colonial medical activities and social conditions under semicolonialism, and no example illustrates this better than that of the most famous contributor to the *Medical Reports*, Patrick Manson.

In 1866, Manson (1844–1922), a Scottish physician, secured an appointment as a port surgeon in the Imperial Maritime Customs Service. While in China he made important discoveries in parasitology and eventually came to be known as the founder of the field of tropical medicine, especially after establishing the London School of Tropical Medicine in 1898.[55] Among his notable medical achievements during a career of more than ten years in Xiamen (Amoy) was the discovery in 1877 that mosquitoes carried *Filaria bancrofti* (now *Wucheria bancrofti*).[56] In addition, Manson's research on the elephantiasis of the legs led to his discovery of the bacteria he called *Filaria sanguinis hominis*.[57]

Wong and Wu's *History of Chinese Medicine* includes a detailed description of Manson's work, based on the twenty-two reports he submitted to the *Customs Medical Reports* from 1871 through 1883. Manson's first great achievement in Xiamen was an exhaustive description of a modified operation for elephantiasis of the scrotum illustrated by some drawings and short histories of ten cases, with his treatment method published in *Medical Report No. 3* in 1872.[58] In addition to the regular half-year health reports, Manson also wrote several monographs about his research interests, scientific practice, microscopic demonstrations, as well as his discoveries. He trained and utilized Chinese assistants, on whom he relied to procure ample amounts of research material and observational data, which then enabled Manson to enlarge the scale of his research and eventually led to his discovery of filarial periodicity. In 1875 Manson examined the apparently dissimilar diseases such as what he had previously called "lymph scrotum," tropical chyluria, and elephantiasis, and drew the conclusion that "they are not only similar diseases, but that they are the same disease in slightly different forms, or at different steps."[59]

In an extensive follow-up report, Manson first suggested that blood-sucking insects may have played a most important role in the transmission of disease—in this case the *Filaria* disease called elephantiasis.[60] In 1879, he proved his speculation by actual observation, showing some satisfaction that "the parasitic theory of the causation of elephantiasis has been subjected during the past eighteen months to a considerable amount of criticism, favorable and unfavorable." By tapping the lymphatic gland, often many times and of the same patient, he proved that the parent *filariea* live in the lymphatics and not in the inguino-femoral glands.[61] To add credibility to his discovery, Manson invited his friend Dr. Myers and his brother David to observe the cases of *Filaria sanguinis hominis* in South Formosa.[62]

In addition to his monographs and numerous health reports, Manson published thirteen research papers in the *Medical Reports*, not including his regular half-year health reports of Amoy, which are listed in table 2.4.

Table 2.4: Patrick Manson's papers published in the *Medical Reports*

Issue and year	Title
No. 10, 1875	Remarks on lymph scrotum, elephantiasis, and chyluria
No. 13, 1876	Report on haematozoa
No. 14, 1877	Further observation on *Filaria sanguinis hominis*
No. 16, 1878	Notes on *Tinea imbricata*, an undescribed species of body ringworm
No. 18, 1879	Additional notes on *Filaria sanguinis hominis* and filaria disease
No. 19, 1880	Notes on sprue
No. 20, 1880	*Distoma ringeri*
No. 21, 1881	*Trichina spiralis* in Chinese pork
	Notes on some skin disease
No. 22, 1881	*Distoma ringeri* and parasitical hemoptysis
	The periodicity of filarial migrations to and from the circulation
No. 23, 1882	Notes on filaria disease
No. 26, 1883	On the operative treatment of hepatitis and hepatic abscess

The discoveries of diseases constitute an important contribution of the *Medical Reports*, furnished through their detailed descriptions of major epidemics. By the order of Inspector-General Hart, medical officers paid special attention to the observation of leprosy.[63] Some officers reported leprosy was not found in their ports, while others explored incidences and manifestations of this disease carefully. For example, an 1871 report from Hankou had a specific feature on leprosy that extensively discussed fourteen cases;[64] and in 1873, Chinese medical officer Dr. F. Wong submitted another memorandum on his experience dealing with leprosy.[65] John Dudgeon of Beijing and G. Barbezieux also reported on the disease based on their clinical experience and research with Chinese medical texts. More typically, customs medical officers focused their interest on diseases prevalent at their ports of residence. The nationwide circulation of the *Medical Reports* of the Imperial Maritime Customs not only disseminated to every customs port including those in Japan and Korea the news of epidemics taking place in the most remote corners of China,[66] these stations also collected scientific information on the epidemics relative to the causes, course, and treatment as well as data on fatalities. The *Medical Reports* helped build a communication platform, making it possible for scientific discussion among medical officers of China, Japan, and Korea in their discovery of diseases in Asia.

Beriberi is an important disease in the modern history of medicine. August Hirsch described different types of beriberi in his *Handbuch der Historisch-geographischen Pathologie* in 1883, and the name "beriberi" was first applied to the disease by physicians in Malabar, India, who described symptoms such as "anesthesia of the skin, hyperaesthesia and paralysis of the muscles, anasarca, palpitation, cardiac and arterial murmurs."[67] The disease occurred during the summer months, especially in the seaport towns and southern coasts of Japan. Native physicians of Japan described patients with a heavy or tired feeling in their legs, which they called *kakké*. In 1885, Takaki Kanehiro, a British-trained Japanese navy physician, observed that beriberi was endemic among low-ranking crew members who were provided nothing but rice, but not among crews and officers of Western navies who consumed a Western-style diet. Takaki acknowledged that he "regarded the Japanese disease *kakké* as being 'beriberi,' the name he used for it in his English-language article."[68] *Customs Medical Report No. 10* in 1875 presented a short history of seven beriberi cases illustrated with drawings, demonstrating that research interest in the disease of beriberi began among Western physicians living in Japan in the 1870s, much earlier than the work of Takaki. Five years later, and still before Takaki's published work, Duane B. Simmons, an American director and surgeon-in-chief at the prefectural hospital of Yokohama, wrote an extensive report connecting beriberi and *kakké*, defining the disease based on observations of his clinic practice in Japan.[69] After an exhaustive exploration of common patterns of disease etiology under the categories of age, sex, occupation and social condition, diet, relapse of the disease, nonacclimatization, season, and temperature changes, as well as comparison with the case study by the British physicians in India, he stated that many cases that consisted of these symptoms were actually beriberi, no matter what terminology was presently being used. "I am quite certain that these are masked cases of beriberi, as I have not infrequently seen them later on, develop other symptoms, which left no doubt as to their nature. Further investigation will doubtless lead to the discovery of other masked forms of this disease."[70]

Simmons's report included definitions of the disease, a historical account, and geographical distribution, as well as the literature on beriberi, its etiology, and clinical history. Simmons found that those suffering from this disease found rice of "the better quality" difficult to bear, while at the same time it was the chief food of those most liable to contract beriberi, but he was nonetheless unable to explain this as the cause of beriberi.[71] Rather than being able to identify it as a disease of deficiency linked to a diet heavy in polished white rice—a high-status food—his investigations of the causes of beriberi came to the conclusion that it was a specific miasma or ground exhalation, thus comparing beriberi to marsh malarial disease.[72]

Interactive studies can be seen in every issue of the *Medical Reports*, as ambitious medical officers collected and shared infectious disease information in their pursuit of making discoveries. In *Medical Report No. 1*, John Dudgeon announced that Beijing had an epidemic of diphtheria in 1871, while the report from Xiamen in the next issue mentioned that diphtheria was rare in the southern part of the city.[73] Dudgeon reported that diphtheria was recognized as a new disease, was known only in the last fifty years, and seemed to be almost entirely confined to Beijing.[74] The report *Plague in China* offers another good example of accumulating knowledge. In 1884, when the plague disappeared from Egypt and Turkey, Western physicians living in Asia congratulated themselves on being finally rid of the most terrible of all epidemic diseases. But then it broke out once more in Mesopotamia (Iraq) in 1873. At this time, according to investigations by medical officers and medical missionaries published in the *Medical Reports*, bubonic plague also existed in China. In 1878, Dr. E. Rocher drew a map of the course pursued by the plague in 1871, 1872, and 1873 based on medical reports and official documents.[75] This map (fig. 2.1) shows the districts where it was most fatal and those through which it merely passed, demonstrating its Chinese origin in Yunnan Province, but also that it had originally passed into China from Burma. In addition, thirty years before the discovery of the rat flea vector of bubonic plague, Rocher noted a link between plague and rats.[76]

In 1879, Dr. Simmons published his findings on the prevalence of cholera in Japan in the previous three years.[77] For a century and a half, cholera had been a stigmatizing disease. Although the entire world was susceptible to cholera, Europeans nevertheless associated it with Asia, even calling it Asiatic cholera, particularly with regard to Bengal and its people. That stigma was the product of epistemic practice within an interdisciplinary and Orientalist cholera science that took shape in the 1860s and 1870s.[78] Those practices involved an overinterpretation of the historical epidemiological work of John Macpherson by his colleague N. C. Macnamara.[79] After reviewing Macpherson's writing about eastern Asia in his *Epidemic Cholera*, Simmons made note of "the small number of widespread epidemics which are reordered as having penetrated thither from early times, as compared with those which travelled in an opposite direction, and often arrived even in the heart of Europe."[80] Simmons asked why China and Japan, situated eastward of the Indian source of the scourge, were not affected by cholera even when it ravaged Belochistan, Persia, Arabia, and other countries to the west.[81] He thought that there were good grounds for the belief that lack of evidence of numerous visits of the disease confirmed the infrequency of its appearance, especially in countries so rich in historical records as China and Japan. So he first briefly reviewed what had been chronicled about epidemics in China and Japan.[82]

In order to ascertain the source of the visitation and the probable means by which the disease was imported into Japan in 1877, Dr. Simmons referred to what was known of its existence and progress in China immediately beforehand. He believed that this research was especially important because the questions raised at the time—whether the disease was really Asiatic, or

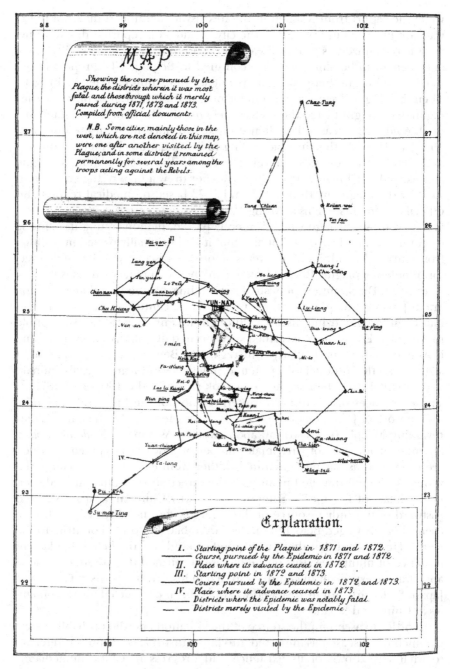

Figure 2.1. Map of plague from 1871 to 1873. Source: "Dr. Manson's Report on the Health of Amoy for the Half-Year Ended 31st March 1878," *Medical Report* no. 15 (1878): 26.

epidemic, cholera—were the first attempts to research the prevalence of the disease in China. Dr. Simmons was able to publish his findings in *Medical Report No. 14*, in which he found that the first cases of the disease on the coast of China manifested in Xiamen, based on a report communicated by David Manson:

> The first intimation of cholera was a request by the Spanish Consul General to examine the body of a Manilaman [Filipino] who had died suddenly . . . on the 20th June. . . . The first week in June, many deaths had occurred from a similar affection. . . . The first week in July the Chinese reported the mortality at from 10 to 100 daily. . . . The disease was no longer confined to one part of the town, it had spread over the whole native city.[83]

In tracing the epidemic situation of cholera in China, Simmons also referenced Jamieson's report on Shanghai and Somerville's report on Pagoda Anchorage.[84] He described the epidemics of 1877, 1878, and 1879 in Japan by the tables of the cholera returns and a map of the track of the epidemic in eastern Asia. He analyzed the general considerations of the character of the epidemic and its treatment. In addition, Simmons wrote a monograph on the influence of the habits and customs of various "races" on the epidemic prevalence of cholera among the Japanese. The observations by the residential medical officers in reference to the habits of life, the cultural influence, and the indigenous treatments deserve particular attention. The history of most of these factors has not yet been thoroughly studied.

The Globalization of Medical Knowledge: A Historical Perspective on Discovering Diseases

As has been mentioned above, there were no official statistical reports of morbidity and mortality in China before those of the *Customs Medical Reports*. In 1861, a medical officer was appointed by the Shanghai Municipal Council to be in charge of the health administration in terms of disease, epidemic, birth, and death statistics. Such reports emerged gradually in the Chinese Concessions in Shanghai, Xiamen, and Tianjin,[85] but those files were limited to foreign residents. The *Medical Reports* broke the boundary between Chinese and foreigners by extending their view to Chinese patients in the mission hospitals and in Chinese residential areas. An important requirement of the *Customs Medical Reports* was that the records of deaths from a disease and its morbidity be collected on a sustained and systematic basis. The result was that the efforts of the customs medical officers built up a database of public health and disease statistics in nineteenth-century China, in effect establishing what would later be considered the responsibility of the Chinese government.

The *Medical Reports* lasted nearly half a century, thereby providing a comprehensive survey and research of the ecological environment and disease geography of many cities and regions of China. They tracked the spread of epidemics throughout the whole Chinese empire, and even to neighboring Asian societies like Korea and Japan. The network of disease observation offered a communication platform with Shanghai at the center for the collection and delivery of epidemic information. The observations and reports by the medical officers contributed to the progress and development of scientific medicine via their discovery and description of new diseases in China with the support and encouragement of Robert Hart.

By recording the epidemics in Chinese coastal cities, the *Medical Reports* provide information for historians of nineteenth-century China and Japan as well as for comparative studies. In addition, according to John Dudgeon, there were at least seventy thousand foreigners living in Chinese Concessions, who, far away from their home countries, lived in a strange new world with climate, diet, and conditions and ways of life completely different from Europe and America.[86] Climate was the first challenge for missionaries and their dependents who also had to face the sudden change and the unexpected diseases in unfamiliar environments. How to deal with this environment and plague attacks were two serious challenges that made missionaries deeply anxious. The *Medical Reports* kept historical documents of diseases by recording Western residents' adaptations to the environment and their methods of surviving their struggles with diseases, including the management and treatment of foreign children who became ill in China.[87]

Germ theory, validated in the late nineteenth century and now a fundamental part of modern medicine and clinical microbiology, led to important innovations such as hygienic practices among medical professionals and the general public, and eventually to antibiotics. In the nineteenth century, when scientists in European laboratories devised tests to assess the germ theory of diseases, other scientists followed European colonists, leaving their laboratories for Asia and Africa in an attempt to discover new and rare diseases worldwide and then return to their labs to analyze their collected data. Patrick Manson's contributions to the development of tropical medicine is an illustrative example. The eighty volumes of *Medical Reports* show the history of how Western doctors applied germ theory in their observation of diseases in China. Their remarkable record of scientific research and contributions to global medical development from Asia to the West is of the highest interest. They expanded research connecting Chinese medical theory and the ecological environment. From the perspective of a wide variety of nationalities and cultures, medical scientists from America and Europe who went to Asia and Africa built up a global, interactive scientific network to investigate diseases and develop medicines, beginning in the 1870s. The *Medical Reports* makes it possible for scholars to evaluate Western

physicians—particularly their methods of observation and their achievement of research and treatment, and to explore those doctors' research ability and interest in nineteenth-century Asia.

From October through December 1884, the International Health
Exhibition was held in London—the biggest public health exhibition in
nineteenth-century Europe.[88] There was no doubt that tackling diseases,
particularly those spread through international trade networks, had become
a primary concern. Promoters of the concept of health in the nineteenth
century sought to improve the life of human beings—in terms of their food,
dwellings, dress, water supply, streetlights—through the inventions of science and technology to change people's social behavior and even moral
values. Ernest Hart, chairman of the exhibition, explained in his lecture
that "the health exhibition means that health was accepted as a synonym of
hygiene." He further said that the exhibition of Chinese health and hygiene
was worthy of international attention.[89] The Chinese Imperial Maritime
Customs, on behalf of the Chinese government, took part in the exhibition,
displaying such curiosities as Qing court dress, a wedding chair, Chinese
books, and Chinese musical instruments.[90] Among more than one hundred
books there were two regarding the health of the Chinese people—one was
Diet, Dress, and Dwellings of the Chinese in Relation to Health by John Dudgeon,
the medical officer of Peking; the other one was *An Epitome of the Reports of
the Medical Officers to the Chinese Imperial Maritime Customs Service*, arranged
by Surgeon General C. A. Gordon. To compile this collection, Gordon had
reedited the *Medical Reports* of the previous ten years and divided them into
three parts: the first on local conditions in relation to public health, the
second on historical notices of medicine and epidemics in China, and the
third on therapeutics and drugs. Dr. Gordon emphasized: "It will thus be
seen that the Reports submitted by those medical officers contain not only a
survey of matters more purely medical in their nature, but also many which
bear upon physical geography, climate, agriculture, commerce, natural history etc."[91]

The importance of the *Medical Reports* in the modern history of medicine
in China cannot be overemphasized. Several journals, such as the *Chinese
Repository*, the *Chinese Recorder*, and the *Bulletin of the Royal Asiatic Society*, published hospital reports and medical knowledge but were unwilling to publish academic articles. Hence, it is no surprise that the *Medical Reports* was
the first medical periodical in China from which the *Lancet* quoted articles.
When that journal introduced the *Medical Reports* in November 30, 1872, it
stated that the reports "contain matter of much novelty—indeed some of
them are not only interesting in the facts they narrate, but excellent specimens of medical reports."[92] Wong and Wu, in their history of medicine
in China, commented that "the references in this volume clearly show to
what high degree even the modern historiographer and epidemiologist is

indebted to the enterprise instituted by Jamieson and Hart."[93] Taken as a corpus, the *Medical Reports* are a remarkable record of the history of medicine, while also providing a unique point of view to observe Asian society.

As the concepts of disease geography and medical ecology emerged in nineteenth-century Europe, physicians and scientists followed colonizers to Asia and Africa to explore the history of disease from regional and social perspectives and find evidence for pathological research. This kind of multicultural and multiethnic exploration of diseases broadened the historical perspective of medical scientists and developed a global configuration of cooperation. International cooperation from Asia to Europe to Africa created circuits of global medical knowledge transmission. As much as any other example explored in the present volume, the *Medical Reports* demonstrate the globalization of medical knowledge between China and the rest of the world in the nineteenth century.

Notes

1. Robert Hart, "Inspector General's Circular No. 19 of 1870," *Customs Gazette Medical Reports for the Half-year Ended 31st March*, no. 10 (April–June 1871): 3.

2. Ibid.

3. Korea was a tributary state of the Qing dynasty until 1895 when China and Japan signed the Treaty of Shimonoseki to dissolve this relationship. So the inspector-general of the Imperial Maritime Customs took charge of the Korea Customs and appointed a medical officer there before the year of 1895.

4. Archive.org has digitized *An Epitome of the Reports of the Medical Officers of the Chinese Imperial Maritime Customs Service*, available at https://archive.org/details/cu31924023644234/page/n9 (accessed October 13, 2018).

5. Wu Songdi, "Cognition and Utilization of Chinese Traditional Maritime Customs Trade Return," *Journal of Historical Science*, no. 7 (2007): 33.

6. John K. Fairbank, *Trade and Diplomacy on the China Coast: The Opening of the Treaty Ports, 1842–1854* (Stanford, CA: Stanford University Press, 1953); Takeshi Hamashita, *Trade and Finance in Late Imperial China: Maritime Customs and Open Port Market Zones* (Singapore: Singapore University Press, 1989). Both Fairbank and Hamashita used this database to finish their remarkable books in English and Japanese, respectively. See also Donna Brunero, *Britain's Imperial Cornerstone in China: The Chinese Maritime Customs Service, 1854–1949* (London: Routledge, 2006); and Thomas P. Lyons, *China Maritime Customs and China's Trade Statistics, 1859–1948* (Trumansburg, NY: Willow Creek of Trumansburg, 2003). For Chinese research, see Wu Shongdi, "An Essay on the Publications of the Chinese Imperial Maritime Customs," *Journal of Historical Science*, no. 12 (2011): 54–63. Since 1951, the trade returns and annual and decennial reports of the Customs Service have been gradually published. The Second Historical Archives of China and the Chinese Customs has together published *The Imperial Maritime Customs Historical Resource* 70 (2001), which is considered the most important resource for research. The Chinese Maritime Customs Project at Bristol

University links resources from Cambridge University and the Second Historical Archives of China in Nanjing. For more on this project, see http://www.bristol. ac.uk/history/customs/about.html.

7. K. Chi-min Wong and Wu Lien-teh, *History of Chinese Medicine* (Shanghai: National Quarantine Service, 1936).

8. Ibid., 302–4.

9. W. Scarborough, "Medical Missions," *Chinese Recorder* 5, no. 3 (1874): 138.

10. Hosea Ballou Morse, *The Chronicles of the East India Company, Trading to China 1635–1834*, vol. 4 (Oxford: Clarendon Press, 1926–29), 226.

11. Charles Alexander Gordon, *China from a Medical Point of View in 1860 and 1861* (London: John Churchill, 1863), describes a military doctor's medical activities in China.

12. The "Treaty of Tien-tsin" was signed in Tianjin (Tientsin) in June 1858, ending the first part of the Second Opium War (1856–60). The Second French Empire, United Kingdom, Russian Empire, and United States were the parties involved. Such treaties opened more Chinese ports to foreigners, permitted foreign legations in the Chinese capital Beijing (Peking), allowed Christian missionary activity, and legalized the import of opium.

13. For detailed research see Gao Xi, *Dezhen zhuan: Yige Yingguo chuanjiaoshi yu wan Qing yixue jindai hua* [A biography of John Dudgeon: An English missionary and the modernization of late Qing medicine] (Shanghai: Fudan University Press, 2009).

14. Hart, "Inspector General's Circular No. 19."

15. Ibid. J. Dudgeon of Peking, J. Watson of Newchwang, J. Frazer of Tientsin, Carmichael and Meyers of Chefoo, A. G. Reid of Hankow, G. Shearer of Kiukiang, Somerville of Pagoda Anchorage, C. M. Scott of Swatow and F. Wong of Canton were medical missionaries and medical officers; the nonmissionary contributors were Barton and Galle of Shanghai, R. Meadows of Ningpo, J. M. Beaumont of Foochow, Sherwin of Pagoda Anchorage, Jones and Muller of Amoy, L. H. Franklyn of Tamsui, P. Manson of Takow, and R. Shillitoe of Whampo are medical officers.

16. *Medical Reports*, no. 10 (April–June 1871): 3.

17. Yung Wing, *My life in China and America* (New York: Henry Holt, 1909), 32.

18. According to Hart, the semiannual report should have ended October 31 for the winter season, but it actually ended September 30. *Medical Reports*, no. 10 (April–June 1871): 5.

19. *Medical Reports*, no. 22 (September 1881): 55–62.

20. *Medical Reports*, no. 18 (September 1879): 1–55.

21. H. W. B., "Notices of Books, China Imperial Maritimes Customs Medical Reports," *China Medical Missionary Journal* 4, no. 1 (January 1890): 18.

22. *China Medical Journal* 44, no. 12 (December 1930): 1137.

23. A complete list of cities with the Chinese postal spellings is as follows: Peking, Shanghai, Canton, Hankow, Newchwang, Tientsin, Ninpo, Amoy, Swatow, Kiukiang, Chefoo, Pagoda Anchorage, Foochow, Takow and Formosa, Tamsui and Kelung, Tainan, Chingkiang, Wenchow, Kiungchow, Ichang, Pakhoi, Wuchow, Szemao, Nanking, Chungking, Kongmoon, Mengtzu, Soochow, Wuhu, Lapa, Changsha, Lungchow, Tengyueh.

24. *China Imperial Maritime Customs: Customs Publications: Free List* (Shanghai: Statistics Department of the Inspectorate General, 1882). See note 4 above for URLs for all reports.

25. *Medical Reports,* no. 10 (April–June 1871): 3

26. C. A. Gordon, *An Epitome of the Reports of the Medical Officers to the Chinese Imperial Maritime Customs Service from 1871–1882* (London: Baillere, Tindall, and Cox, 1884), xv. This aspect of the *Reports* is of great interest for the comparative study of disease nosology, but a full examination falls outside the scope of this chapter.

27. G. Alter and A. Carmichael, "Studying Causes of Death in the Past: Problems and Models," *Historical Methods* 29 (1996): 44–48.

28. Rev. Peter Parker, "Ophthalmic Hospital at Canton: The First-Quarterly Report from the 4th of November 1835 to the 4th of February 1836," *Chinese Repository* 4 (February 1836): 461–73.

29. Ibid.

30. B. Hobson, "Report of the Medical Missionary Society's Operations at Macao in 1840–1841," in *The First and Second Report of the Medical Missionary Society in China with Minutes of Proceedings Hospital Reports & C.* (Macao: S. Wells Williams, 1841), 39–40.

31. J. C. Hepburn, MD, "Report of the Dispensary at Amoy from 1st of February 1841 to 1st of June 1845," *Report of the Medical Missionary Society in China for the Year 1845* (Victoria, Hong Kong: Hongkong Register Press, 1846), 16.

32. W. Lockhart divided his reports into general and constitutional diseases, cutaneous diseases, general surgical affections, and diseases of the ear. See his article "Diseases of the Eye and Its Appendages: Report of the Medical Missionary Society's Operations at Chusan in 1840–41," in *First and Second Report . . .* , 31–33.

33. B. Hobson, "Report of the medical missionary society's operations at Macao in 1840–1841," in *First and Second Report . . .* , 39–40.

34. "Drs. Muller and Manson's Report on the Health of Amoy for the Half-year Ended September 30," *Medical Reports,* no. 11 (July–September 1871): 12–13.

35. "Dr. Scott's Report on the Health of Swatow for the Half-year Ended September 30," *Medical Reports,* no. 11 (July–September 1871): 7.

36. For the relevant research concerning Will Farr, see Mervyn Susser and Abraham Adelstein, "An Introduction to the Work of William Farr," *American Journal of Epidemiology* 101, no. 6 (1975): 469–76; and John M. Eyler, *Victorian Social Medicine: The Ideas and Methods of William Farr* (Baltimore: Johns Hopkins University Press, 1979).

37. Eyler, *Victorian Social Medicine.*

38. "Letter to registrar-general from William Farr, Esq.," in *First Annual Report of the Registrar-General of Births, Deaths, and Marriages in England, Registrar-General's Reports for England and Wales* (London: Clowes and Son, 1839), 71.

39. I. M. Moriyama, R. M. Loy, and A. H. T. Robb-Smith, *History of the Statistical Classification of Diseases and Causes of Death* (Hyattsville, MD: National Center for Health Statistics, 2011), 11.

40. John M. Eyler, *Sir Arthur Newsholme and State Medicine, 1885–1935* (Cambridge: Cambridge University Press, 2002), 34.

41. On the introduction of germ theory in China, see Bridie Andrews, "Tuberculosis and the Assimilation of Germ Theory in China, 1895–1937," *Journal of the History of Medicine* 52 (1997): 114–57.

42. "Dr. Robert Meadows's Report on the Health of Ningpo for the Half-year Ended 31st March 1871," *Medical Reports,* no. 10 (April–June 1871): 34.

43. "Dr. J. R. Somerville's Report on the Health of Foochow (Pagoda Anchorage) for the Half-year Ended 30th September," *Medical Reports*, no. 11 (July–September 1871): 26.

44. Dr. Somerville submitted nine reports during 1871–77.

45. For Farr, see Susser and Adelstein, "Introduction," 472.

46. University of Oxford, Wellcome Unit for the History of Medicine, "Disease in the Royal Navy during the Nineteenth Century, 1856–1898," by Miles Dutton, accessed October 14, 2018, https://beta.ukdataservice.ac.uk/datacatalogue/studies/study?id=7390 (registration required).

47. R. Alex Jamieson, *Medical Reports*, no. 11 (July–September 1871): 3.

48. "Dr. A. G. Reid's Report on the Health of Hankow for the Half-year Ended 30th September," *Medical Reports*, no. 4 (September 1872): 72–73.

49. Moriyama, Loy, and Robb-Smith, *History of the Statistical Classification*.

50. Gordon, *Reports*, xv.

51. "Dr. Jamieson's Report on the Health of Shanghai for the Half-year Ended 31st March 1872," *Medical Reports*, no. 13 (January–March 1872): 82.

52. Ibid., 86.

53. "Dr. John Dudgeon's Report on the Health of Peking for the Half-year Ended 30th September 1871," *Medical Reports*, no. 13 (January–March 1872): 7–8.

54. Ibid.

55. On Manson, see Phillip Manson-Bahr, *Patrick Manson, the Father of Tropical Medicine* (London: Nelson, 1962); Gordon Cook, *Tropical Medicine: An Illustrated History of the Pioneers* (New York: Academic Press, 2007); Douglas M. Haynes, *Imperial Medicine: Patrick Manson and the Conquest of Tropical Disease* (Philadelphia: University of Pennsylvania Press, 2001); and Shang-Jen Li, "British Imperial Medicine in Late Nineteenth-Century China and the Early Career of Patrick Manson" (PhD diss., University of London, 1999).

56. Kenneth F. Kiple, *The Cambridge World History of Human Disease* (Cambridge: Cambridge University Press, 1993), 1127. See also Ka-che Yip, *Disease, Colonialism, and the State: Malaria in Modern East Asian History* (Hong Kong: Hong Kong University Press, 2009), 4.

57. Wong and Wu, *History of Chinese Medicine*, 263–72.

58. "Drs. Muller and Manson's Report on the Health of Amoy for the Half-year Ended 31st March 1872," *Medical Reports*, no. 13 (January–March 1872): 25–33.

59. P. Manson, "Remarks on Lymph Scrotum, Elephantiasis, and Chyluria," *Medical Reports*, no. 10 (July–September 1875): 3.

60. P. Manson, "Further Observations on Filaria Sanguinis Hominis," *Medical Reports*, no. 14 (1877): 1–26; Wong and Wu, *History of Chinese Medicine*, 269.

61. P. Manson, "Additional Notes on Filaria Sanguinis Hominis and Filaria Disease," *Medical Reports*, no. 18 (September 1879): 31–51; P. Manson, "Additional Notes on Filaria Sanguinis Hominis and Filaria Disease," no. 20 (July–September 1880): 13–15.

62. W. Wykeham Myers, "Observations on Filaria Sanguinis Hominis in South Formosa," *Medical Reports*, no. 21 (March 1881): 1–25.

63. For the relevant research, see Angela Ki Che Leung, *Leprosy in China: A History* (New York: Columbia University Press, 2009).

64. "Case of Leprosy, Indicating the Muscular Condition of the Subjects: A Continuation of Those Narrated by Dr. Shearer in Last Report, Dr. A. G. Reid's

Report on the Health of Hankow for the Half-year Ended 30th September," *Medical Reports*, no. 11 (July–September 1871): 49–60.

65. "Dr. F. Wong's Memorandum on Leprosy," *Medical Reports*, no. 6 (September 1873): 41–47.

66. The circulation of the *Medical Reports* in China shows that they were distributed to more than one hundred regions nationwide. See note 23 above.

67. Duane B. Simmons, "Beriberi, or the 'Kakke' of Japan," *Medical Reports*, no. 19 (March 1881): 38.

68. Kenneth J. Carpenter, *Beriberi, White Rice, and Vitamin B: A Disease, a Cause, and a Cure* (Berkeley: University of California Press, 2000), 10.

69. Simmons, "Beriberi," 38–61.

70. Ibid., 67.

71. Ibid., 45.

72. See also Alexander R. Bay, *Beriberi in Modern Japan: The Making of a National Disease* (Rochester, NY: University of Rochester Press, 2012), 22–24.

73. "Drs. Muller and Manson's Report," 11.

74. "Dr. John Dudgeon's Report on the Health of Peking for the Half-year Ended 31st March 1871," *Medical Reports*, no. 10 (April–June 1871): 13.

75. "Dr. Manson's Report on the Health of Amoy for the Half-year Ended 31st March 1878," *Medical Reports*, no. 15 (March 1878): 25–27.

76. Ibid., 26.

77. D. B. Simmons, "Cholera Epidemics in Japan," *Medical Reports*, no. 18 (July–September 1879): 1–30. There are eight chapters in Simmons's report that describe observations and treatment, including "Epidemics Prior to That of 1877," "History of the Arrival of the Epidemic of 1877," "Appearance and Progress of Cholera among Natives in Yokohama in 1877," "History of the Epidemic of 1877 among Foreigners in Yokohama," "General Character of the Epidemic of 1877," "The Epidemic of 1878, the Epidemic of 1879," "General Considerations on the Character of the Epidemic of 1879," and" Treatment." In addition, he wrote a short monograph discussing the relationship between national habits and customs (what he calls "races") and the spread of cholera: "Cholera Epidemics in Japan: With a Monograph on the Influence of the Habits and Customs of Races on the Prevalence of Cholera," which included sections describing the management of drinking water and human sewage in Western countries and theories about the role of the atmosphere in the dissemination of cholera. D. B. Simmons, *Medical Reports*, no. 18 (July–September 1879): 27–30.

78. Christopher Hamlin, *The Cholera Stigma and the Challenge of Interdisciplinary Epistemology: From Bengal to Haiti* (London: Routledge, 2010).

79. John Macpherson, *Epidemic Cholera: Its Mission and Mystery, Haunts and Havocs, Pathology and Treatment* (New York: Carleton, 1866).

80. Simmons, "Cholera Epidemics in Japan," 1.

81. Ibid.

82. Ibid., 2–6.

83. "Dr. David Manson's Report on the Health of Amoy for the Half-year Ended 30th September," *Medical Reports*, no. 14 (July–September 1877): 27.

84. "Dr. Alexander Jamieson's Report on the Health of Shanghai for the Half-year Ended 30th September," *Medical Reports*, no. 14 (July–September 1877): 38–39;

"Dr. J. R. Somerville's Report on the Health of Foochow (Pagoda Anchorage) for the Half-year Ended 30th September," *Medical Reports*, no. 14 (September 1877): 85. Pagoda Anchorage was a name of a stone temple located near the Ming River in the Mawei district of Fuzhou that used to be used as a lighthouse of the Customs Service.

85. Concessions in China were territories within China governed and occupied by foreign powers that are frequently associated with colonialism. Most had extraterritoriality and were enclaves within key cities that were treaty ports, such as Shanghai Municipal Council.

86. "Dr. John Dudgeon Reports on the Health of Peking for the Half-year Ended 30th September," *Medical Reports*, no. 8 (September 1874): 31.

87. Gordon, *Reports*, xv.

88. Ernest Hart, "Abstract of a Lecture on the International Health Exhibition of 1884: Its Influence and Possible Sequels," *British Medical Journal* 1249, no. 2 (1884): 1115.

89. Ibid., 1116.

90. *Illustrated Catalogue of the Chinese Collection of Exhibits for the International Health Exhibition, London, 1884* (London: Clowes and Son, 1884).

91. Ibid., xv.

92. Unsigned review, "Medicine in China," *Lancet*, no. 30 (1872): 784.

93. Wong and Wu, *History of Chinese Medicine*, 253.

Part Two

The Indigenization of Biomedicine in Republican China

Chapter Three

Globalizing Biomedicine through Sino-Japanese Networks

The Case of National Medical College, Beijing, 1912–1937

Daniel Asen and David Luesink

... the Japanese have, indirectly and without any spirit of altruism, accomplished more in the introduction of modern medicine [to China] than any other nation.

—E. V. Cowdry

Dr. Tang Erhe (1878–1940) could not keep silent at the meeting of the National Education Assembly in Beijing late in 1912 when he heard that the top educational priority of the new Republic of China was to establish more schools of politics and law. China would not save itself from the forces that threatened it merely by training politicians, lawyers, and diplomats, Tang argued—science was needed to save the nation, and science could only be established by building institutions for training and research.[1]

Tang had recently graduated from Kanazawa Medical Technical College (Kanazawa igaku senmon gakkō) in Japan and returned to his native Hangzhou to set up a modern hospital and medical school while also becoming drawn into the provincial and national politics of the Xinhai Revolution.[2] The revolutionary medical doctor, Sun Yat-sen, became the Republic's first president, while Tang Erhe filled in as speaker of the provisional national assembly that elected Sun. When people took note of how remarkable it was that two modern-style physicians played prominent roles in the provisional Republican government, a saying became popular that remarked on the singularity that both the speaker of the assembly and the president of the Republic were both physicians.[3] China had become known as "the Sick Man of East Asia" (*dongya bingfu*), but neither physician seemed able to implement his prescription to save China. Sun Yat-sen was forced to resign within six weeks in favor of strongman Yuan Shikai, while Tang resigned as speaker and returned to his medical work in Hangzhou. Medical science itself was a form of politics for Tang Erhe, and the reproduction of like-minded professionals combined with establishment of institutions of scientific research was his solution to China's failed revolution. But when asked to become an official adviser to the Ministry of Education, and soon thereafter to start a central government–administered medical school in the capital, Tang accepted and left for Beijing.

On that day in 1912 at the meeting of the National Education Assembly, Tang asked his colleagues to consider the fact that schools of politics and law were already numerous throughout China, but there were only a small number of government positions, so what would so many officials do? A bloated bureaucracy would be a strain on the common people, whose taxes paid their salaries. An education system, Tang argued, should ensure that China strengthen both the state and the people, not weaken one at the expense of the other. Certainly well-trained bureaucrats were needed, but what China really required, according to Tang, were modern physicians. Advanced nations had an average of one modern physician per 200 to 500 persons. Yet for China to reach the far more modest rate of only one physician per 10,000 persons, it would need 40,000 physicians. According to the draft proposal in front of the assembly, only eight government medical schools would be established for all of China, so if each year approximately 800 physicians could graduate, it would still take fifty years before there would be 40,000 physicians. In the meantime all the new institutions of a modern republic would need physicians: the army, the courts, the schools, the cities, epidemic prevention services, the police, and the maritime customs.[4] The army had one good medical school in Tianjin, but China's civilian population was practically untouched by the power of the new medicine to reshape society. What China needed, according to Tang Erhe, was a medical school system that would produce a large number of physicians as fast as possible.

Tang's fiery speech was not ignored, and the result was the formation of the National Medical College. Immediately after the meeting, he was invited to the house of Fan Yuanlian (1876–1927), the minister of education.[5] Fan explained his intention to establish a model medical school in Beijing that would be second to none, and asked Tang Erhe to lead it. Tang replied that he would do so only if he could establish a medical school that

Table 3.1. National Medical School: Official Chinese name changes and affiliation with Peking University

Year	Name (direct translation)
1912	National Beijing Medical Technical College
1923	National Beijing Medical University
1927	★National Beijing University, Medical Section❖
1928	★National Beiping University Medical School
1938	★Beijing University Medical School (Occupied Beijing)
1945	Beiping Provisional University Training School, Section #6
1946	★Beijing University Medical School
1953	Beijing Medical School (separate from Beijing University)
1985	Beijing University of Medical Sciences
2000	★Beijing University Health Sciences Center

★ Formal affiliation with Peking University
❖ Despite the PRC's insistence on the use of pinyin for Chinese words and place-names, in English, Beijing University was and still is spelled Peking University; When Nanjing was the capital of China, the city was renamed as Beiping in Mandarin,

focused exclusively on Western medicine without any instruction in Chinese medicine, thus avoiding the syncretism that shaped the curriculum of the small-scale government medical school that Tang's new institution was to displace.[6] The result was the founding of Beijing Medical Technical College (Beijing yixue zhuanmen xuexiao), a school that spent much of the early Republican period as an independent national-level medical college before becoming the medical school of Peking University, an affiliation that has been maintained, with some oscillation, into the present (see table 3.1). Given that a standard English translation for the school's name was never established, in this chapter we will refer to it as National Medical College (NMC), an English moniker that was used by Tang Erhe himself and that is suggestive of the important status the school held as a leading government institution of medical education. While the official name of the school did change over the 1920s and 1930s, the result of a shift away from the "technical college" model, we refer to it as National Medical College throughout this period, a convention that allows us to acknowledge continuity in the school's identity despite changes to its curriculum.[7]

Despite the challenges of being a public institution during a period of acute political and economic crisis, the NMC did successfully implement a four-year medical program, which produced its first class of graduates in 1917. The impact of the school was significant not only for the establishment of the modern Western scientific medicine profession in China but also for the broader activities in education, public hygiene, and even administration of justice in which faculty and school alumni were actively engaged. Moreover, during a period in which the quality of Chinese medical education emerged as a pressing question, the NMC effectively prepared its students to participate in international medical networks that extended to Japan and Germany.

Students of modern Chinese history, even specialists, could be forgiven for believing that the impact of the NMC was negligible and that its curriculum and training were inferior to those offered at other institutions of Western scientific medicine, especially the Rockefeller-funded Peking Union Medical College (PUMC). Historians of Western medicine in China tend to adopt the assumptions of the China Medical Commission (1913–14) in judging the quality of medical education in China on the eve of the establishment of PUMC, an institution that was meant to radically transform China's medical landscape through the influx of Rockefeller capital. The goal associated with this new model was to create centers of global excellence, or "make the peaks higher," thereby developing a small core of elite physicians who would eventually form the faculty for the rest of China's medical schools.[8] In comparison to this model of medical education, which focused on establishing "high standards" for the medical profession without consideration of cost or constraint, the very different Japanese-German "medical technical college" model that was initially adopted for the NMC was viewed by some to be inferior, a perception that has left a lasting legacy in the English-language historiography on medicine in early twentieth-century China.[9]

While China did participate in the globalization of biomedicine during the first decades of the twentieth century, this process was not exclusively centered on Anglo-American models of medical education, research, and expertise. German and, especially, Japanese models played a significant role in establishing the patterns that Western scientific medicine would take in pre-Maoist China.[10] Japanese practices of medical education provided a blueprint—validated by Japan's recent historical experience—for rapidly building a functional corps of physicians, one of Tang's major goals. As implemented at the NMC, the model of the four-year "medical technical college" formed the basis for what might be referred to as a "sliding scale" model of medical education: begin sensibly, improvise with what is available, and improve and expand when possible.[11] Thus, rather than pursuing the highest standards from the outset, NMC faculty and administrators used limited resources to support targeted actions that promoted the careers of particular students, often with considerable impact for both the school and the medical profession. Under the financial limitations inherent in China's semicolonial status, the NMC provided a standard of medical education that was realistic, if not sustainable, for public institutions during a period of crisis.

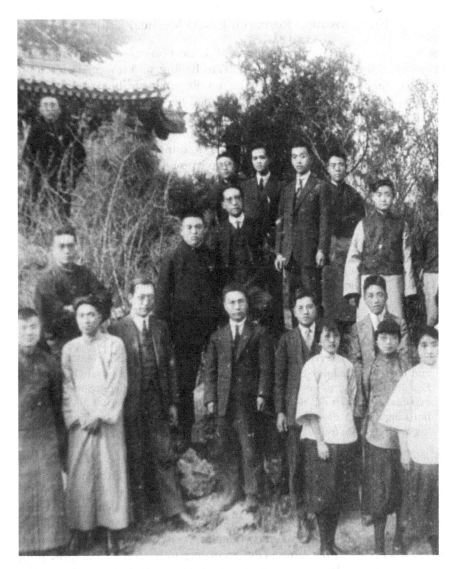

Figure 3.1. Image of participants in National Medical College investigative delegation to Japan, n.d. (ca. 1930). Courtesy permission of Archives of Peking University Health Science Center.

Improvising a Research-Based Medical College

On October 16, 1912, the Ministry of Education appointed Tang Erhe principal of the newly established NMC in Beijing, and it was chartered on October 26, within the first year of the new Republic of China. According to Bao Jianqing, a previous medical school had been established in 1903 and became a medical academy (*yixue guan*) in 1905, but "the academy's equipment was simple and crude, and it was not considered good in the eyes of contemporary foreign physicians."[12] The account by Bao, one of the first NMC graduates, successor to Tang Erhe as histology teacher, and director of the medical school from 1938 to 1945, is worth quoting in some detail for its juxtaposition of the meager resources bequeathed to Director Tang with Tang's determination to overcome these limitations:

> When the Qing dynasty was destroyed and the Republic was established, but the results were still far from certain, a national medical college was established, with Tang Erhe taking responsibility as president of National Beijing Medical Technical College, [but] this truly national medical college was limited in its funding, and was not able to develop properly. When it was established, the scale was truly small. Speaking of buildings, several dozen rooms from private houses of old style buildings were used—it did not deserve to be even an elementary school. Speaking of equipment, it had only two damaged microscopes, several thousand books of old medicine, and several models and charts of the human body—greatly inferior to that of a private hospital. Equally trifling funds were transferred from the medical academy. Speaking of expenses, startup funds were only 800 *yuan,* and each month only 1000 *yuan,* but Tang did not allow this to dishearten his resolution, and he continued laying the long-term foundation for the medical field.[13]

The equipment was basic, but sufficient for decent work, as is clear from a photograph from the National Medical College depicting the pathological histology laboratory where microscopes line the windows, blackboards and wall charts line the walls, and students experiment with specimens and dyes that will make clear the cellular level anatomy (see figure 3.2).

Faced with such financial limits, Tang improvised to provide for both the medical school and his own needs. According to his son's biography, Tang was above reproach in all his financial dealings, although a corrupt business manager found ways to embezzle money when following up on some of Tang's real estate dealings (he was later discovered and fired).[14] During his time as director, Tang Erhe lived inexpensively in Beijing without his family, looking for every possible way to avoid wasting public money and keeping careful account of each expense. He personally scouted, bought, and sold real estate as a way to both stretch a limited budget and expand facilities for teaching, research, and accommodation, as well as purchase an essential ceremonial burial plot for cadavers outside the city gates. Like the

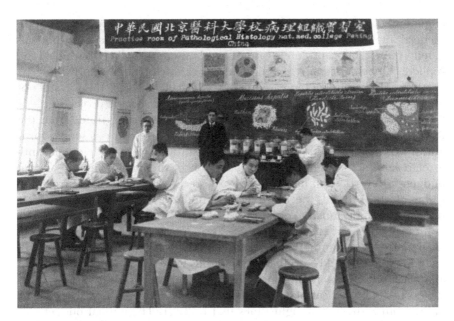

Figure 3.2. Practice room of Pathological Histology, National Medical College, Peking. Courtesy of Archives of Peking University Health Science Center.

Confucian gentleman he had originally trained to be, Tang supplemented his income with literary work by translating Japanese books on medicine and biology.[15] Under these conditions of uncertain income, Tang worked himself so hard that he aged in appearance, not getting enough sleep and not eating enough. The Japanese had a phrase for this, translated into Chinese by his son: *yizhe luanbao*, perhaps translated best as "overworked physician's syndrome."[16] By his mid-forties, Tang looked substantially older, and Rockefeller employees referred to him as "an elderly man."[17]

The NMC was not fully supported financially throughout the 1910s and 1920s for a variety of reasons: weak central government that could not collect taxes in most provinces; massive indemnities owed to imperialist powers; new loans for railroads and for the purchase of weapons for a warlord arms race. This situation forced Tang Erhe and his staff to be flexible and improvise, like many other educators in China at this time. Tang was, at times, embarrassed in front of his Japanese colleagues by the fact that the government did not support the medical school more appropriately. In 1917, Tang traveled for a month touring Japanese medical schools in Manchuria, Korea, and the home islands. In Seoul, Tang learned that the colonial Keijo Medical School had an annual budget of 330,000 *yuan*, more than three times that of his own school's budget of only 100,000. The Japanese director, Dr. Sato, commented, "Your distinguished country's government is quite stingy in medical affairs to not grant sufficient funding. . . . If finances are not sufficient, these affairs absolutely cannot be planned carefully." To which Tang replied, "Our finances are not enough, nor can we obtain more."[18]

Although the budget increased to MXN$140,000 in 1921, this was still not enough, so Tang sought further funding grants for specific projects quietly through back channels, and he was not above requesting funds from the Rockefeller Foundation. But he sought to keep these requests secret, for if grants from foreign sources for a national institution were made public, anti-foreign sentiment might lead to a reduction in the already limited annual budget.[19] Nevertheless, in 1921 the NMC received MXN$12,000 from the China Medical Board, the Rockefeller Foundation's main China organization, to purchase much-needed new property, while in 1922 it received a grant to acquire an X-ray machine, used not only for live anatomical diagnosis, but also for radiation therapy. Perhaps Tang was thinking of such improvisations when he told Sato that public funds were not the only way to keep a medical school functioning.[20] It is worth pointing out in this context that the cost of the physical plant of the PUMC was budgeted in 1915 at US$1 million but actually cost eight times that by 1921. The annual budget had been set at five times that of the NMC, at MXN$493,000, but actually more than doubled.[21] It is important to take into account this enormous disparity in funding when assessing what was accomplished during the first decade of the NMC's history. As we will see, the financial challenges faced by the NMC made it all the more essential to utilize existing networks and prioritize resources according to the most immediate needs and opportunities.

Japanese Connections

During the first ten years of NMC history, Japanese models were important for every aspect of school life. The school itself was originally conceived along the lines of the Japanese "medical technical college" (*igaku senmon gakkō*), a kind of medical institution that admitted secondary school graduates without any premedical education for a four-year medical program that incorporated training in basic sciences and German. Beginning in the 1870s, Japan had begun to put into place a system of state-regulated medical education that drew deeply on German models and expertise.[22] The exigencies of rapidly training physicians and of providing for Japanese-language medical education outside of the German-dominated medical programs of the elite imperial universities gave rise to a need for preparatory medical training programs. Early on, this institutional lacuna was filled by a number of different medical programs, some of which were affiliated with university and Higher School programs (*Kōtō gakkō*), elitist "feeder" schools for the imperial university system. By the first decade of the twentieth century, at the exact moment when Chinese students began to study in Japan en masse, a number of these programs were reorganized as "medical technical colleges" that would provide a terminal professional education and would not culminate in entrance to the elite imperial universities.[23] These institutions trained more of Japan's physicians than did the imperial university medical schools, a point of some significance for understanding the crucial role that they played in Japan's rapid development of a modern medical education system.[24]

It was along the lines of this very same model of the "medical technical college" that Tang Erhe planned and established the NMC in Beijing. From major questions of curriculum and faculty to myriad other organizational details, the NMC was deeply influenced in design and implementation by the model of the Japanese *igaku senmon gakkō*.[25] Even the illustrated template for the NMC student uniform included in the school's early regulations made use of an image that had appeared in the school regulations of the medical college at Kanazawa, the source of numerous other organizational details that defined the NMC's institutional life during its early years.[26] The selection of this model had implications for the organization of the school's curriculum, discussed below, as well as for the strong Japanese influence on instruction and institutional culture more generally.

A number of the Chinese faculty members who established the NMC and guided it through its first decade had been trained at this tier of Japanese medical technical colleges. Tang Erhe himself had been trained in medicine at Kanazawa, an institution that also trained two other early members of the faculty: physiologist Zhou Songsheng and Zhang Fuqing, an expert in ophthalmology and dermatology.[27] Zhang Kai, who taught physics and chemistry, had been trained at Nagasaki Medical Technical College. Otolaryngologist Sun Liuxi had been trained at Okayama Technical Medical College. Zhu Qihui, a specialist in internal medicine and psychopathy, was a graduate of Chiba Technical Medical College. Surgeon Ge Chengxun, one of the NMC's early founders, had been trained at the Technical College of Medicine of the Tokyo Charity Association, a private school that carried the status of a medical technical college.[28] Faculty who had received medical training in China were the exception. These included, for example, Ge Chenghui, an expert in midwifery who had been trained at Shanghai Women's Technical Medical College (Shanghai nüzi zhuanmen yixuexiao) and Zhou Ruilin, who taught obstetrics and gynecology and was a graduate of Tongji German Medical School, forerunner of National Tongji University Medical College.

Affiliates of Rockefeller medicine in China, as they planned to reform medical education in China along American lines, criticized China's existing public medical schools because their faculty had been trained at Japanese technical colleges, which they considered to be second-rate schools.[29] The relatively lower entrance requirements of these schools undoubtedly played a role in making them more accessible to the first groups of Chinese students than would have been the elite imperial universities. Yet it is worth pointing out that there were several NMC faculty who had been trained in Japan's imperial university medical schools. Xu Songming, a pathologist and expert in legal medicine, had received his *igakushi* degree from Kyūshū Imperial University College of Medicine.[30] Rong Zhaomin, who taught surgery and otolaryngology at the NMC, had completed his training at this institution as well. Yan Zhizhong, an expert in bacteriology, had received his *igakushi* from Tokyo Imperial University.

The Sino-Japanese medical networks that played such an important role in the early history of the NMC also brought Japanese faculty to Beijing. In 1913, Tang returned to Kanazawa to recruit faculty to teach at the school, and several soon joined, including anatomist Ishikawa Yoshinao, pathologist Murakami Shōta, and anatomy assistant Nakano Chūtarō.[31] Ishikawa became fatally ill soon after taking up this position, reportedly from overworking himself in Beijing.[32] During Ishikawa's time in Beijing, Tang Erhe completed a Chinese translation of his *Topographical Anatomy*, while Qian Daosun, who seems to have worked at the NMC during these years as a translator as well as an instructional assistant in anatomy, collaborated on a Chinese translation of Ishikawa's *Human Anatomy*.[33] After the latter's death, Tang Erhe reportedly established Ishikawa's portrait, as well as his instruments, in a commemorative display in the NMC Anatomy Department.[34] An anatomist from Nagasaki Medical Technical College, Ikegami Keiichi, joined the faculty soon after.[35]

Amid the networks that connected the NMC to Japan's medical education system, the school's faculty would have encountered shared backgrounds, experiences, and connections. For example, faculty member Zhou Songsheng, who might have encountered Ishikawa Yoshinao during his own time at Kanazawa, translated the preface for Ishikawa's *Topographical Anatomy*, which was written in Beijing in September 1914. It appears as though Tang met Qian Daosun, the translator of Ishikawa's *Human Anatomy*, while he was attending the preparatory military school Seijō gakkō in Tokyo.[36] In informal transnational connections and deliberate decisions of school policy, the NMC's institutional culture was deeply cosmopolitan, lying at the intersection of cultures and languages of science drawn from Japan, Germany, and China, and tied to medical institutions, experts, and instructional materials produced in all of these countries.[37] What we see at the NMC, then, is a particular way of globalizing Western scientific medicine, one that resulted from Chinese engagements with Japan's earlier appropriation and improvisation of German models of medical education, reorganized yet again to suit the needs of Republican China.

Curriculum and Coursework

The fact that the NMC initially followed the "medical technical college" model shaped the instructional curriculum that it implemented during its first decade. One of the consequences of the selection of this model was that entering students pursued study in the basic sciences and German as part of their four-year curriculum. Thus, much of the first year and significant time during following years were spent on foundational subjects instead of more specialized instruction in medicine or clinical experience. In Japan, the requirements surrounding premedical training constituted a crucial difference between the tier of imperial university medical schools, which required several years of preparatory education prior to admission, and the medical technical colleges, which did not. The curriculum established at the NMC in 1912 was modified in 1923, when the school changed its status from a "medical technical college" to a "medical university" (*yike daxue*). From this point until it was incorporated into Beijing University in 1927–28 (see table 3.1), the school was called National Beijing Medical University (Guoli Beijing yike daxue), and the four-year program was changed into a six-year program that combined two years of premedical training with four years of advanced training in medicine.

The curriculum that was implemented during the first decade of NMC's history was formulated by Tang Erhe in accordance with regulations on medical education promulgated by the Ministry of Education in November 1912.[38] In fact, Tang himself had largely written and promoted these laws through his connections in this agency.[39] These regulations were clearly based on laws that regulated technical colleges in Japan, possibly the "Regulations on Government Medical Technical Colleges" (Kanritsu igaku senmon gakkō kitei), which had been promulgated in 1907.[40] As in the Japanese regulations, medical technical colleges in China were to follow a four-year curriculum covering a range of basic and specialized medical subjects as well as German. The NMC's initial curriculum was formulated in accordance with the Ministry of Education's regulations, establishing a four-year curriculum with each year of instruction divided into three terms.[41] NMC school regulations also included a timetable of student coursework that closely resembled the regulations governing medical technical colleges in Japan.

Of course, actually implementing the four-year curriculum delineated in the NMC's early regulations presented numerous challenges. In implementing a model of medical education that incorporated instruction in all of the foundational and specialized fields of medical science, the NMC required diverse faculty and instructional resources. Achieving satisfactory levels in these areas was an unending challenge during the first decade of the school's history. As the fall semester of 1914 was about to commence, Tang Erhe contemplated various shortcomings in the school's available resources.[42] These included a shortage of necessary instruments and insufficient facilities to support the growing student population. By implication, there was a need to cut costs, use existing resources for purposes for which they were not designed, prioritize which facilities and resources were most essential, and move facilities to newly available spaces. Students' practical training saw serious setbacks due to a lack of human tissue specimens in histology (requiring temporary substitution of animal material), cadavers in anatomy, and pathological specimens. Bringing these fields of practical training up to standard would require additional efforts to procure unclaimed cadavers and establish a school-run clinic.

At least on paper, the NMC was providing a standard of medical education that matched what one could expect to receive at certain medical schools in Japan. One can understand why Chinese proponents of modern medical education like Tang might have seen particular value in a curricular model that provided students with the necessary training in German and the basic sciences "in house"—that is, as part of their medical education at the NMC rather than as premed requirements to be completed prior to enrollment in the college. This arrangement would have provided a way of compensating for the uneven preparation of incoming students while facilitating the rapid production of relatively large numbers of professional physicians who had received adequate, albeit not superior, training.

In fact, the issue of premed requirements and training became one of the areas in which proponents of Rockefeller medicine would assert the superiority of their own model of medical education in comparison to the purportedly less rigorous curricular models of China's existing medical colleges. For example, the First Medical Commission noted of the NMC curriculum in 1914 that "during the greater part of the first year nonmedical studies (German, chemistry, physics, ethics, Chinese literature, and gymnastics) take up twenty out of the thirty-six hours of formal work prescribed, leaving inadequate time for the strictly professional studies."[43] Rockefeller commissions that convened in 1914 and 1916 upheld that students entering a medical program should have completed at least two years of premedical training prior to admission, a standard that informed the planning of PUMC.[44] In the end, however, even PUMC faced difficulties in enforcing the requirement that all incoming students complete premed requirements prior to enrollment in the school, a standard that, in retrospect, was unrealistic in the context of late 1910s and early 1920s China.[45]

As it would turn out, by the mid-1920s even the NMC had moved away from a four-year curriculum that included preparatory training. This shift, which occurred in 1923, coincided with a trend in Japanese medical education that saw the earliest "medical technical colleges" transform, en masse, into medical universities (*ika daigaku*).[46] Kanazawa Medical Technical

College, for example, became Kanazawa Medical University (Kanazawa ika daigaku) in 1923. This seems to have been part of a broader reorganization of Japanese medical education begun in the early 1920s that by the mid-1930s had transformed the initial "medical technical colleges" into university programs requiring premedical education as a condition of enrollment while establishing a new group of "C-grade" medical technical colleges without this requirement.[47] That the NMC's own transformation into a medical university in 1923 coincided with this trend suggests that Chinese standards of medical education could be improved organically from within the "medical technical college" model itself.

School Traditions

Beyond the school curriculum, students' experience at the NMC was also shaped by annual events of commemoration and celebration, rituals that played a role in their professional education. Early regulations governing various aspects of school life, issued in 1912, established a kind of "ritual calendar" that divided up the school year. Almost identical to the calendar found in Kanazawa's school regulations, the NMC calendar simply substituted Chinese holidays for Japanese ones. Aside from spring, summer, and New Year breaks, these included National Commemoration Day (*Guoqing jinian ri*, October 10), Unification Commemoration Day (*Tongyi jinian ri*, February 12), Confucius's Birthday (October 17), and commemoration of the founding of the school, which would be celebrated annually on October 26.[48] In subsequent years, students themselves became involved in organizing commemorative events to celebrate this occasion.[49]

An important ritual of school life at the NMC was the annual offering to those whose bodies were dissected for purposes of medical research or students' training. Ceremonies to commemorate the dissected dead and acknowledge their service to medicine were conducted in colonial Taiwan as early as 1902 and continued in subsequent decades, including after 1949.[50] Similar ceremonies were carried out at the NMC, almost certainly at the urging of Tang Erhe. In an important petition sent to the Ministry of Education in November 1912 that preceded the legalization of dissection in China and proposed a system for ensuring medical schools' access to corpses, Tang included in a proposed set of anatomy regulations that "each year the head of a school will lead staff and students in an offering to demonstrate their solemnity."[51] Such ceremonies were dutifully carried out at the NMC throughout the Republican period, often receiving coverage in newspapers and constituting one element of the school's public image in the city. Aside from morally legitimizing the procurement of dead bodies for medical education, these ceremonies also served as collective rituals in which faculty and students participated as a group.

The first of these ceremonies was carried out on April 30, 1915, at a graveyard just beyond the southwestern edge of Beijing's Outer City that had been purchased during the previous year for the purpose of burying dead bodies that had undergone dissection.[52] Personnel from the entire school as well as relatives of the deceased whose bodies had been dissected were invited to attend. An undated prospectus describing these ceremonies, almost certainly from the mid-1910s, lists the steps that were to be followed.[53] First, students and staff were to assemble, followed by bowing rites (*jugong li*) performed by faculty and then students. A prayer would be read followed by another series of bowing by staff and students. After this a burnt offering would be made and commemorative trees would be planted. The ceremony would conclude with refreshments.

Four photographs and a brief description of these ceremonies were published on a single page of *Beiping Medical Journal* (*Beiping yikan*) in June 1933.[54] The photographs show members of the school faculty as well as unidentified participants taking part in a ceremony occurring in a small clearing. The largest of the photographs depicts the assembled group standing at attention, seemingly at the moment that the elegiac prayer (*jiwen*) was being read by an unnamed officiant. Wu Xiangfeng, president of the medical school, appears at the edge of the clearing with an "X" drawn under his figure to indicate his identity. Several other unidentified figures, including a child, appear behind him gathered around the site of the ceremony. To the left of this photograph is an image of Wu himself at the time of the reading of the prayer. The last two images feature Bao Jianqing, at that time director of the Anatomy Department, and Wu Xiangfeng standing, sequentially, in the same spot and assisting in the planting of commemorative trees.

Another tradition in which students participated was the organizing of annual anatomical specimen exhibitions at the school, multiday public events that attracted crowds of city dwellers and that commonly received coverage in Beijing newspapers.[55] In 1921, for example, such an exhibition was held to support the establishment of a clinic bearing the name "Aiyou," which referenced the seal of the school—two leaves of Artemisia argyi (*ai ye*) surrounding the character *you*.[56] Proceeds from the exhibition were also meant to support the publication of *Tongsu yishi yuekan*, titled *Popular Medical Journal* in English, which was published by NMC graduates through the Aiyou Society (Aiyou xuehui), of which they were a part.[57] The goal of the journal, as explained in its first issue, was to "instill common knowledge in medicine among our countrymen and arouse common consciousness of hygiene." The journal combined articles of interest to professional physicians with accessible treatments of medical subjects targeted to a nonspecialist readership. Not only did students play a role in organizing the annual anatomical specimen exhibitions, but particular students also served as docents (*shuoming yuan*) in order to educate members of urban society about what they were viewing. For example, in an exhibition held in early February 1932, sponsored by the body of fourth-year students, certain "outstanding students with deep knowledge in medicine" were tasked with providing these explanations.[58] Such exhibitions thus allowed students to play the role of professional expert—that is, to speak authoritatively about a body of specialist knowledge for which the soon-to-be graduates would be held accountable.

From Alma Mater to Profession

Understanding the full impact of the NMC on the establishment of a modern Western medicine profession in Republican China would require a detailed investigation of the careers of the school's alumni of the kind that Mary Bullock has done for PUMC and Karen Minden for West China Union University in Chengdu.[59] While a comprehensive study of this kind is beyond the scope of this chapter, there are a couple of ways in which we might begin to gauge this impact. For example, we are fortunate to have comparable statistics on the training of medical students for most Chinese medical schools in 1932 and 1933, and these provide a sense of the relative numbers of medical students who were graduating from the NMC and other schools.[60] What is remarkable about these statistics is not simply the numbers of NMC graduates, but the cost-effectiveness with which they were trained. Compared with PUMC, which had a 1932 budget of over US$2 million for a total of ninety-eight medical students, the NMC had a budget that was roughly one-tenth as much, having risen to US$228,000, but with almost double the number of students. This meant that for each PUMC student, eighteen NMC students were being trained. And although all institutions subsidized tuition with other sources of income, NMC students paid only one-fifth that of students at PUMC (see table 3.2).[61]

The much newer National Shanghai Medical College had a similar tuition and budget as its northern public counterpart, but only half as many students in 1932 and almost double the number of full-time faculty.[62] We can compare these figures with those of Qilu University Medical College, a private missionary institution in the capital of Shandong Province. With a slightly smaller budget and just more than half the number of students, Qilu was able to train students at a similar cost to that of the National Medical College, at about one-fourteenth the cost at PUMC. One final statistic about the National Medical College is revealing—the number of women being trained as physicians. Of the 113 women studying

Table 3.2 Comparison of four Chinese medical colleges, 1933

	Institution (year established)	Full-time faculty	Part-time faculty	Female students	Male students	Total students	Total graduates	Budget (in US$)	Tuition
Public	National Medical College (1912)	18	16	55	130	185	465	160,000	20
Public	National Shanghai Medical College (1927)	33	12	16	76	92	12	240,000	20
Private	Qilu University Medical College (1909)*	29	0	16	83	99	67	230,000	80
Private	Peking Union Medical College (1915)	116	5	26	77	103	78	2,130,000	100

Sources: Mu Jingqiang, *Minguo xiyi gaodeng jiaoyu* (1912–1949) [Advanced medical education in Republican China, 1912–1949] (Hangzhou: Zhejiang Gongshang University Press, 2012), 174–75; Chinese Medical Association, *Chinese Medical Guide* 1932 (Shanghai: Chinese Medical Association, 1933), 30–34.

*Also known in English as Cheeloo University Medical College, or Shantung Christian University Medical College. This was a purely private, missionary institution formed by a union of several Protestant missions from Canada, Great Britain, and the United States.

for a medical degree at these four institutions, half, or 55, were studying at the NMC, and about one in three NMC students in 1933 was female. In fact, of 601 female medical students in China in 1932, 55, or 9.2 percent, were studying at the NMC. As He Xiaolian explores elsewhere in this volume, medicine opened up a new and high-status profession for women in the Republic, even if they faced challenges their male counterparts did not (see figure 3.3).

For some who received their medical education at the NMC, the school itself continued to provide the setting in which their professional careers played out after graduation. Early on, the school followed a policy of retaining a small number of graduates and grooming them for faculty positions. Between 1917 and 1922, at least sixteen NMC graduates were retained at the school as assistants in various departments or as instructors in the school of midwifery.[63] Bao Jianqing, for example, remained as an assistant in anatomy after graduating in 1917, became a faculty member after studying abroad in Germany, and went on to serve as president of the school during the Japanese occupation of Beijing (1938–45). Hong Shilü, who remained as an assistant in pathology after graduation, also became a faculty member and served as president of the school from 1924 to 1925. Lin Zhen'gang and Lin Ji, both of whom graduated in 1922, were employed at the school as pathology assistants. Over the course of the 1920s and 1930s, both would become faculty members in pathology and legal medicine, respectively, with administrative responsibility over these departments.

The case of Lin Ji gives a sense of the opportunities that the NMC afforded some of its graduates as well as the impact that the unique institutional culture of the school had on the development of China's professional and state medical infrastructure during this period.[64] Lin's career path was shaped by the NMC in a number of ways. After a short period of postgraduate employment as an assistant in the school's Pathology Department, in 1924 Lin Ji was sent by the school to Germany, where he pursued his MD at Würzburg University. After returning to China in 1928 and spending a short period with the Nationalists' new Ministry of Health, Lin Ji returned to the NMC—now the medical school of Beiping University—to serve as director of the Legal Medicine Department. In 1932, Lin Ji was appointed as director of a new medico-legal testing and research facility, subordinate to the Ministry of Judicial Administration, that was established in northwestern Shanghai. Within three years of taking this position, however, Lin Ji stepped down and returned, once again, to the medical school of Beiping University, where he continued to pursue his longstanding goal of expanding judicial officials' access to laboratory testing services. Lin Ji remained in Beiping until 1937, at which point he took up a series of positions under the Nationalists in northwestern and central China, where he remained for the duration of the Pacific War.

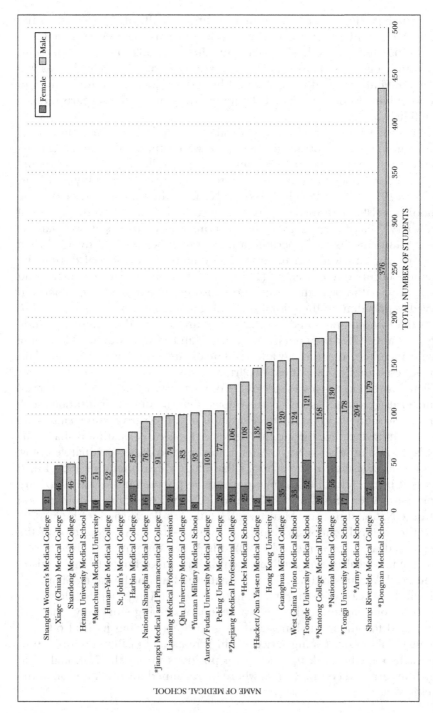

Figure 3.3. Number of male and female students at Chinese medical schools, 1933.

During Lin Ji's time as an NMC student, legal medicine was already a well-established subject of instruction at the school. Murakami Shōta, who taught courses in pathology, pathological anatomy, and histology, had taught "forensic medicine" in 1916 as part of the curriculum for fourth-year students. Xu Songming taught "forensic medicine" and "legal medicine," as well as pathology, from at least 1919 to 1922.[65] Tang Erhe himself was interested in promoting an expanded role for physicians and medical knowledge in the judicial system and in modern Chinese government administration more generally; this was the subject of a speech that he delivered at National Beijing Technical College of Law and Politics in early December 1919, one year after Lin Ji began his studies at the NMC.[66] For several years, as Tang described in his speech, NMC faculty had already been providing forensic assistance to Chinese judicial officials in their investigations into suspected homicide cases, an indication of the significant and early commitment of the school and its faculty to this area of medicine-state relations. This was the context in which Lin Ji began his medical training.

It is perhaps not coincidental, in this sense, that so many of Lin Ji's subsequent professional activities addressed goals articulated by Tang Erhe during the first decade of the Republic, whether it was Tang's vision of a state bureaucracy staffed by physicians—a goal congruent with Lin Ji's own proposals during the 1920s and 1930s to establish a national infrastructure of medico-legal officials who could assist in forensic investigations and other state-related medical matters—or Tang's criticisms of the *Records on the Washing Away of Wrongs* (*Xiyuanlu*), the Qing-era forensic handbook that continued to be used by judicial officials during the Republican period.[67] During the 1930s, for example, Lin Ji devoted considerable time to publicly criticizing judicial officials' practice of using needles and other silver objects to test for poison in the body of suspected homicide victims, an established method in the *Washing Away of Wrongs* that was of questionable validity from the perspective of modern chemistry. In fact, this was a forensic technique that Tang himself had denounced in his speech in 1919, in part on the basis of simple experiments that demonstrated that the appearance of discoloration on the needles—accepted as evidence of poisoning in the *Washing Away of Wrongs*—would occur whenever silver objects came into contact with the chemical byproducts of decomposition and, specifically, sulfur.[68] Over ten years later, Lin Ji too urged officials of the state's judicial system to abandon this technique, using his own series of experimental demonstrations to prove the exact same point.

One wonders whether Lin Ji's career trajectory would have followed the path that it did if he had not experienced the Sino-Japanese institutional culture of the NMC or the value that school affiliates placed on the capacity of medicine to serve and strengthen the modern Chinese state. The example of Lin Ji indicates some of the ways in which strengthening the school, strengthening the profession, and strengthening the state could be construed as interrelated, not easily separated, projects; it suggests some of the ways in which an ongoing affiliation with one's "alma mater" (*muxiao*) was, for some physicians in Republican China, a very real element of professional activities and identity, one that was at least as important as membership in local or national associations.[69] Finally, the case of Lin Ji demonstrates that the NMC as an institution was capable of pursuing the pragmatic goal of rapidly training a large number of physicians at the same time as it intensively supported a smaller number of graduates as they took leadership roles within the school and, more broadly, the professional community of physicians of Western medicine.

In January 1920, Tang Erhe arrived in Berlin, where he began research in the laboratories of anatomist Professor Krause.[70] Many of Tang's former students were already studying in Berlin, and they held a dinner to welcome him. When the drinking was at its height, Tang stood up to thank them while encouraging them to capitalize on the foreign connections and networks that they already had as a practical strategy for strengthening the Chinese medical profession: "China's new medicine has only arisen for a single day. When you gentlemen return to China, decide to invite a foreign professional to return with you. When he returns to his country, you gentlemen should again return overseas to study. Two to three years later, you will not need to invite another foreigner. At that time you gentlemen will be truly independent. This is my plan."[71] As the Japanese had done fifty years earlier with their German teachers, the Chinese were now to learn as much as possible from their foreign teachers, and then become independent.

This chapter has argued that we must take seriously the "sliding scale" model of medical education that defined the early history of the NMC. We would like to highlight the remarkable improvisation that is evident in the early history of the school and the significant fortitude of people like Tang Erhe and Lin Ji who pushed forward ambitious visions of school, profession, and state in the context of limited resources and political uncertainty. Like the staff of the medical school in Malawi described by Claire Wendland, those who worked at, and built, the NMC can be viewed as "good doctors [who] had to use flexibility and creativity to make do with inadequate resources . . . to secure any available tools, equipment, social networks, and funds."[72] The process of improvising, we have argued, leant itself to a remarkable esprit de corps among graduates who built and deepened their alma mater networks.

Anglo-American medicine loomed large in Beijing in the 1910s and 1920s: only some four miles northeast of the National Medical College, John D. Rockefeller Jr. dedicated Peking Union Medical College in 1921, claiming that the state-of-the-art facility had already begun to set standards for China and beyond.[73] With bottomless pockets, PUMC inflated expectations in Beijing and throughout Republican China, while the NMC faculty and students made do with what they had at hand. In the process, the NMC impacted the medical scene in Republican China in many different ways, whether by training a large number of professional physicians or by fostering relationships between physicians, urban society, and the state.

While biomedicine may appear at first glance to be standardized in its knowledge and practice, it is in fact different in every context. As Julie Livingston argues, "Everywhere, doctors, patients, nurses, and relatives tailor biomedical knowledge and practices to suit their specific situations."[74] To understand how biomedicine was established and grew in China, historians must look carefully at the full range of experiences, especially those that were far from ideal. And we must also remember that most of the 40,000 modern trained physicians in China in 1949 had been trained in conditions more like those found at the NMC than at PUMC or the wealthy missionary schools. There were at least twenty-seven medical schools in China by 1933, and many more were established during Japan's wartime occupation when many medical professors migrated to the far west of the country and established medical schools in "Free China" in places like Guizhou, Yunnan, Sichuan, and Shaanxi. All public medical colleges in China suffered from a lack of ideal conditions and sought to strike a balance between adequate training, limited resources, and the task of providing enough physicians to establish a modern medical infrastructure in China. Foreign institutions certainly contributed many physicians to meet this need, but they were targets of anti-imperialist nationalism in the 1920s—for good reason: they served the goals of their foreign funders rather than those of the nation-state.

It now seems ironic that it was Japan, "indirectly and without any spirit of altruism," that "accomplished more in the introduction of modern medicine [to China] than any other nation."[75] Today in China the history of Anglo-American imperialism is downplayed while Japan's imperialism and invasions remain fresh in the collective memory, so missionary or Rockefeller medicine is no longer condemned, but celebrated, while Japanese connections are elided. In the 1930s, Tang Erhe—founder of the National Medical College—became one of the top Japanese collaborators, serving as minister of education, president of Peking University, and head of the East Asia Cultural Cooperation Association, shuttling constantly between Beijing and Tokyo between 1937 and his death in 1940. The NMC, by then long incorporated into Beijing University, saw its own "return" to Japanese influence with a new group of Japanese faculty at the school. In the ongoing context of anti-Japanese nationalism in China, it is understandable that such history has been ignored, but as historians we cannot ignore overwhelming evidence that, at least for a time in the 1910s and 1920s, Chinese elites' state-building goals aligned more closely with those of the Japan-influenced NMC and its efforts to produce a large number of moderately well trained physicians than with the elitist vision of medical education put forward by the China Medical Board.

Notes

Epigraph: "Japanese Influence in Chinese Medical Education," *Scientific Monthly* 14, no. 3 (1922): 289.

1. This account comes from a biography of Tang Erhe penned by his son, Tang Yousong (Tang Qi), titled *Tang Erhe xiansheng* [Mr. Tang Erhe] (Beijing: Jinhua yinshuju, 1942), 49–50. The details are repeated in Mu Jingjiang, *Minguo xiyi gaodeng jiaoyu (1912–1949)* [Advanced medical education in Republican China, 1912–1949] (Hangzhou: Zhejiang Gongshang University Press, 2012), 85–86. Potentially controversial points in Tang Yousong's biography of his father are here confirmed with other sources, either government documents in the Beijing Municipal Archives [hereafter cited as BMA] or in the voluminous published record.

2. Tang, *Tang Erhe xiansheng,* 23–47. The hospital was the Zhejiang Hospital (Zhejian bingyuan), and the medical school was the Zhejiang Medical Technical College (Zhejiang yiyao zhuanmen xuexiao).

3. Ibid., 39.

4. Ibid., 49–50.

5. Fan Yuanlian was adviser to the Qing Ministry of Education from 1910, vice minister of education for the Republic from April 1912, and minister of education from July 1912 until November 1913. Through the many political intrigues of the following years, he was sometimes minister of education or minister of the interior or was touring the United States and Europe on educational fact-finding missions. Xu Youchun, *Minguo renwu da cidian* [Biographical dictionary of Republican China] (Shijiazhuang: Hebei renmin chubanshe, 1991), 592.

6. Tang made it a condition that the new medical school be a school of *exclusively* Western medicine with no attempt made to mix aspects of Chinese and Western medicine, as had become popular in China since the late nineteenth century. He reportedly wanted a free hand to ensure that the school would not continue the policy of "Chinese medicine for internal ailments and Western medicine merely for surgery." Tang, *Tang Erhe xiansheng,* 50–51.

7. "National Medical College," one of several English-language names of the school at the time, will be used throughout for the sake of consistency. Two important references are a series of photographs in the Peking University Health Science Center Archives and an English letter from Tang Erhe to E. V. Cowdry wherein he calls the school "the National Medical College at Peking." Subsequent correspondence in the Rockefeller China Medical Board archives is filed under this name (Tang to Cowdry, November 15, 1922), Record Group (RG) 4, Chinese Medical Bureau (CMB), folder 1969, box 85, Rockefeller Foundation Archives, Sleepy Hollow, New York [hereafter cited as RFA]. However, K. Chimin Wong and Wu Lien-teh, in *History of Chinese Medicine* (Shanghai: National Quarantine Service, 1936), call it "Peking Medical Special College" (627, a direct translation; see table 3.1), a practice followed in the influential report of the Rockefeller Foundation, *Medicine in China* (Chicago: University of Chicago Press, 1914); E. V. Cowdry, in "Anatomy in China," *Anatomical Record* 19–20, no. 1 (1920), calls it "Government Medical School" (41); and Tang's 1922 German article on the histology of the heart lists it as "Medizeinschule in Peking," in line with Boorman's biography, which names the school Peking Medical College. Howard L. Boorman, *Biographical*

Dictionary of Republican China, vol. 3: *Mao-Wu* (New York: Columbia University Press, 1970), 229.

8. Raymond B. Fosdick, "Introduction," in George W. Gray, *Education on an International Scale: A History of the International Education Board, 1923–1938* (New York: Harcourt, Brace and Company, 1941), vii.

9. For "high standards" rhetoric in relation to the Rockefeller Foundation's medical work in China, see Roger S. Greene's lecture given before the First Annual Conference of the National Medical Association of China (Shanghai, February 1916):

> Here in China where modern medicine is in its beginnings as far as the Chinese people themselves are concerned, it is most important to set a high standard and to establish the best possible traditions for the future. While it takes longer to train a good doctor than a poor one, the experience of European countries has shown that a sufficient number will take the thorough training that is necessary if the facilities are provided and if they are protected against the unfair competition of the poorly trained. (*National Medical Journal of China* 2, no. 1 (March 1916): 18–31)

For more on the assumption that medical education should be based on the principle of "quality, not quantity," see S. P. Chen, "Medical Education in China," *National Medical Journal of China* 2, no. 2 (June 1916): 13.

10. On the larger German influence, see William Kirby, *Germany and Republican China* (Stanford, CA: Stanford University Press, 1984); on Japanese influence on public health, see Ruth Rogaski, *Hygienic Modernity: Meanings of Health and Disease in Treaty-Port China* (Berkeley: University of California Press, 2004); see also Douglas Reynolds, *China, 1898–1912: The Xinzheng Revolution and Japan* (Cambridge, MA: Council on East Asian Studies, Harvard University, 1993); see also Keishū Sanetō, *Zhongguo ren liuxue riben shi* [History of Chinese students in Japan], trans. Lin Qiyan and Tan Ruqian (Beijing: Beijing University Press, 2012).

11. On improvising high-tech medicine when machines are often broken, and drugs are out of stock, in Botswana, see Julie Livingston, *Improvising Medicine: An African Oncology Ward in an Emerging Cancer Epidemic* (Durham, NC: Duke University Press, 2012); for an excellent account of the improvising of medical education in contemporary Malawi, see Claire Wendland, *A Heart for the Work: Journeys through an African Medical School* (Chicago: University of Chicago Press, 2010).

12. Bao Jianqing, "Woguo xinyi zhi jiepouxue shi" [A history of anatomy in our country's new medicine], *Ziran kexue jikan* [Natural science quarterly] 2, no. 3 (1935): 4–5.

13. Ibid.

14. Tang, *Tang Erhe xiansheng*, 69–70.

15. A full list of works that Tang translated includes the following (listed by English translated titles and year of publication): *Topographical Anatomy* (1915), *Embryology* (1919), *Diagnostics* (1919), *Outline of Anatomy* (1924), *Adolescent Psychology* (1924), *The Borders of Biology and Philosophy* (1926), *Medicine and Philosophy* (1926), *Recent Studies in Gynecology* (1928), *Recent Studies of Immunology and Microscopic Pathology* (1928), *Introduction to Biology* (1929), *Outline of Physical Anthropology* (1930), *Psychiatry* (1930),

Parasitic Diseases (1930), *Dental Pathology and Therapy* (1934), and *Selected Studies in Anatomy* (1938).

16. Tang, *Tang Erhe xiansheng*, 75.

17. Cowdry to Eggleston, January 25, 1922, RG 4, CMB, I, II, folder 1969, box 85, RFA.

18. Tang Erhe. "Dong you riji" (Diary of a journey to the East), Zhonghua minguo yiyao xuehui huiboa (1) 11–48.

19. E. V. Cowdry, "Anatomy in China," *Anatomical Record* 20, no. 1 (1920): 37.

20. David Nanson Luesink, "Dissecting Modernity: Anatomy and Power in the Language of Science in China" (PhD diss., University of British Columbia–Vancouver, 2012), 265–66.

21. Mary Brown Bullock, *An American Transplant: The Rockefeller Foundation and Peking Union Medical College* (Berkeley: University of California Press, 1980), 10.

22. English-language overviews of Western scientific medicine in Japan during this period include John Z. Bowers, *Medical Education in Japan: From Chinese Medicine to Western Medicine* (New York: Hoeber Medical Division, Harper & Row, 1965); Y. Fujikawa, *Japanese Medicine*, translated from the German by John Ruhräh (1934; reprint, New York: AMS Press, 1978). For an overview of the system of medical education and relevant regulations that existed as of 1914, see Sanitary Bureau Home Department, *The Present State of the Medical Administration of the Japanese Empire* (Tokyo, 1914). For the complex networks that bound German and Japanese medicine during the late nineteenth and early twentieth centuries, see Hoi-eun Kim, *Doctors of Empire: Medical and Cultural Encounters between Imperial Germany and Meiji Japan* (Toronto: University of Toronto Press, 2014).

23. The rise of these institutions can be followed in Amano Ikuo, *Kyūsei senmon gakkō ron* [On the old system of technical colleges] (Machida: Tamagawa Daigaku shuppanbu, 1993).

24. For an assessment of the relative impact of these two kinds of institutions in Japanese medical education before the Pacific War, see Bowers, *Medical Education in Japan*, 40–42. In 1911, there were three imperial university medical colleges and eleven public and private institutions with the status of "technical medical college" (Fujikawa, *Japanese Medicine*, 65). As of 1912, approximately 30 percent of licensed physicians in Japan were graduates of public and private technical medical colleges, as compared to the 8 percent who had been trained at the imperial universities. The rest of physicians had received licenses by passing government-run examinations (without having attained a degree from one of the schools) or by having received a medical degree at a foreign institution. Sanitary Bureau, *State of the Medical Administration*, 26–28.

25. It is noteworthy that Mu Jingjiang's recent history of medical education in Republican China completely elides this Japanese influence in its substantial account of the NMC (*Minguo xiyi gaodeng jiaoyu*, 85–93); however, he does focus on the Japanese influence with a case study of Manchuria (160–93).

26. For clothing regulations in the early NMC regulations, see National Medical College, "Regulations of Beijing Medical Technical College" [*Beijing yixue zhuanmen xuexiao zhangcheng*] (Beijing: Beijing yixue zhuanmen xuexiao, 1912), 8a–9a. For regulations of Kanazawa Medical Technical College, see *Catalog of Kanazawa Medical Technical College, 1910–1913* [Kanazawa igaku senmon gakkō ichiran] (Kanazawa: Kanazawa Medical Technical College, 1912), 66–67; 83–84; 86.

27. Records pertaining to the educational background of NMC faculty can be found in lists of faculty and staff submitted to the Ministry of Education in 1918–22. "Register of teaching and administrative staff of Beijing Medical Technical College" [*Beijing yixue zhuanmen xuexiao zhiyuan mingce*], 1918–1922, 11–13, 96–100, BMA J29-1-9; "List of teaching and administrative staff of Beijing Medical Technical College" [*Beijing yixue zhuanmen xuexiao jiaozhiyuan mingce*], 1919–1921, 17–22, 149–55, 174–80, BMA J29-1-11. See also "Tables from general survey of Beiping University Medical School and teaching and administrative staff, 1933" [*Beida yixueyuan Minguo ershi-er nian jingkuang diaocha biao ji jiaozhiyuan diaocha biao*], 1933, BMA J29-3-124.

28. See Sanitary Bureau, *State of the Medical Administration*, 15–19.

29. See, for example, China Medical Commission of the Rockefeller Foundation (CMCRF), *Medicine in China* (Chicago, 1914), 9–10.

30. The Kyūshū Imperial University College of Medicine had been established in 1903 as the Fukuoka Medical College and had become part of the university in 1910. Sanitary Bureau, *State of the Medical Administration*, 2.

31. Tang, *Tang Erhe xiansheng*, 58. For a contemporary list of Kanazawa Medical Technical College faculty and staff with entries for all three scientists, see *Catalog of Kanazawa Medical Technical College, 1910–1913* [Kanazawa igaku senmon gakkō ichi-ran] (Kanazawa: Kanazawa Medical Technical College, 1912), 83–84, 86.

32. This is the assessment in Tang, *Tang Erhe xiansheng*, 59.

33. Ishikawa Yoshinao, *Topographical Anatomy* [*Jubu jiepouxue*], trans. Tang Erhe (Tokyo: Tohōdō Shoten, 1915). This publication includes an advertisement for Tohōdō Shoten's line of Chinese-language medical publications—including Tang Erhe's own *Histology* [*Zuzhixue*].

34. Tang, *Tang Erhe xiansheng*, 59.

35. Ibid., 60.

36. Tang Yousong mentions that at the time that Tang Erhe studied at this school, he was classmates with "Mr. Qian," current president (as of 1942) of Beijing University. This would seem to be Qian Daosun (Ibid., 19).

37. During the first decade of the institution's history, for example, it would have been common for students to receive instruction in anatomy, histology, pathology, and forensic medicine from Japanese faculty members. For more on their instruction, see the brief descriptions of course content for the classes they taught included in "Courses of Study in the Various Fields of Instruction at Beijing Medical Technical College, 1914–5" [*Beijing yixue zhuanmen xuexiao Minguo san zhi si nian ge ke jiaoshou chengxu biao*], 1914, BMA J29-1-21; and "Courses of Study in the Various Fields of Instruction at Beijing Medical Technical College" [*Beijing yixue zhuanmen xuexiao Minguo wu, shiyi nian geke jiaoshou chengxu biao*], 1916–22, BMA J29-1-22. Descriptions of these instructors' courses submitted to the Ministry of Education were often written in Japanese. See, for example, descriptions of Murakami Shōta's pathology labs held for third-year students and Ishikawa Yoshinao's topographical anatomy classes for second- and third-year students, histology lab for second-year students, and anatomy lecture for first-year students in BMA J29-1-21, 53–74. For faculty members' use of German (and to a lesser extent English) as a research language, see various articles included in issues of *Collected Research Articles of National Beijing University Medical School* [*Guoli Beijing daxue yixueyuan lunwen ji*], published in Beijing between 1939 and 1941.

38. "Regulations on Medical Technical Colleges" [*Yixue zhuanmen xuexiao guicheng*], Ministry of Education Order No. 25, promulgated November 22, 1912. For an English translation, see CMCRF, *Medicine in China*, 103–4.

39. See the laws published in *Zhonghua minguo yiyao xuehui huibao* [Journal of the Republic of China Medico-Pharmaceutical Association] 1, no. 1 (1917): 1, and no. 2 (1917): misc. pp.

40. These regulations are reproduced in *Catalog of Kanazawa Medical Technical College* (1912), 13–18. For a partial English translation of the regulations, see Sanitary Bureau, *State of the Medical Administration*, 6–10.

41. Instruction proceeded during two yearly semesters: September–December, during which one term of teaching could be covered; and January–July, which included enough time for the completion of two terms. For the curriculum and timetable included in the regulations, see "Regulations of Beijing Medical Technical College," 3a–4b.

42. "Beijing Medical Technical College 1914 Administrative Plan and Expansion Plan" [Beijing yixue zhuanmen xuexiao san nian du xiao wu jihua shu ji kuangzhang jihua shu], 1914–19, BMA J29-1-23.

43. CMCRF, *Medicine in China*, 12.

44. The history of these commissions can be followed in John Z. Bowers, *Western Medicine in a Chinese Palace: Peking Union Medical College, 1917–1951* (Philadelphia: Josiah Macy Jr. Foundation, 1972), 29–61.

45. The Second China Medical Commission, for example, recommended a program of funding to existing Chinese and missionary institutions in order to strengthen their training in the basic sciences. Moreover, in recognition of the unfeasibility of requiring that entering students complete premedical education in advance, PUMC itself established a two-year premed training program to prepare students to enroll in its medical program. This program closed in 1925, after it became feasible to actually require that incoming students complete their premed training at other institutions. Ibid., 56, 64, 78.

46. Amano, *Kyūsei senmon gakkō ron*, 26.

47. See Fujikawa, *Japanese Medicine*, 70–73. The number of technical medical colleges seems to have skyrocketed during the Pacific War in order to meet wartime needs for producing physicians. As those "technical medical colleges" that remained after the war were reorganized under the auspices of a Council of Medical Education formed in March 1946, this category of institution disappeared from the Japanese medical landscape. See Yoshio Kusama, "Medical Education in Japan," *Journal of Medical Education* 31, no. 6 (June 1956): 393–98, which forms the basis of Bowers's discussion (*Medical Education in Japan*, 40–42).

48. "Regulations of Beijing Medical Technical College," 5a.

49. See, for example, "National Medical College's Thirteenth-Anniversary Commemorative Gathering" [*Yida shisan zhounian jinian hui*], *Chenbao*, November 25, 1925, 6/186. Peking University Health Science Center held its centenary celebrations in October 2012, culminating in ceremonies on October 26, 2012. See http://www100.bjmu.edu.cn/xsgc/fzlc/353.htm.

50. For a brief overview, see Kao Tien and Ha Hongchien, "Taiwan jiepou ji kao" (Anatomy Cadaver Ceremonies in Taiwan), *Zhonghua yishi zazhi* 29, no. 3 (1999): 175–77.

51. "Announcements Regarding the Ministry of Interior Issuing Revised Regulations on Dissection" [*Neizhengbu gongbu xiuzheng jiepou fabu de guanggao*], 1912–15, 15, BMA J29-1-16.

52. "Brief Account of the Development of National Beijing Medical Technical College" [*Guoli Beijing yixue zhuanmen xuexiao yange lüe*], in *Guoli Beijing yixue zhuanmen xuexiao shizhou jinian lunwenji* [Collection of essays commemorating the tenth anniversary of National Beijing Medical Technical College] (Beijing: National Beijing Medical Technical College, 1922), 4.

53. "Announcements Regarding the Ministry of Interior," 98–101.

54. National Medical College, "Dissection Rites." National Medical College, "Dissection Rites of National Beiping University Medical College" (illustration), *Beiping yikan* 1, no. 6 (June 10, 1933): n.p.

55. See, for example, "Medical Specimen Exhibition Has Set a Fixed Time Period," *Chenbao*, December 28, 1921, 7/651; "Anatomical Specimen Exhibition at the Medical University," *Chenbao*, Feburary 1, 1927, 6/240; "The Medical School Displays Anatomical Specimens," *Chenbao*, February 9, 1927, 6/256; "The Anatomical Specimen Exhibition Will Remain Open for Another Three Days," *Chenbao*, February 13, 1927, 6/288; "The Anatomical Specimen Exhibition Closes," *Chenbao*, February 14, 1927, 6/296.

56. See "Regulations of Beijing Medical Technical College."

57. *Tongsu yishi yuekan*, issue no. 1 (1919). The journal was renamed *Yishi yuekan* (The Medical Journal) in 1923 after the sixth issue.

58. "Correspondence Pertaining to Beiping University Medical School Holding Anatomical Specimen Exhibitions, Fundraising and Visitors, and Measures for Collecting Human Skulls" 1931–39, 12–15, BMA J29-3-552.

59. Bullock, *American Transplant*; Karen Minden, *Bamboo Stone: The Evolution of a Chinese Medical Elite* (Toronto: University of Toronto Press, 1994).

60. Chinese Medical Association, *The Chinese Medical Directory 1932*, 3rd ed. (Shanghai: Chinese Medical Association, 1932), 30–34; Mu, *Minguo xiyi gaodeng jiaoyu*, 174–75.

61. There were important reasons for the large cost-per-student gap between PUMC and NMC. PUMC's paid salaries were equivalent to those at top American institutions and came with expatriate benefits, while faculty salaries at most public and missionary medical schools were much lower.

62. This can be explained by two factors: that the Shanghai institution had been established only five years earlier, in 1927, and that salaries and living expenses were higher than in Beijing.

63. See Tang, *Tang Erhe xiansheng*, 74.

64. The following account of Lin Ji's career and professional activities is derived from Daniel Asen, *Death in Beijing: Murder and Forensic Science in Republican China* (Cambridge: Cambridge University Press, 2016). See also Huang Ruiting, *Fayi qingtian: Lin Ji fayi shengya lu* [A righteous medico-legal expert: A record of the career of the medico-legal expert Lin Ji] (Beijing: Shijie tushu chuban gongsi, 1995).

65. See "Courses of Study," 1916–22, BMA J29-1-22.

66. Tang Erhe, "Xue fazheng de ren keyi budong xie yixue ma?" [Can those who study law and politics not also understand a bit about medicine?], *Xin jiaoyu* [New Education] 2, no. 3 (1919): 295–303.

67. For these aspects of Lin Ji's professional activities, see Asen, *Death in Beijing*, chap. 7.

68. Tang, "Xue fazheng de ren keyi budong xie yixue ma?," 298–99.

69. For a usage of this term in the context of the NMC and its graduates, see "Special announcement of Aiyou Society," *Tongsu yishi yuekan*, no. 1 (1919). For the role of associations in the lives of professionals, see Xiaoqun Xu, *Chinese Professionals and the Republican State: The Rise of Professional Associations in Shanghai, 1912–1937* (Cambridge: Cambridge University Press, 2001).

70. This professor is almost certainly the son of Wilhelm Krause (1832–1909), anatomist of Gottingen and Berlin, and grandson of Karl Freidrich Theodor Krause (1797–1868). Tang's research publications in histology came out of this research.

71. Tang, *Tang Erhe xiansheng*, 94.

72. Wendland, *Heart for the Work*, 173.

73. Bullock, *American Transplant*, 1

74. Livingston, *Improvising Medicine*, 6.

75. Cowdry, "Japanese Influence," 289.

Chapter Four

An Abortive Amalgamation

Multiple Western-Style Doctors in Republican China, 1927–1937

SHI YAN

In 1934, two of China's largest nationwide medical organizations, the Chinese Medical Association (CMA) and the China Medical and Pharmaceutical Association (CMPA), tried to amalgamate, but then failed, due to a series of impolitic articles in the Chinese section of the *Chinese Medical Journal* in 1933. This chapter will examine this incident, revealing the underlying reasons in order to emphasize that the development of modern medicine in Republican China was seriously impeded by the contradictions between multiple groups of Western-style doctors. The appearance of these distinct groups of physicians can be attributed not only to the impact of different colonial powers on China, but also to the different experiences of development and group interests that led these different groups to diverge from each other. When the contradiction between modern Western-style medicine and Chinese native medicine intensified after 1929, the relationship between these groups of Western-style doctors worsened, and as a result, Western-style doctors failed to merge or even find agreement on many issues to improve the state of Western-style medicine in China.

In the past few decades significant research has been done on medicine in Republican China, particularly the massive transformation of Chinese medicine. As a variation of the impact-response model, many studies emphasized Chinese native doctors' resistance or adjustment to the transformation. Comparatively less attention has been paid to Western-style doctors, especially as groups or associations, due perhaps to the influence of

China-centered history since the 1980s. Some scholars have pointed out the different opinions among Western-style physicians on the issues of abolishing Chinese native medicine and building a modern style of medicine. Memoirs of various physicians have also mentioned that there were different factions among Western-style doctors; they had conflicts in either the bureaucracy or various medical institutions. However, some basic questions have not yet been answered: When and how were these groups formed? What were the differences among them? How did these differences affect their nature? Understanding the nature of Western-style doctors is essential for us to understand medicine in Republican China; they were, after all, primary advocates and promoters in the development of modern medicine in China. In this chapter, I will explore the divergence between two leading Western-style doctors' associations by focusing on the failed merger incident in 1934, and then discuss the reason behind this divergence and the influence it had on the medical field.

Abortive Amalgamation

After the Nationalists (Guomindang) established themselves in Nanjing, the government undertook a program of national reconstruction, a part of which was the founding of a separate Ministry of Health, which aimed to improve modern medicine and public health conditions in China.[1] Under these circumstances, Western-style doctors believed it was necessary to unify a truly national medical association for China. One of the leading Western-style medical associations, the Japanese-oriented China Medical and Pharmaceutical Association (Zhonghua Minguo Yiyao Xuehui), appointed a committee to devise ways and means for the formation of a national association as early as 1927. This committee actively conferred with another noticeable Western-style medical association, the Anglo-American-oriented National Medical Association of China (Zhonghua Yixuehui, or NMAC), and obtained a favorable response.[2] Several presidents of the NMAC made speeches to support and implement this idea.[3] Apart from the CMPA, they communicated with other medical associations too, and received a grant-in-aid from the Rockefeller Foundation for the amalgamation. A general secretary was secured to visit the larger cities, maintain contact between the different associations, and investigate the situation of all physicians, hospitals, dispensary clinics, medical organization, and medical schools in the country.[4] When Chinese native physicians organized the National Federation of Medical and Pharmaceutical Associations (Quanguo Yiyao Tuanti Zonglianhehui), the issue of Western-style doctors' unification became more fraught. In April 1932, the NMAC merged with the missionary China Medical Association,[5] under the name of the Chinese Medical

Association, and the two organizations combined their journals as the *Chinese Medical Journal.*[6] This demonstrated a great step forward in the unification of Western-style medical associations and made the next amalgamation on the agreed agenda very promising—that between the CMA, the CMPA, and a third group, the Medical Practitioners Association (Quanguo Yishi Gonghui).[7] In addition, after the situation in northeastern China became tense in 1931,[8] many members of the CMPA joined the CMA; the CMPA then had to give up its main source of financial support, the Japanese Boxer Indemnity.[9] These early signs of amalgamation were apparently looked on favorably by all, but then the merger was aborted unexpectedly in 1934.

This failure was caused directly by the publication in 1933 of two articles in the Chinese section of the *Chinese Medical Journal*, the CMA's official organ. One of the articles carried no byline and rebuked Japanese-style doctors and schools for their poor quality and irresponsibility.[10] The other criticized German-Japanese medical schools indirectly by presenting some statistics comparing medical schools, revealing that German-Japanese-style medical schools had lower admission requirements and required fewer courses and a shorter hospital residency. In addition, these schools admitted a great number of students with a very high student-to-teacher ratio, as can be seen in the previous chapter.[11]

The second article was written by Lee Tao (Li Tao), the chief editor of the *Chinese Medical Journal*'s Chinese section and a teacher at Peiping Union Medical College (PUMC); but there is reason to believe that the first article was also by Lee Tao. Since these two articles touched on the sensitive issues of language and training for CMPA members,[12] they created conflict with the Anglo-American group, the CMA.[13]

Immediately, both the Medical Practitioners Association and the CMA demonstrated their deep disappointment about the failed merger. Niu Huisheng, the president of the CMA, expressed his opinion on this incident in the Medical Practitioners Association's journal *Yishi Huikan.* He said that the amalgamation had been unconditionally welcomed by all the leaders of the three associations at first, but that the negotiations ended unexpectedly with the appearance of the two articles in the *Chinese Medical Journal.*[14] As a result, Lee Tao resigned as chief editor two months later, but his interventions had already incited bad blood between the two groups.[15] Some other people also wrote about the unfriendly atmosphere prevailing between German-Japanese and Anglo-American groups.[16] In order to relieve this tension, the CMA secured the famous doctor Yu Yan (Yu Yunxiu), who had completed his studies in Japan, to take the position of Chinese chief editor of its journal in 1934. The journal's Chinese editorial board was also enlarged to include members who had graduated from Japan, Germany, and France.[17] But this brief account only begins to explain the differences between the two groups and explain why their promising cooperation in the early 1930s was eventually broken.

The Forming of Different Groups in China's Medical Profession

As modern Western-style medicine was not born in China, all of the first generation of Chinese Western-style doctors were trained by foreigners.[18] At first, some learned medicine as the apprentices of medical missionaries; others received more-formal training from medical missionaries and were sent abroad to complete their educations. In 1872, the Chinese government started to send students to study in the United States and Europe.[19] Although this plan was not sustained, an awareness of studying scientific technology abroad was fostered; some people chose to study medicine in Western countries. Later, some missionary hospitals became medical schools, and the Beiyang Army Medical School was also founded to teach modern Western-style medicine in the 1880s. Most of those who learned medicine in this period were taught in English.

A cohort of German-Japanese-style physicians emerged after 1895. Impressed by the achievements of the Meiji Restoration, especially after the First Sino-Japanese War (1894–95), numerous Chinese preferred to go to Japan to learn Western technology. It was thought that the expense would be cheaper, communication would be easier, and culture shock would be less in Japan. Both the central and provincial governments encouraged young people to study in Japan; the Guangxu emperor and key officials like Zhang Zhidong and Liu Kunyi all talked about the advantages of studying in Japan. From its perspective, Japan attempted to promote mutual understanding and communication between China and Japan in order to extend its own growing influence.[20] Japan invited more Chinese to study in its schools, offering to pay the expenses of two hundred Chinese students, and several schools were established especially for Chinese.[21] Compared to those who had studied earlier in the United States and Europe, a larger number among these students chose to study medicine, because they believed that national prosperity and power depended on racial strengthening—the production of strong and healthy people.

When the civil service examinations were abolished in China in 1904, studying abroad became a shortcut to officialdom, and many returned students could be sure of official jobs and promotions upon their return to China. Meanwhile, the Japanese victory over Russia in the Russo-Japanese War (1904–5) attracted even more Chinese to Japan to learn the secrets of its success.[22] As modern medicine in Japan adopted the German model, this great number of returned physicians together with a few who came home from Germany gathered to be the German-Japanese group. Many of them held prominent positions in the army or the Beiyang government after 1912.

Sino-Japanese relations became more complicated in the 1910s. After the 1911 Revolution, the number of Chinese students in Japan declined, especially after Japan's Twenty-One Demands and the Shandong Problem ignited anti-Japanese nationalism.[23] Around this time, US-China educational exchanges drastically expanded, and the United States replaced Japan as the most popular destination among Chinese students, owing to America's ambitions to spread its power through education.[24] Large sums of money, from the Boxer Indemnity and the Rockefeller Foundation, were invested in Chinese education and many students were trained. As a result, a significant group of English-speaking physicians began to cluster together in large urban centers like Beijing, Shanghai, and Guangzhou.

Although Chinese students learned modern Western-style medicine in different countries, the medical knowledge they gained was similar. We might call this either "modern medicine" or "scientific medicine," and it dated from the nineteenth-century turn to clinical medicine in hospitals combined with allied laboratory sciences. Since the latter half of the nineteenth century, Germany's medical establishment took the lead due to its great laboratories and attracted students from all over Europe and North America.[25] After the Meiji Restoration in 1868, Japan decided to embrace Western-style medicine by adopting German medicine, the most advanced model at that time. For many years, most of the foreign teachers in Japanese medical schools and institutions came from Germany, and a number of Japanese medical leaders had studied in Germany, so it made sense that the languages of medical education in Japan were German and Japanese.[26] The German model influenced the United States too, as with Johns Hopkins, but there were nonetheless significant differences in curriculum arrangements. German medical education concentrated on basic medical science by preferring research, and deferring major clinical experience until after graduation. While medicine in Britain had a "tenacious clinical culture," the learning of medicine by "walking the wards" and making contact with cases held an important position in British medical education.[27] American medical education combined Germany's laboratory-centered approach and Britain's clinical medicine as it innovated at the turn of the twentieth century. Thus, Japanese medical education had a closer relationship with the German model while American medicine was more closely aligned with the British example.[28]

Inevitably, Chinese physicians learning modern Western-style medicine in a particular country would be inclined toward the particular nature of that system. Due to the newness of modern Western-style medicine as a discipline to China, returned Western-style doctors had to take the medicine that they were taught as a model. Once they were in position to administer medical schools or hospitals, they followed curriculum arrangements and service systems they had learned abroad. The number of Chinese textbooks was limited, and the translation of medical terminology into Chinese took a long time to standardize and become widely accepted in the Republican period.[29] Foreign languages were used in teaching students, recording cases in hospitals, publishing papers, and so on. As a Western-style doctor, Tao Shan-min explained, "Our medical schools, being started either by foreigners, or by our graduates trained abroad, have been based upon the system of medical education of the countries where our teachers derived their medical education. Thus English, American, German, Japanese and French methods of medical education are met with here."[30] As a result, Chinese physicians who had returned from either Germany or Japan and the Anglo-American group rarely engaged in mutual academic exchange and were constrained by their language of medical education in their choice of jobs.[31] Most medical schools modeled their program as either German-Japanese style or Anglo-American style as a marketing tool to attract students.[32] This resulted in the divisions in the medical field being passed on to a generation of Chinese-trained medical students.

Besides, the custom of traditional Chinese intellectuals was to develop a teacher-disciple or patron-client relationship, such as *tongnian*.[33] This relationship was considered not only helpful in academic research, but also very important to their career life or even livelihood. After the civil service examination was abolished, the old exam-based relationships were replaced by new schoolmate ties. People often secured jobs and advancements in bureaucratic or medical positions, or got involved in various controversies, due to these relationships.[34] This kind of tie was strengthened by regionalism. Because communication was limited, people from the same place could more easily share similar information and apply for the same schools or jobs. Thus the internal bonds of the German-Japanese group and the Anglo-American group were much stronger than any intergroup bonds. The many frictions between these two groups are recorded in numerous memoirs.[35] And so it is not surprising that a survey from Medical College of Peiping University (i.e., the National Medical College of chapter 3) said that the majority of its Chinese professors were of the German-Japanese group, among whom half came from Zhejiang Province, and who dominated the school while marginalizing other professors.[36]

Prejudices about Quality and Superiority in Quantity

The German-Japanese-style and Anglo-American-style physicians not only distinguished themselves from each other based on where they were educated. They also continued to differentiate when different Western-style models were intentionally or unintentionally applied to Chinese medical education. The discrepancy of the camps became more marked when Western-style physicians began to compete in China's bureaucratic jungle and workplaces. As each group fought for its own benefits, various conflicts and arguments occurred between the different groups. The most important argument between the German-Japanese group and the Anglo-American group was about physician quality. As the articles in the *Chinese Medical Journal* by Lee Tao and the anonymous author claimed, many in the Anglo-American group considered the qualifications of many German-Japanese physicians inferior.

Although Anglo-American medicine was greatly influenced by German medicine, which was the most advanced in the Western countries at that time, the number of Germany-returned Chinese physicians was small among the German-Japanese group.[37] Since the 1870s, German medical schools required students to have a solid background in chemistry, biology, and other basic sciences.[38] Admission standards for medical students were strict and narrow, which made it difficult for Chinese students to study in Germany, given the poor state of science education in China's secondary schools, not to mention the language barrier. Then World War I led to a long period of stagnation for German medicine, and in China, physicians who had studied in Germany became fewer and thus the superiority of German medicine was reduced.[39] The German-Japanese group, therefore, mainly contained Japan-returned students and graduates of the German-Japanese-style schools in China. According to the statistics on graduates from foreign medical schools registered with National Health Administration in 1933, there were only 42 Germany-returned doctors among a total of 367 returned graduates.[40] Another survey published in 1935 by the Japanese-oriented Dōjinkai Association (Tongren Association, Association of Universal Benevolence); there were about 4,800 Western-style doctors in China, only 104 of whom had studied medicine in Germany.[41]

In the late Qing era, one unique feature of the Chinese students who studied in Japan was what they termed "instant education" (*sucheng jiaoyu*), which meant the dramatic reduction in the length of education programs. On the demand side, Chinese students felt deeply anxious about the slow progress of national prosperity and power and also began to see studying abroad as a shortcut to officialdom. This led to many schools in Japan vying with one another to shorten the time to degree of their programs in order to attract Chinese students.[42] The Chinese ambassador to Japan, Yang Shu, wrote in 1904 that 60 percent of Chinese students in Japan were trained by this method of "instant education," 30 percent entered institutions of higher education, and less than 1 percent were admitted by Japanese universities.[43] In 1905, just as the Confucian examinations were abolished, the Qing government created a special exam to select officials. One result was that the scores of Japan-returned graduates were far below those of returnees from other countries.[44] Japan copied the German model in which students acquired a science education in secondary schools, so that medical schools did not have to teach basic science.[45] Medical schools did require a competitive examination for the applicants. However, because few Chinese students learned chemistry, physics, and biology in Chinese middle schools until the 1920s, it was difficult for Chinese students to learn medicine in Japan. As Daniel Asen and David Luesink explain in chapter 3, many medical schools in Japan began as medical technical colleges (*igaku senmon gakkō*), rather than full imperial university medical schools. By the early 1920s, however, many of these started to reorganize and formed university medical schools providing a longer curriculum and higher quality of training.[46] But until such time as all Chinese physicians graduated from the higher status Japanese medical schools, Japan-returned doctors were open to the charge of being less qualified and might be criticized by Anglo-American-style doctors for being poor at academic research and ill-prepared to teach students.[47]

Following the tradition of deferring internship until after graduation and preferring theory, most German-Japanese medical schools in China also had a short curriculum without an internship. Moreover, many German-Japanese medical schools were poorly equipped, in contrast to Anglo-American medical schools that received financial support from the Boxer Indemnity or the Rockefeller Foundation.[48] Accordingly, some Anglo-American-trained physicians like Lee Tao criticized that China's German-Japanese medical schools produced inferior students.[49] This opinion was even sometimes voiced by medical students in German-Japanese-style schools. Hou Zonglian was a famous graduate of Manchurian Medical University, where he was trained by well-known Japanese physiologist Yas Kuno. Yet when Hou became the president of Northwest National Medical College in Xi'an, he chose to adopt the Anglo-American style instead of the Japanese one to arrange the college's curriculum. In his opinion, German-Japanese-style medical education could not foster a qualified doctor with enough clinical skill.[50] In 1942, PUMC was forced to close; some PUMC professors joined the German-Japanese-oriented Medical College of Peiping University. These professors received high praise by the students, while many German-Japanese-style professors in the college were criticized sharply either for their deficiency in knowledge or their lack of enterprise and ambition.[51]

In contrast, more and more Chinese middle school students learned English, making it easier for them to study in English-speaking countries rather than in Germany. At the same time, American medical universities paid more attention to basic science training because of the discrepancy between the secondary educations of incoming students,[52] and this made US schools more suitable for Chinese students who arrived with less chemistry, physics, and biology knowledge. More importantly, Anglo-American-style medical education, which tried to balance preclinical science and clinical study, emphasized both research and "walking the wards" in training teachers and specialists in hospitals; these factors made many Anglo-American-style doctors believe that their abilities were superior to those of the German-Japanese group.[53]

Apart from these various accounts, it is difficult to evaluate whether the educational and professional attainments of the Anglo-American group were generally higher than those of the German-Japanese group, but we do know that prevailing prejudices about the quality of the German-Japanese group favored the Anglo-American group in competing for patients and top hospital positions.

In addition to the general competition among groups of Western-style physicians, there was another important cause for the criticism of the quality of the German-Japanese group. Beginning in the early 1900s, the Rockefeller family began to show great interest in philanthropy in China, choosing public health and medicine as the medium for a larger project. Medicine was a wedge for the newly formed Rockefeller Foundation to "offer to the people of China the best that is known to Western civilization not only in medical science but in mental development and spiritual culture."[54] The Rockefellers' interest in China also accorded with American foreign policy and was encouraged by the US government.[55] In 1914, the Rockefeller Foundation sent out a commission to China to do a survey on medicine. This commission found that "the Chinese government and private medical schools in China are almost exclusively under Japanese influence, practically all their staff having been trained in Japan or by Japanese teachers in China."[56] Then the commission commented that "most of the Chinese who have studied medicine [in Japan] have attended second-grade schools, on account of the difficult entrance requirement of the University medical schools." Chinese applicants for medical schools were only admitted by "technical medical colleges" in Japan that dispensed with the entrance examination, but provided a shorter curriculum and lower quality of training without what the commission considered proper premedical training. Upon completion of their course, Chinese graduates of these medical colleges received a certificate without having to pass the same examination as Japanese graduates of the same colleges and were not granted the same degree.[57] In order to impress Chinese people with the advantage of American medicine, the Rockefeller Foundation was determined to build its medical enterprises in China at the highest possible global standard. In 1915, the Rockefeller Foundation bought and then reorganized the hitherto missionary establishment, the Peking Union Medical College, modeling it on the Johns Hopkins Medical School, one of the preeminent medical schools in the United States.[58] Under Rockefeller patronage, PUMC became not only the best equipped and staffed medical school in China, but by some accounts the best in all of Asia, including Japan. This imbalance of investment in medical education created the conditions for prejudice of those associated with PUMC and other elite Anglo-American establishments against graduates of the German-Japanese-style medical schools.

The National Medical Association of China had as one of its principal objects to "preserve the honor and to uphold the interests of the Profession."

The NMAC believed that maintaining the high quality of Western-style physicians would both show the advantage of modern Western-style medicine to the general population and maintain prestige in the eyes of the foreign doctors. NMAC membership was restricted to "graduates in medicine of foreign universities or colleges" or graduates of medical colleges in China with a good reading and writing knowledge of at least one Western language. If a person did not know a Western language, he or she usually would only be associate members without eligibility as officers.[59] It followed that the physicians who joined the association were considered to be better-trained Western-style physicians. The NMAC never expected to recruit only Anglo-American-style doctors, although it was seen as an Anglo-American Oriental association due to most of its members being graduates from British and/or American universities or Anglo-American-related medical schools in China.[60] Therefore, as with Lee Tao, many senior members in the NMAC and CMA judged most of the German-Japanese group to be inferior, even when they decided to unite with CMPA. For example, the president of the CMA, Niu Huisheng, expressed his opinion in private that he wanted to invite the better members of the CMPA instead of merging with the whole association. He did not feel that it would be advisable from the point of view of standards of the new association to take in all of the Japanese-trained students. "Many of them are extremely inferior both in their medical education and in their medical ethics," he said.[61]

Despite this, the NMAC and CMA never expressed their prejudices openly toward the German-Japanese group when they criticized the poor quality of Western-style doctors before the 1930s, because the NMAC and CMA aimed to first combine all Chinese Western-style doctors in order to improve the overall position of China's modern Western-style medical profession.[62] Since the German-Japanese group was a substantial part of China's Western-style medical profession, to attain its unification goal, the NMAC and CMA believed they must cooperate with the German-Japanese group.

According to the 1914 Rockefeller Foundation's report, China's Western-style medicine up to that point was largely under Japanese influence.[63] The League of Nations surveyed medicine in China around 1926, rendering a similar judgment: "The majority of reside [sic] in big cities and a large proportion are considerably under a low European or Japanese standard."[64] The National Health Administration of China also gathered some statistics on medical practitioners registered during 1929–32. Among 367 registered doctors who had graduated abroad, 53 percent were Japanese-trained doctors; American-trained doctors were the second-largest group, with 20 percent; and German-trained physicians were third, with 11 percent (see fig. 4.1). Among 2,557 registered doctors graduated from medical schools in China, 67 percent were from German-Japanese-style schools, compared to 22 percent from Anglo-American-style schools (see fig. 4.2).

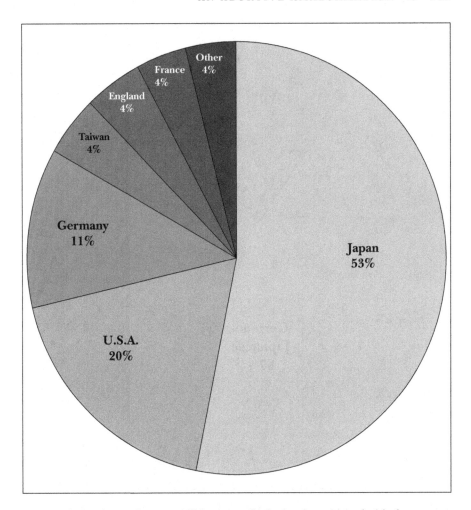

Figure 4.1. Graduates from non-Chinese medical schools registered with the National Health Administration by Country, 1929–32. Source: Xu Shijin, "Quanguo dengji yishi tongji" [Statistics on medical practitioners registered with National Health Administration of China], *Zhonghua yixue zazhi* 19, no. 5 (1933): 746–54.

In 1937, another survey also showed that 5,358 people graduated from twenty-one medical schools in China. Dong Nan Medical School ranked first, with 692; the College of Medicine in National Peiping University was second, with 622 (National Medical College, Beiping, see chapter 3); and Zhejiang Provincial Medical and Pharmaceutical School third, with 570. All three were German-Japanese-style medical schools, and together they comprised 35 percent of all the graduates in the country.[65]

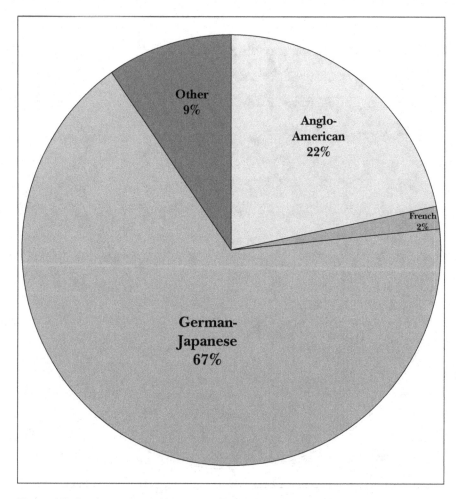

Figure 4.2. Graduates from Chinese medical schools registered with the National Health Administration according to affiliation, 1929–32. Source: Xu Shijin, "Quanguo dengji yishi tongji" [Statistics on medical practitioners registered with the National Health Administration of China], *Zhonghua yixue zazhi* 19, no. 5 (1933): 746–54.

The German-Japanese group was overwhelmingly more influential than other groups. The CMPA, composed largely of doctors trained in Japan many of whom served in army, was particularly significant, not to mention that its founder and president, Tang Erhe, occupied an important position in the Peking government and was prominent in both the medical profession and the wider academic scene at that time.[66] In addition, a series of new educational regulations followed the Japanese model from 1904 to 1922, as did medical regulations.[67] When the NMAC decided to implement the unification of medical associations by cooperating with the German-Japanese group, the CMPA was one of its best partners.

When the CMA, CMPA, and Medical Practitioners Association decided to cooperate, why did the CMA openly publish articles that criticized the German-Japanese physicians? The motivation had much to do with conditions for modern Western-style medicine being less than hopeful, and in fact quite harsh in the late 1920s and early 1930s.

Problems for Modern Western-Style Medicine in the Nanjing Decade

In the progress toward national reconstruction, a new Ministry of Health, led and dominated largely by Anglo-American-trained physicians with strong ties to PUMC and the Rockefeller Foundation, was established in 1928 at the beginning of the Nanjing Decade. This new ministry was greatly influenced by institutions of the Anglo-American group, such as CMA. When it started to build a modern medical system for the country, decades-long contradictions between modern Western-style medicine and Chinese traditional medicine intensified.[68]

Unlike other Western-style doctors, members of the NMAC rarely talked about abolishing Chinese traditional medicine before 1932. Yu Fengbin, the president of the association, once talked about the value of Chinese traditional medicine. He believed it was worth keeping because it was part of China's national essence that had survived for thousands of years.[69] Beginning in 1919, a series on the history of Chinese medicine was published in the *National Medical Journal of China* by Chen Bangxian and K. Chimin Wong (Wang Jimin). Most members of the association had unshakable faith in modern Western-style medicine, believing that traditional medicine, as the inferior approach, was doomed to extinction. But they nevertheless adopted a tolerant attitude toward traditional medicine because of the shortage of modern physicians.[70] They saw their most urgent task as upholding the standard of modern Western-style medicine and denouncing quackery or unqualified Western-style practitioners.[71] But they did not target any of the major Western-style physician groups.

When native doctors successfully organized a national federation and achieved the right to call their form of medicine "National Medicine," Western-style doctors came to the realization that modern medicine was progressing too slowly to defeat traditional medicine or to win completely the trust of the public for at least several decades.

When proposals were made that the Nanjing government adopt "National Medicine Regulations" and establish an Institute of National Medicine (Guo Yi Guan) that would allow native medicine to acquire an equal official status with biomedicine at the end of 1932, the *Chinese Medical Journal* published articles deploring these proposals. Concerned that only Western-style medicine have an official status, the writers were afraid that "the use of the title Kuo I [*Guo yi*, or National medicine] by practitioners of the old system of medicine, implying as it does official connection with the State, is derogatory to the dignity of our country and misleading to the public."[72] In 1933, the proposal that entrusted the Institute of National Medicine to administer Chinese traditional medicine finally made the Chinese Medical Association move beyond criticism and take action.[73] President Niu and the former president of the Chinese Medical Association, Yan Fuqing, went to see the presidents of the Executive Yuan and Legislative Yuan to express their strong opposition to the regulations on the institute.[74] After that, the Chinese Medical Association's attitude toward native medicine appeared hostile;[75] however, the eagerness to eliminate obstructions to promoting modern Western-style medicine was heightened.

In the view of the Anglo-American group, after several years' development, the number of Western-style physicians was not small, nor was the amount of annual expenditures on medical education considered inadequate. But the vast interior and rural districts could not support qualified modern doctors' practices with living expenses and equipment owing to their poverty. Western-style doctors thus tended to reside disproportionately in big port cities.[76] In Canton, for example, the doctor-patient ratio was higher than Germany's in the 1930s: "There are more than enough doctors and hospitals in the city to adequately care for the population; but it does not follow that the people are adequately cared for."[77] Excessive competition among doctors to earn a livelihood inevitably resulted in quackery and low quality of some practitioners. Although graduates from most medical schools did not possess a level of training that would permit them to compete legitimately with those who had superior training, some resorted to unethical practices to prey on the ignorant public.[78] However, sometimes these "half-Western-style" practitioners were able, by offering flexible treatment methods and lower fees, to compete with highly qualified scientific doctors. and if they lied or conducted malpractice, they would further lower the standard of modern medical practice in the eyes of the public.[79]

Niu Huisheng of the Anglo-American group blamed this situation partly on the inferior quality and medical ethics of the German-Japanese group. Lee Tao's 1933 survey revealed that German-Japanese-style schools had the most graduates and the lowest teacher-student ratios. For instance, the German-Japanese Dongnan Medical School had a teacher-student ratio of 1 to 19, yet its total number of medical graduates ranked second among medical colleges (see fig. 4.5).[80] These Chinese medical graduates were considered ill-prepared to practice their profession. For all of these reasons, representatives of the Chinese Medical Association finally voiced their dissatisfaction, and cooperation between the two groups largely ended, leaving China's Western-style medical profession disunited for the rest of the Republican era.

The Influence of the Abortive Amalgamation: Divergence in Regulating Medical Education

After the failure of the amalgamation of CMA and CMPA, the relationship between the German-Japanese and Anglo-American groups worsened. They turned bitterly suspicious of each other regarding many aspects of the development of modern Western-style medicine in China. One example is disagreements on how to standardize medical education.

In 1935, Robert K. S. Lim (Lin Kesheng), the head of the Physiology Department of Peiping Union Medical College, submitted his proposed curriculum for Chinese medical colleges. The opinion of the Anglo-American group was that the curriculum struck a successful balance to achieve both quality and quantity of physicians needed in China,[81] and they were able to get it adopted by the Ministry of Education.[82] Once this provisional curriculum was promulgated, it provoked harsh criticism from the German-Japanese group, who had not been consulted. The most contentious issue was that of foreign-language requirements. In the provisional curriculum, 270 hours were required to learn a first and second foreign language; and hours spent on the first language should not be less than two-thirds of the total hours. As English was the most popular foreign language in middle schools, most students did not have enough credit hours to become proficient in other foreign languages such as Japanese or German. The German-Japanese group claimed that this requirement was used by the Anglo-American group to intentionally oppress the German-Japanese-style medical schools.[83] Their second charge against the new curriculum was that it laid too much emphasis on practice and maintained too little emphasis on the theory of medicine. Some German-Japanese-style physicians said theory was the soul of medicine; the medical colleges were the place to foster medical scientists rather than private practitioners—so most of the hours should be spent on theory. It was the lower-level technical medical colleges instead that were to train practitioners.[84] This article also argued that the Anglo-American group intended to mold China's medical education into their own style and exclude the German-Japanese group. Aside from foreign language and theory, there were lots of disagreements on names, hours, and arrangement of various courses, even including disagreements about essential teaching equipment. These critics even attacked the Committee of Medical Education in the Ministry of Education, of which most members were Anglo-American-style physicians, and predicted that the provisional curriculum, which represented only the interests of the Anglo-American group, would never be accepted nationwide.[85] As a result of this fundamental disagreement, the Ministry of Education was never able to promulgate a permanent curriculum for medical colleges, and medical education in China therefore failed to achieve a recognized standard.

The China Medical and Pharmaceutical Association and the Chinese Medical Association were the two leading associations in China and represented the largest two identifiable groups among Western-style medical doctors: the German-Japanese group and the Anglo-American group. The appearance of different Western-style practitioners due to different nationalities' educational backgrounds can be considered to be the result of competing colonial interests in China. Because modern Western-style medicine was not born in China, the governments of Britain, the United States, and Japan wielded influence through their systems of medical education by educating Chinese students and offering financial support. But the formation of these groups was not purely the result of external pressures; it was also influenced by conditions in China. Several factors strengthened the relationship within different groups, such as career restrictions and preexisting tendencies toward factions in Chinese tradition. The divergence of approaches was consciously fostered among different groups as Western-style physicians labored in China. After the Nationalists established themselves in Nanjing, unification became a common desire among Western-style physicians. While latent prejudices were never expressed openly and broadly, modern Western-style medicine did not develop well, and the influence of native doctors seemed to be more powerful in the 1930s. The struggle between the German-Japanese group and the Anglo-American group resulted in further hindrances to the development of modern Western-style medicine. This episode in cooperative failure involving the two competing groups reveals that there were multiple Western-style doctors in Republican China. The friction between them was one of the important factors impeding their common goal of modernizing medicine in China.

Notes

1. Ka-che Yip has described this matter in some detail in *Health and National Reconstruction in Nationalist China: The Development of Modern Health Services, 1928–1937* (Ann Arbor, MI: Association for Asian Studies, 1995). Ye Xiaoqing also has examined what the government actually achieved in terms of regulating the medical profession and the difficulties of policy implementation. Ye Xiaoqing, "Regulating

the Medical Profession in China: Health Policies of the Nationalist Government," in Alan K. L. Chan, Gregory K. Clancey, and Hui-Chieh Loy, eds., *Historical Perspectives on East Asian Science, Technology, and Medicine* (Singapore: Singapore University Press: World Scientific, 2001), 198–213.

2. F. C. Yen, "The Significance of Having One National Medical Association for China with Suggestion for Its Formation," *National Medical Journal of China* 15, no. 1 (1928): 24.

3. Ibid., 23; J. Heng Liu, "President's Address," *National Medical Journal of China* 15, no. 1 (1928): 29; Wu Lien-teh, "The Future Status of the Chinese Medical Profession," *National Medical Journal of China* 15, no. 2 (1929): 196–97; Robert K. S. Lim, "Presidential Address," *National Medical Journal of China* 16, no. 1 (1930): 115–16; W. S. New (Niu Huisheng), "Presidential Address," *Chinese Medical Journal* 46, no. 9 (1932): 1028.

4. Lim, "Presidential Address," 115–16.

5. The China Medical Missionary Association, founded in 1886, was one of the earliest nationwide medical missionary organizations in China. Since 1925, it was renamed the China Medical Association and allowed physicians who were not engaged as missionaries to join. New, "Presidential Address," 1028.

6. Ibid., 1025–26.

7. The Medical Practitioners Association is different from CMA or CMPA; it was a guild concerned mainly with the rights and interests of medical practitioners. Formed in 1929, the majority of its membership came from the Shanghai Physicians Guild, the core members of which were also Japan-returned physicians, such as Yu Yan and Wang Qizhang. "Quanguo yishi lianhehui duiyu bu dengjitiaoli xuanyan" [Claim of Medical Practitioners Association for the regulation of medical profession], *Yishi huikan* 2 (1930): 1; "Quanguo yishi lianhehui zhangcheng" [Constitution of Medical Practitioners Association], *Yishi huikan* 2 (1930): 1.

8. On September 18, 1931, Japan invaded northeastern China, known as Manchuria.

9. Gist Gee to W. S. Carter, April 4, 1932, folder 21, box 2, series 601, Record Group (RG) 1, Rockefeller Foundation Archives, Sleepy Hollow, NY [hereafter cited as RFA].

10. "Zhongguo de yixue jiaoyu" [Medical education in China], *Zhonghua yixue zazhi* 19, no. 2 (1933): 197–216.

11. Lee Tao, "Minguo ershiyi niandu yixue jiaoyu" [Medical education in China for the year 1932–1933], *Zhonghua yixue zazhi* 19, no. 5 (1933): 681–700.

12. The China Medical and Pharmaceutical Association was founded in April 1915. This association was an ambitious one, because it included not only physicians but also pharmacists without any language requirement. The association's original membership drew mostly from medical special colleges and army medical institutions and hospitals, such as Tianjin Army Medical School (Tianjin Lujun Junyi Xuexiao), Peiyang Medical School (Beiyang Yixue Xiao), Guangdong Medical and Pharmaceutical Special College (Guangdong Gongli Yiyao Zhuanmen Xuexiao), and Jiangsu Medical Special College (Jiangsu Yixue Zhuanmen Xuexiao). "Minguo sinian bayue wuri diyici chenglihui jiyao" [Minutes of inaugural meeting on April 5], *Zhanghua minguo yiyao xuehui huibao* 1 (1917): 6. The majority of the members shared in common that they were trained in Japanese- or German-style medical schools.

13. The National Medical Association of China (NMAC) was founded in January 1915 by Chinese members of the China Medical Missionary Association. Although the members were required to know at least "one western language," a 1932 survey of the membership revealed that 84.7 percent members in the association were graduates from British or American universities or Anglo-American-related medical schools in China, not to mention that all NMAC presidents had studied in Britain or the United States. Editorial, "Ourselves," *National Medical Journal of China* 1, no. 1 (1915): 15; Editorial, "Zhonghua yixuehui gaikuo baogao" [General report of the National Medical Association of China], *Zhonghua yixue zazhi* 18, no. 1 (1932): 181–83.

14. Niu Huisheng, "Quanguo yijie ying xiangjianyicheng" [Medical professionals should be frank to each other], *Yishi Huikan* 18 (1934): 15.

15. Lee Tao, "Congcong wunian" [Five years passed], *Zhonghua yixue zazhi* 19, no. 6 (1933): 959–60.

16. Yu Yunxiu, "Song Pang Jing-zhou yishi beixing xu" [Seeing Dr. Pang Jingzhou off], *Zhonghua yixue zazhi* 20, no. 4 (1934): 651.

17. H. P. Chu, "Conference Proceedings: Chinese Medical Association," *Chinese Medical Journal* 48, no. 5 (1934): 490–91.

18. In this chapter, "modern Western-style medicine" refers to biomedicine that came to China firstly from Western countries in the nineteenth century.

19. Yi Chu Wang, *Chinese Intellectuals and the West, 1872–1949* (Chapel Hill: University of North Carolina Press, 1966), 42.

20. Nakajima Chieko, "Medicine, Philanthropy, and Imperialism: The Dōjinkai in China, 1902–1945," *Sino-Japanese Studies* 17 (2010): 56.

21. Sanetou Keishuu, *History of Chinese Students in Japan*, trans. Lin Qiyan and Tan Ruqian (Beijing: SDX Joint Publishing Company, 1983), 23–27, 59–61; Wang, *Chinese Intellectuals and the West*, 59.

22. Wang, *Chinese Intellectuals and the West*, 64.

23. Chieko, "Medicine, Philanthropy, and Imperialism," 60.

24. Hongshan Li, *U.S.-China Educational Exchange: State, Society, and Intercultural Relations, 1905–1950* (New Brunswick, NJ: Rutgers University Press, 2008), 1.

25. Roy Porter, ed., *The Cambridge Illustrated History of Medicine* (Cambridge: Cambridge University Press, 1996), 181.

26. Sugimoto Isao, ed., *History of Science in Japan*, trans. Zheng Pengnian (Beijing: Commercial Press, 1999), 333–48.

27. Thomas Neville Bonner, *Becoming a Physician: Medical Education in Britain, France, Germany, and the United States, 1750–1945* (New York: Oxford University Press, 1995), 275, 292; George E. Vincent, "The Medical Profession from an Inter-National Point of View," *American Journal of Psychiatry* 83, no. 2 (1926): 297.

28. John M. Barry, *Great Influenza: The Story of the Deadliest Pandemic in History* (New York: Penguin Books, 2005), 33–34; Bonner, *Becoming a Physician*, 292.

29. Knud Faber, *Report on Medical Schools in China* (Geneva: League of Nations Health Organization, 1931), 20; David Nanson Luesink, "Dissecting Modernity: Anatomy and Power in the Language of Science in China" (PhD diss., University of British Columbia–Vancouver, 2012), 42–209.

30. S. M. Tao, "Medical Education of Chinese Women," *Chinese Medical Journal* 47, no. 10 (1933): 1019–20.

31. Zhu Hengbi, "Zhongguo yixue jiaoyu yingyong yuwen zhi wojian" [My opinion on language used in medical education in China], *Zhonghua yixue zazhi* 17, no. 5 (1931): 491.

32. Chen Zhiqian, "Gongyi yu yixue jiaoyu" [State medicine and medical education], *Duli pinglun* 138 (1935): 9.

33. Originally *tongnian* included those who passed the civil service examination and become candidates in the same year.

34. Yeh Wen-Hsin has studied this transition in her book *The Alienated Academy: Culture and Politics in Republican China, 1919–1937* (Cambridge, MA: Harvard University East Asian Studies, Harvard University Press, 1990).

35. "Report of the China Medical Commission to the Rockefeller Foundation," October 21, 1914, 17, folder 243, box 27, series 601, RG 1, RFA; J. Heng Liu to Roger S. Greene, November 14, 1928, and J. Heng Liu to Roger S. Greene, April 16, 1930, both in *Dr. J. Heng Liu and Medical and Health Development in China*, ed. Liu Sijin (Taipei: Commercial Press, 1989), 328–30; Jin Baoshan, "Jiu Zhongguo de xiyi paibie he weisheng shiye de yanbian" [Western-style groups and the development of medical affairs in Republican China], in Wenshi ziliao xuanji bianjibu, *Wenshi ziliao xuanji*, vol. 101 (Beijing: Zhongguo Wenshi Chubanshe, 1985), 125–38. Fu Hui and Deng Zongyu, "Yixuejie de yingmeipai yu deripai zhi zheng" [The struggle between the German-Japanese group and Anglo-American group], in Wenshi ziliao xuanji bianjibu, *Wenshi ziliao xuanji*, vol. 119 (Beijing: Zhongguo Wenshi Chubanshe, 1989), 64–74.

36. "Shibianhou banianlai zhi yixueyuan" [The situation of medical schools during World War II], October 1945, Zhu Jiahua Archive, 301-01-09-088, Institute of Modern History, Academia Sinica, Taipei.

37. Jin, "Jiu Zhongguo de xiyi paibie he weisheng shiye de yanbian," 127.

38. Barry, *Great Influenza*, 6; Bonner, *Becoming a Physician*, 254.

39. Robert K. S. Lim to Roger S. Greene, August 28, 1923, folder 890, box 123, CMB, RFA; Bonner, *Becoming a Physician*, 330.

40. Xu Shijin, "Quanguo dengji yishi tongji" [Statistics on medical practitioners registered with National Health Administration of China], *Zhonghua yixue zazhi* 19, no. 5 (1933): 749–50.

41. Dōjinkai Association, ed., *The Overview of Chinese Medical Issue* [*Zhonghua Minguo Yishi Zonglan*] (Tokyo: Dōjinkai, 1935), 136–406.

42. Keishuu, *History of Chinese Students in Japan*, 58–60.

43. Yang Shu, "Plans for Studying in Japan," in *Zhongguo jindai jiaoyushi jiaoxue cankao ziliao* [Resources for the history of Chinese modern education], ed. Chen Xueyun, vol. 1 (Beijing: People's Education Press, 1987), 710–11.

44. Ruth Hayhoe, *China's Education and the Industrialized World: Studies in Cultural Transfer* (Shanghai: Shanghai People's Publishing House, 1990), 116.

45. Barry, *Great Influenza*, 6.

46. Editorial, "Medical Education in Japan," *National Medical Journal of China* 18, no. 6 (1932): 1029, 1034–35.

47. Editorial, "Riben de yixue jiaoyu" [Medical Education in China], *Zhonghua yixue zazhi* 19, no. 2 (1933): 205–6; Dr. Rajchman, "Report to League of Nations," *National Medical Journal of China* 13, no. 3 (1927): 291.

48. At this time, both American and Chinese governments were willing to provide strong administrative and financial support for education. The Rockefeller Foundation

contributed greatly as well, not only to the PUMC, but also to public health training and medical education in China, as research has showed. The amount of British indemnity funds rated fourth with 11 percent of the total Indemnity, behind Russia (28 percent), Germany (20 percent), and France (15 percent). After the Russian share was canceled, by arrangement with the Soviet government, and as the payment of Germany's portion ceased in 1914 and a large portion of the French indemnity was used as capital for the *Banque Franco-Chinoise pour l'Industrie* leaving only US$250,000 in gold as interest from the investment to be used yearly for educational and cultural purposes, Britain's portion therefore then ranked first in importance and amount. Grants were given from this money annually to applicants from the medical field. "British Boxer Indemnity," *Chinese Medical Journal* 51, no. 4 (1937): 558; "News and Notes: Scholarships for Study in England," *Chinese Medical Journal* 48, no. 10 (1934): 1091.

49. Lee Tao, "Medical Schools in China for 1932–1933," *Chinese Medical Journal* 47, no. 10 (1933): 1031.

50. Hou Zonglian to Zhu Jiahua, May 16, 1945, Zhu Jiahua Archive, 301-01-09-157, Institute of Modern History, Academia Sinica.

51. "Shibianhou banianlai zhi yixueyuan" [The situation of medical schools during World War II], October 1945, Zhu Jiahua Archive, 301-01-09-088, Institute of Modern History, Academia Sinica.

52. Barry, *Great Influenza*, 6.

53. Wu Lien-teh, "Yixue xianzai zhi qudi ji jianglai zhi wanjiu shangqueshu" [Discussion on abolishing medicine now and preserving medicine in the future], *Zhonghua yixue zazhi* 1, no. 1 (1915): 9; W. S. Carter interview with Way Sung New (Niu Huisheng), January 3, 1933, folder 22, box 2, series 601, RG 1, RFA; J. Heng Liu to Helen K. Stevens, September 19, 1947, folder "Liu, J. Heng: July–Dec. 1947," box 16, Permanent File J. Heng Liu (July 1947–December 1951), American Bureau for Medical Aid to China Records, 1937–1979, Columbia University Rare Book & Manuscript Library, New York.

54. John D. Rockefeller, "Response for the Rockefeller Foundation," in *Addresses and Papers: Dedication Ceremonies and Medical Conference, Peking Union Medical College, September 15–22, 1921* (Peking, 1922), 64–65.

55. China Medical Commission of the Rockefeller Foundation (CMCRF), *Medicine in China* (New York, 1914), v; Ma Qiusha, *Gaibian Zhongguo: Luokefeilei jijinhui zaihua bainian* [*To Change China: The Rockefeller Foundation's Century-Long Journey in China*] (Guilin: Guangxi Normal University Press, 2013), 132–45.

56. CMCRF, *Medicine in China*, 9.

57. "Report of the China Medical Commission to the Rockefeller Foundation," October 21, 1914, 12–14, folder 243, box 27, series 601, RG 1, RFA.

58. CMCRF, *Medicine in China*, 91; Mary E. Ferguson, *China Medical Board and Peking Union Medical College: A Chronicle of Fruitful Collaboration, 1914–1951* (New York: China Medical Board of New York, 1970), 25.

59. "The National Medical Association of China," *National Medical Journal of China* 1, no. 1 (1915): 23; "Constitution and By-Laws," *National Medical Journal of China* 1, no. 1 (1915): 26.

60. "Zhonghua yixuehui dahui jiyao" [General report of the National Medical Association of China], *Zhonghua yixue zazhi* 18, no. 1 (1932): 181–83.

61. Carter interview with Way Sung New, January 3, 1933.

62. "National Medical Association of China," 23.

63. CMCRF, *Medicine in China*, 9.

64. Rajchman, "Report to League of Nations," 291.

65. "Woguo yixue yuanxiao zuijin gaikuang" [Recent situation of medical schools in China], *Zhonghua yixue zazhi* 23, no. 8 (1937): 1130. Compare figure 3.3 for 1933 data.

66. Ye, "Regulating the Medical Profession," 207; Timothy B. Weston, *The Power of Position: Beijing University, Intellectuals, and Chinese Political Culture, 1898–1929* (Berkeley: University of California Press, 2004), 108.

67. Wang, *Chinese Intellectuals and the West*, 99.

68. Sean Hsiang-lin Lei (*Neither Donkey nor Horse: Medicine in the Struggle over China's Modernity* [Chicago: University of Chicago Press, 2014]) and Bridie Andrews (*The Making of Modern Chinese Medicine, 1850–1960* [Vancouver: University of British Columbia Press, 2015]) have contributed greatly to the research about the contradictions of Western-style medicine and Chinese native medicine during Republican China.

69. Yu Fengbin, "Baocun guyixue zhi shangque" [Discussion on preserving Chinese traditional medicine], *Zhonghua yixue zazhi* 2, no. 1 (1916): 4.

70. Wu, "Yixue xianzai zhi qudi ji jianglai zhi wanjiu shangqueshu," 9–11.

71. Ibid., 11; E. S. Tyau, "The Demand of Modern Medicine upon the Profession, the College and the Government," *National Medical Journal of China* 1, no. 1 (1915): 2–3; Yen, "Having One National Medical Association for China," 23–24; F. C. Yen, "Medicine and Public Health Service under Nationalist Government," *National Medical Journal of China* 15, no. 1 (1929): 114.

72. "Conference Reports: Resolution at Final Session of Conference," *Chinese Medical Journal* 46, no. 11 (1932): 1137.

73. H. P. Chu, "Conference Proceedings: Chinese Medical Association," *Chinese Medical Journal* 48, no. 5 (1934): 494.

74. H. P. Chu, "Yinianlai benhui gongzuo zhi huigu" [Review for works in last year], *Zhonghua yixue zazhi* 20, no. 1 (1934): 166.

75. Chu, "Conference Proceedings," 494; H. P. Chu, "Practitioners of Native Medicine," *Chinese Medical Journal* 49, no. 5 (1935): 495; Jiang Huiming, "Cunhu feihu: guanyu zhongguo jiuyixue cunfei wenti de jiantao" [Preserve or not, the review of abolishing Chinese old nedicine issue], *Zhonghua yixue zazhi* 21, no. 7 (1935): 762; "Herb Medicine," *Chinese Medical Journal* 51, no. 4 (1937): 552.

76. His-Ju Chu and Daniel G. Lai, "Distribution of Modern-Trained Physicians in China," *Chinese Medical Journal* 49, no. 6 (1935): 543–52; C. C. Chen, "State Medicine and Medical Education," *Chinese Medical Journal* 49, no. 9 (1935): 953; C. C. Chen, "A Proposed Basic Medical Curriculum," *Chinese Medical Journal* 49, no. 6 (1935): 862; Lin Jingcheng, "Zhongguo gonggong weisheng xingzheng zhi zhengjie" [The crux of Chinese public health administration], *Zhonghua yixue zazhi* 22, no. 10 (1936): 959.

77. Frank Oldt, "Scientific Medicine in Kwangtung," *Chinese Medical Journal* 48, no. 7 (1934): 670.

78. Yen, "Medicine and Public Health Service," 114.

79. Chen, "State Medicine and Medical Education," 953; C. C. Chen, "Some Problems of Medical Organization in Rural China," *Chinese Medical Journal* 51, no. 6 (1937): 813. Lei discusses the wide variation of practitioners in Republican Shanghai in *Neither Donkey nor Horse*, chap. 6.

80. Lee, "Minguo ershiyi niandu yixue jiaoyu," 681–700.

81. R. S. Greene, "Proposed Curriculum for Medical Colleges Offering A Six-Year Course," *Chinese Medical Journal* 49, no. 9 (1935): 847–60.

82. "Daxue yixueyuan ji yike zanxing kemubiao" [Provisional curriculum for medical colleges], *Zhonghua yixue zazhi* 21, no. 7 (1935): 802–7.

83. "Xijing yishigonghui duiyu nanjing yixue jiaoyu weiyuanhui suoni yixueyuan kechengdagang pingyidian dayao" [Xijing Medical Practitioners Association's main opinions as to the provisional curriculum for medical colleges], *Yishi huikan* 7, no. 23 (1935): 164; Li Fujing and Zhang Jingwu, "Duiyu nanjin yixue jiaoyu weiyuanhui suoni yixue kechengdagang zhi yijian" [Our opinions as to provisional curriculum for medical colleges], *Yishi huikan* 7, no. 23 (1935): 152.

84. Li Fujing, "Zhongguo yixue jiaoyu de huayi ji zhang'ai fasheng de yuanyin" [Unifying China's medical education and the barriers to it], *Xin yiyao* 3, no. 2 (1935): 191; "Tang nizhou yishi zhi yijian" [Opinion of Dr. L. C. Tang], *Yishi huikan* 7, no. 23 (1935): 165–66.

85. Li and Zhang, "Duiyu nanjin yixue jiaoyu weiyuanhui suoni yixue kechengdagang zhi yijian," 151; Wang Qizhang, "Yixiao shebei gebiaozhun de shangque" [Question about the standard of teaching equipment in provisional curriculum for medical colleges], *Xin yiyao* 3, no. 8 (1935): 645.

Chapter Five

Shanghai's Female Doctors

A Discussion of the Gendered Politics of Modern Medical Professionalization

HE XIAOLIAN

A common feature of medical practice in Shanghai before 1949 was the dominance of male physicians; the only exception was in the field of obstetrics, in which female practitioners predominated. Investigations of the status of the Western medical profession in Shanghai have done much to reveal the social complexity of the profession, but the subject of female doctors in China has been largely unexamined by historians.[1] Perhaps this is because although the careers of Shanghai's top woman physicians were dramatic and influential, in a male-dominated medical world these women nevertheless appear as exceptions, and although they are sometimes mentioned in passing, sustained historical analysis of gender in the study of Chinese medicine is lacking. We might compare the situation in China to a 1904 account of the limited participation of female physicians in the American Medical Association's annual meeting: "Twenty years ago, they stood together outside the door. Now they sit in isolation on the inside; their influence nil."[2] Within such a framework of male dominance, what accounted for women's progress in medicine in modern Shanghai? What was the professional status of modern woman physicians? How was their professional domain fashioned? How did this compare to the women who were also entering into medical careers as traditional physicians? When women entered into male-dominated domains, gender differences and gender relations became a focus of patriarchal attention and control. Thus, at the same time that women were becoming liberated on the professional front, they suffered gender-specific political restrictions. On the one hand, in areas such as professional status, income, marriage, and family, their inferior position in comparison to males stood out. On the other hand, the cachet of being a female doctor set them apart from other women as well as from their male medical peers, so once female physicians broke into the public sphere, they were very active in social, cultural, and political affairs. This chapter aims to elucidate the professional liberation and hardships of modern female physicians, their professional values, and the gender-specific body politics that they experienced.

Gender as a Factor in Medical Careers

Before the opening of Shanghai as a treaty port, most women working in traditional medicine were midwives, sometimes called "medicine women" (*yaopo*) or "matrons" (*wenpo*), but just as often dismissed by literate male physicians with derogatory phrases such as "three aunties and six grannies" (*sangu liupo*). What female herbal doctors there were did not, for the most part, enter the ranks of regular physicians. In general, women in late imperial China were limited to the "inner quarters" of the home by neo-Confucian notions of female virtue, and those medical grannies and midwives who were exceptions were seen as something of a threat to the social order.[3] Yet male physicians saw any difficult childbirth as completely preventable, and thus derided the "active management and intervention" of the illiterate female midwives.[4] With the decay of neo-Confucian norms in the semicolonial space of Shanghai and the arrival of the Western medical profession, opportunities increased for female healers to enter the public sphere. In the early Republican period, before professional organizations or the state were able to monitor the medical field, there was a wide variety of persons practicing medicine, and this was also the case with female practitioners.[5] Some came from traditional Chinese medical families and learned Chinese *fuke* (women's medicine) through apprenticeship, while others from such backgrounds abandoned Chinese medicine and began to study Western medicine. Some claimed to be Western medical doctors after being assistants to missionary doctors in Christian hospitals, but others studied abroad and, by the twentieth century, increasingly were graduates of domestic medical schools; some went on to pursue further studies abroad. This variety reflects the changing urban society and culture of Shanghai at that time: more and more female physicians appeared and advertised in popular dailies such as *Shenbao*, like male physicians, soliciting patients with their marks of status.

In the early Republican period up to the 1920s, woman physicians were still rare, yet from the mid-1930s on, the number of female graduates of domestic medical schools significantly increased every year. Some female physicians were listed in the *Shanghai Business Directory*, including several celebrated modern figures, such as Shi Meiyu (Mary Stone), Zhang Zhujun, and Zhang Xiangwen, all rigorously trained medical specialists. Zhang Zhujun was the first listed of just four Chinese-nationality Western physicians in the 1909 *Guide to Shanghai*, an indication that women had already begun making their mark in the field at that early date. Female medical doctors, both traditional Chinese and Western, mainly opened their practices in the foreign concessions of Shanghai where the richest residents lived, which provided opportunity to build lucrative practices.[6] But the number of Chinese women in medical practice in Shanghai increased dramatically by the end of the Republican period.

In a 1947 address to a meeting of the Trustees of the American United Board for Christian Higher Education in China, the president of St. John's Medical School of Shanghai, Ni Baochun, said, "Not counting preparatory students, St. John's University Medical School at this time has 154 students, and among them around forty are women, or about one in three." From this he concluded that "women physicians have good prospects in the future of China."[7] This ratio at St. John's University was comparatively high compared to other nations, as well as to Shanghai. In 1944, in England, the proportion of women among medical school students was only 20 percent, and the actual prewar average was 15 percent.[8] In 1947, the Shanghai Medical Association had 1,826 physician members, of whom 310 were women, or 17 percent. In the same year, the medical association took sixty-five new members, of whom twelve were women, an almost identical 18 percent.[9] As shown in a 1947 survey, the proportion of women to men among Western physicians who opened practices in the urban districts of Shanghai was one in ten, which shows a drop from the 17–18 percent rate of female physicians overall. This disparity might be explained through hospitals' employment of woman physicians, and by their either leaving the city or discontinuing practice.[10] Yet if we take the more conservative 10 percent and extrapolate from the overall number of practitioners, we arrive at around 200 female physicians operating private practices at the beginning of 1950.[11] Meanwhile, during the same period, over 150 female physicians of Chinese traditional medicine opened practices in the city,[12] excluding those who had not registered with the municipal Public Health Bureau. From these statistics we can get a general view of the expanding opportunities for female medical practitioners in Shanghai. Growth in their numbers did not occur out of thin air: economic development and the rapid expansion of modern Shanghai increased the value of scarce medical resources, while the growth of feminism and the women's liberation movement played a vital role in the expansion of medical opportunities, imbuing a mental strength and moral courage in the women who joined the movements.

Female medical students generally studied one of four fields: either gynecology, obstetrics, pediatrics, or nursing. During the Republican period, most Chinese obstetricians were women, and men were rare, except among obstetric surgeons. Hsiu-yun Wang has argued that male and female medical practice were gendered differently: "The significance of women receiving medical education and becoming physicians was different than for men; male physicians commonly claimed that physicians were there to save lives [apparently life has no gender], but female physicians were there to save women [to avoid contact with men]."[13] One reason for this difference was that the tradition of men and women not having contact caused some female patients to actually prefer the risk of death over visiting a male doctor since it violated social norms for a woman to be touched by any man other than her husband. Another reason was the example of female medical missionaries, who had more career opportunities overseas than at home.[14] Wang Hsiu-yun's research shows that toward the end of the nineteenth century and into the early twentieth century, as Western imperialism expanded its reach globally, so too did the flow of Western medical influence into the non-Western world, leading to expanded opportunities for female physicians.

From the late Qing period, discerning literati called for women to practice medicine with the specific goal of aiding births. One source says these women would emulate "the example of Western countries," even as they would "concurrently serve as midwives."[15] The use of the term "midwives" is telling, since aiding at birth and dealing with gynecological problems had long been considered the natural purview of women in Chinese society—traditional decorum required females to treat females. Such gender norms around medical care prevailed not only in China, but in Latin America, the Middle East, and the other countries of Asia, where female gynecologists and obstetricians also became necessary for similar cultural reasons. In this era, most Europeans and Americans were against women studying medicine, since it was believed that men's and women's different physiological characteristics determined different roles in the public and private sphere. It was believed that women were unable to compete physically and mentally in medical education and medical practice, and some even believed that women engaged in medical and other intellectual activities would become masculinized and infertile. But in the wake of China's "enlightenment" of the New Culture era after 1915 when women's equality gained prominent proponents, the culture of women studying medicine became established the advantages for female patients of having a female practitioner became clear to all concerned.

During the Republican period, magazines published numerous examples of the merits of women practicing women's medicine. It was claimed, for example, that women were more meticulous than men and, if they could devote themselves to medicine, would become fine doctors. Other arguments sought political legitimacy in accordance with Sun Yat-sen's Principle of the People's Livelihood, saying that women studying medicine would have a profession and be able to generate a living, which would also help establish a foundation of equal rights between men and women. But since medicine also permitted the freedom of working from home, women could still take care of household duties. Moreover, those women studying medicine would be well versed in the methods of nursing hygiene, which would be certain to have positive consequences for the future rearing of the nation's children. But perhaps the most important reason given was that women understood other women on a more intimate level: woman physicians, in diagnosing women patients, because they shared similar psychologies, would more easily understand the sources of illness; and having similar physiologies, they would more easily understand the locations of disease and could explicitly discuss disease symptoms and more easily explicate them. Because of complications related to pregnancy and childbirth, women had more illnesses in general, so having female physicians would make mothers' situations easier when they got sick.[16] "Women handling women's matters" was viewed as natural, reflecting the gender politics of traditional times, and this was the starting point for those writers who argued for the advantages of training a sufficient percentage of female physicians.

However, viewed from a feminist perspective, this kind of gendered medical care also became part of the women's rights movement.[17] Ironically, in the gender-specific health care of "women diagnosing woman" (*nüzi zhen nüzi*)—that is, "women handling women's matters" (*nüren chuli nüren de shiqing*)—traditional gender politics actually legitimized women to study medicine and regulated the gender landscape of the medical profession. Meanwhile, discrimination against females as patients underwent a great change. Formerly women avoided seeing doctors when they were sick. The Chinese had an old saying: "It is better to treat ten men than one infant; it is better to treat ten infants than one woman"—meaning it is difficult to treat infants because they could not speak, and difficult to treat women because female patients commonly avoided physicians. If patients refused face-to-face diagnosis, then diagnosis was impossible. But because these limitations were for male physicians, female Chinese patients had almost no barrier to accepting female physicians. So, for example, when pioneer female doctors like Shi Meiyu (Mary Stone) and Kang Aide (also known as Kang Cheng and Ida Kahn) returned from their studies in the United States in 1896, American missionaries were surprised at how warmly they were welcomed in local communities in Jiangxi Province.[18] As they began to practice, female physicians became the primary medical caregivers to women who were able to access them. And an even larger number of females experienced the care of woman physicians through school examinations, given the requirement that these be administered to female students only by female doctors (female students were to remain clothed if examined by male doctors).[19]

As modern obstetrics became popular for a growing middle class in Shanghai, a number of medical schools focusing on childbirth were established, producing a growing number of female graduates. Some attained their qualifications by graduating from schools of obstetrics in Shanghai, such as those attached to the Tongde, Zhongde, and Dade Obstetrics Hospitals. Those who practiced with a medical degree avoided any association with those who merely assisted women in labor, such as traditional midwives or young women who had completed a short course on modern midwifery, and this created tension between those groups.

Graduates of programs in midwifery at obstetrics hospitals who set up practices were called *chanpo*, or midwife, meaning "matrons who assist in childbirth" (*zuchanpo*), clearly distinguishing them from the old-style midwives, who were identified with the terms *yapo* and *wenpo*. They matriculated at the level of a secondary school degree after three years of study, although a minority were able to finish in two years. Obstetrics became so popular that a good number of women studied it at this basic level, some even taking this limited training and becoming famous.[20]

According to the 1947 survey of medical facilities in the nineteen districts in Shanghai, there were 290 midwives (*zuchanshi*) in hospitals compared to 58 fully qualified obstetricians and gynecologists, and 36 part-time midwives. In addition, there were 19 midwives at various clinics, and the survey found another 55 midwives practicing inside Shanghai's metropolitan districts for a total of about 400 midwives of various kinds.[21] These numbers may not appear significant given greater Shanghai's population of about 3 million by the late 1930s. However, newspapers and magazines described a much greater number of specialists set up to aid women in birth. One account described "a house every three steps and a dwelling every five; at the mouth of every alley hangs between one and five signs for 'So-and-So's Obstetrics,'" while the author estimated in total "at the least there are over a thousand."[22] Although "over a thousand" is certainly not a hard statistic, it nevertheless indicates the ubiquity of these obstetrical clinics. We are on firmer ground looking at government-registered midwives, and we can see that between 1927 and 1936 a total of 555 midwives were approved to open practices by the municipal Public Health Bureau, a number significantly greater than that in the 1947 survey.[23] We can look at these statistics from another angle, that of the number of births managed by midwives. By 1947, more than 65,000 babies were registered, and midwives attended a significant number of those births.[24] But while Western midwifery made advances, traditional midwifery also continued to play a great role as well.

In addition to midwives, there was a separate category of female medical practitioner: trainees of short hospital courses or correspondence programs who sometimes passed themselves as fully qualified Western-trained physicians. These women were able to take advantage of the fact that women patients were often unclear about the qualifications of the clinicians they visited and primarily concerned that they were seeing a female practitioner. Elite Western physicians derided such people—the Western-trained medical doctor Wang Yugang mocked them as "magicians," disparaging them as "a toxic influence on society, who leave a legacy of boundless harm."[25] Gu Shouchun argued that when prospective patients "go to inquire about 'obstetrical clinics,' their first question was, 'Do you have female physicians doing deliveries?' to which the clinic's old matrons of course happily reply, 'we have only female physicians doing deliveries.'" In the absence of strong enforcement of professional qualifications, these clinics "elevate[d] the position of the midwife by appropriating the title of a female physician."[26] Passing as a physician had many upsides and virtually no downsides for such medical practitioners, given the lack of a single, unified professional association or state enforcement. Shi Yan argues elsewhere in this volume that the two major medical associations were unable to unify for most of the Republican period and Bridie Andrews has argued that even when there were licensing regulations, they "were seldom enforced."[27] Rumors circulated about the wealth of obstetrical clinic doctors, and calling oneself a physician could also bring prestige and social status. Sean Hsiang-lin Lei has described such practitioners through the words of Pang Jingzhou in his 1933 survey of the medical environment in Shanghai as "opportunistic practitioners of the New Medicine" and "self-proclaimed experts in both the New and the Old Medicine," among at least forty other categories.[28] From the perspective of Shanghai society, such cases further emphasize the chaos of early medical professionalization illustrated in Shi Yan's contribution in this volume.

Women Physicians' Income and Position

After the introduction of Western medical systems, educational requirements and licensing laws became social norms. The broad social acceptance of the idea of women becoming doctors was directly related to their receipt of medical education and to the social status correlated to their education. Those who possessed the highest positions were those who had studied overseas; in the next tier were those who had formally graduated from domestic medical universities. As one might expect, most of those who graduated from domestic medical schools came from medical schools in Shanghai. There were also students who came from medical schools in other parts of the country, the most famous being Hackett Medical College for Women and National Sun Yat-sen University Medical School in Guangzhou in the south, and Beiping Union Medical College and Cheeloo University Medical College in northern China. Shanghai had become the preferred destination for doctors who were beginning a new practice. The main qualifications to practice Chinese medicine, meanwhile, were registration with the Shanghai Public Health Bureau or membership in a medical lineage; however, for modernizing elites, these were considered far inferior to the growing prestige of a doctorate in medicine.

Those who underwent Western medical training in specialties became the elite among female physicians. Modern medical schools had unified standards for their curricula and for graduation requirements, and women and men had the same entrance qualifications. Yet some suggested that female students' proficiency levels were actually even more demanding than those for men. In 1918, when Wang Shuzhen received a Tsinghua Boxer Indemnity scholarship to study in the United States, only a few women were allowed to enroll. In addition to standard academic requirements, those women who received a scholarship were required to be well-behaved and virtuous, to have natural (unbound) feet, to be unengaged, no older than twenty-three years of age, and graduated from high school, while men had no such extra-academic requirements. Many years later, Wang chaired Shanghai Women's Medical School. The school had high entrance requirements, though less rigorous than the qualifications for obtaining a Boxer Indemnity scholarship: completion of at least two years of college, and fixed grade requirements for main courses, such as chemistry, organic chemistry, biology, physics, and English. Most of the students recruited came from Christian colleges such as Jinling Women's College, Yanjing University, and Huanan Women's College of Literature and Science. The medical schools of Shanghai offered specialized courses taught by English-speaking professors. Most of the full-time faculty were physicians who had graduated abroad, and they engaged professors with joint appointments at St. John's University. Shanghai Women's Medical School was launched on a small scale, with just over ten students, and twenty-two in 1934.[29] This kind of elite education was unattainable for most women. Dr. Ge Chenghui, a graduate of the school, pointed out, "The practice of medicine needs a strong physique, and those who practice it without healthy bodies go halfway and have to give up, especially in this type of matter, because when you are working you have to be especially nimble, and furthermore those who practice medicine must learn fortitude."[30] Even so, in whatever country, whether woman physicians are few or many, these highly qualified female physicians rarely held high positions in clinics, hospitals, or medical schools.[31]

Only a few ranked among the elite of woman physicians who had the wealth and influence to make a name for themselves in Shanghai. For example, Dr. Zhang Xiangwen was also an active figure in Shanghai's women's circles, especially regarding women's issues. After the war against Japan began, in every session of Shanghai's National Salvation Movement, she participated along with distinguished members of the Shanghai cultural scene in the Women's Resistance Support Society. From the fact that she once contributed over twenty gold and silver items to support the resistance effort, we can see that she had considerable economic power. The highly regarded female physician Wang Shuzhen charged patients in American dollars for delivering children (including providing pre- and postnatal care) in the late 1940s, and this amount could be up to one hundred dollars, according to the recollection of her nephew, Cornell professor Tsu Lin Mei.[32] This was a fee earned by a top physician, and Wang could enjoy luxuries such as a car and driver, house, chef, and a nurse. This was the type of lifestyle a well-known physician could attain. Tsu Lin Mei emphasized that the car was just a tool for her work rather than a luxury, and that Wang and her husband, Ni Baochun, a famous orthopedic surgeon in Shanghai, of course needed a chef and nurse. Only wealthy people could afford her care. Mei recalls that as a child, he even wanted to go to his aunt's office to get autographs from some of her famous patients. Another aunt of Mei's, Ni Fengsheng, who was also a doctor who advertised as early as the 1920s. She was devoted to her career, remained single, and was quite successful financially.[33]

Despite such wealth, female physicians alone did not generally approach male physicians' level of upper-class wealth. Fragmentary evidence makes it difficult to piece together the whole picture of the lifestyle of female physicians. But two things are clear: income for Western-style medical doctors was higher than that of Chinese medicine doctors, and male doctors earned more than female doctors. An item from the archives shows that in the beginning of the 1940s, in the first year working at Renji Hospital, a physician's base pay was 70 yuan, the salary for the hospital director was 200 yuan, that for the head of medical affairs was 120–130 yuan, and chief physicians made 95–100 yuan. Residents made 65 yuan in their first year, with annual adjustments.[34] "Base pay" was a new concept in the 1940s; it reflects the characteristics of the times when actual salary was equal to base salary plus various allowances. In accordance with the inflation index, real wages had to be continually adjusted. The president of Renji Hospital, Chen Bangdian, for example, also served concurrently at St. John's Medical School, Tongde Medical School, and South-East Medical School in Shanghai as a professor. In addition to taking a salary from each of these positions, he also ran a private clinic at home for one hour in the afternoon each day. Those like Chen Bangdian who had graduated from a formal medical school and enjoyed a good reputation and social status were comfortable far beyond most middle-class professionals. Yet many physicians worked in hospitals for fixed salaries with additional subsidies, and in the case of Renji Hospital, staff remuneration differed little from that of government workers.[35] In the 1930s, government section chiefs and functionaries had monthly salaries of up to 400 yuan.[36] The most successful physicians, however, on top of what they made in their own practices and joint positions, had salaries comparable to or greater than those of high officials.

From a 1948 Shanghai Police Bureau special household registration survey, data is only available for four female physicians.[37] This "special household registration" refers to professionals, such as physicians, lawyers, engineers, accountants, reporters, and so on. The survey recorded name, age, appearance, occupation, as well as some descriptions of personality. The survey reveals a wealthy, pampered, and even arrogant cohort of male physicians. Few female doctors were mentioned, and those who were worked at Renji and Baolong Hospitals, did not operate private clinics, were unmarried, and were aged twenty-eight to thirty-three.

Baolong Hospital and Renji Hospital were two of the larger hospitals in Shanghai, and employment there generally required an elite educational background. Physicians working in large hospitals could also enjoy additional material benefits such as those offered by Gongji Hospital that aimed to provide "a stable working life and encouragement."[38] Besides disbursements for wage adjustments, meals, and living allowances, the hospital's benefits included leave for childbirth and sickness. Only a small number of female physicians had sufficient social status to allow them to attain the income and stability of appointments at major hospitals. In 1951, there were twenty-two chief physicians at Renji Hospital who had served there three years or more—nineteen men but only three women.[39] All physician salaries depended on their specialty area, with surgeons making the most and ophthalmologists and dentists also making good incomes. Standard monthly salaries eventually reached 2–3 million yuan under the tremendous inflation of the 1940s.[40]

Yet these specialties were male territory, and as has been noted, female physicians tended to thrive primarily in obstetrics and gynecology. Obstetrics developed rapidly, and as new childbirth techniques appeared, the field became increasingly medicalized. However, generally speaking, woman physicians' salaries could not compare to those of specialized surgeons, dentists, or ophthalmologists, or even to the majority of ordinary general and internal medicine physicians who had many joint appointments. Each joint appointment allowed for a significant new income stream for the small number of physicians who had cultivated lucrative specialty practices. Income was thus tied to the number of appointments, and a higher income was generally equated with greater success, with some male specialists holding down five or six joint appointments.[41]

Yet despite the wage gap between the sexes in medicine, the salaries of female physicians were far higher than those of the average female office worker. Physicians who opened private practices mostly relied for their sources of income directly on consultation fees. In 1929, for the first time, the Shanghai Health Bureau issued regulations on medical charges. The onetime delivery charge ranged from between five and fifty *yuan*,[42] which was applicable only to physicians and midwives but not to traditional midwives.

The actual fees that each physician collected, however, were "set according to each person's fame and reputation" so that "those physicians who got their degrees abroad could charge 40–50 *yuan* for a delivery."[43] In order to understand these amounts, it is useful to use figures from Chen Mingyuan's study about the economic life of intellectuals in Republican China. Chen argues that families with an income of 100–200 yuan in Shanghai at that time could be counted as middle class, meaning that these families could live in a house with two or three rooms and hire a housemaid to do the household work.[44]

While some physicians were doing a booming business all the time, others had considerably fewer patients. Some female physicians had a simple home clinic with a few nurses in addition to delivering infants at the local lying-in women's house. Lying-in women could deliver their babies in these clinics, but it is unclear what the clinical delivery fees were. There was one physician who charged up to 150 yuan for ten days of clinical services.[45] Yet most female medical workers were midwives who worked hard but were paid significantly less than physicians. Li Meili, for example, was trained in a hospital for three years, later becoming an assistant doctor, and then a formal one, dealing with everything related to delivering babies except surgery. She earned 20–30 yuan per month, or 40–50 yuan when business was good. She said she could support her single life pretty well but not a family.[46] So those like her would be unable to enjoy the comfortable middle- and upper-class lives of those like Zhang Xiangwen, Wang Shuzhen, or Chen Bangdian described above.

Marriage or Career—a Dilemma

The marital status of female medical workers also directly influenced their economic situation. Generally speaking, those who were married had married male physicians, so their own income was supplementary: "Those who got married are supported financially by their husbands. If they are doing well in the medical business, they can earn extra income through it; if not, they don't have to worry about it."[47] A marriage between two licensed physicians could help the couple step into the upper levels of Shanghai society, as their incomes were combined. The lives of single female physicians who leased clinic space by themselves and put out a sign were not easy, and they worked hard to maintain themselves.[48] An example is Dr. Su Zengxiang, who earned her degree from Germany. As was the case with some other female physicians, her marriage ended in divorce. She had her own clinic, which had only basic amenities due to a lack of funding. But it was said of her that "her exuberance and zeal compensate[d] for the inadequacy of the facility." When asked about her rare leisure time, she said she liked to travel, or watch a movie; however, as a pediatrician she always had too many children to care for. With an extremely busy schedule taking care of inpatients and outpatients, even in her scheduled spare time she could be found providing medical service to patients.[49] According to the reports in *Shenbao*, some female physicians spent part of their weekday practicing Western medicine as charity. Take female physician Zhu Tongzhang, for example; she offered medical services and medicine to patients between nine and ten o'clock every Tuesday, Thursday, and Saturday morning, charging only ten cents for a registration fee.[50] As another female physician explained, "Since Western Medicine spread into China, it gradually won people's trust. At the moment it is usually hard to keep a family going. So if someone in the family is sick, the financial situation is even worse. Therefore we offer a cheap medical service by charging 50 cents for outpatients between 9:00–12:00 a.m. and 1 yuan for home visits between 2:00–9:00 p.m."[51]

What tended to impress people most was that many female physicians chose to remain single. Famous examples of single woman doctors include Lin Qiaozhi and Yang Chongrui from Beijing, Shi Meiyu, Zhang Zhujun, Huang Qiongxian, and Ge Chenghui from Shanghai. Although some remained single, for others late marriage was also common. In the small sample in the 1948 Police Bureau survey, all female physicians between twenty-seven and thirty years old were listed as "having no dependents," or as "living alone." The famous physician Zhang Xiangwen did not marry until she was fifty-two years old, in 1948. Professional women at this time were confronted with a series of contradictions between work and personal life, forcing them to make choices between career and marriage, individual and societal goals, and tradition and modernity: "Any professional woman interviewed will tell you a miserable story of herself and express a series of hopes. Through these stories you can see their courage and determination against the old ethics to step into the society, their resolute and unbending will to face the contempt, ridicule and temptation, and their hearts to seek for progress and serve the community and people."[52] Female physicians, like other educated women, tended to be unmarried because of the practical problem that if they got married and had children, they would be generally unable to go out to work. Some employers even stipulated that married women should resign from their job to avoid the subsequent low productivity and possible losses to the organization when women asked for maternity and sick leave. Therefore, once women got married, their other personal merits were overlooked. One magazine writer opined about this practice: "this is a sheer menace and insult to the married women, and an indirect way to keep women from marriage. Should women sacrifice their youth to profession? Should they marry their profession?"[53] Chen Yongsheng, an educator, affirmed the incompatibility of profession and family for the middle class when she said, "Once women got married, nobody wanted to hire them. . . . Women had no social status at all. That's why I have remained single."[54] These kinds of restrictions on the life choices of women were common throughout middle-class and professional workplaces.

Yet female physicians did face hardships in their lives and in their careers that were specific to the medical profession. According to one survey, the average age of the students in medical colleges and universities was twenty-three, with the oldest being forty. After a few years of study, they generally started their medical practice at the age of thirty, with thirty-five considered the "golden period" for doing so.[55] This "golden period" for opening a practice was a reason for some female physicians to forgo marriage. If a woman began her medical studies at twenty-three and became a physician at twenty-eight, then married that year or later, she would be occupied by professional obligations during her prime childbearing years. If she were to emphasize marriage and childbearing, she may have to give up her career. This raises the question, was the career in medicine still worth the effort with this cost in time, money, and even the sacrifice of marriage and companionship?

Medical careers were arduous; almost every physician had unpleasant experiences. The high tuition fees were another factor that challenged female medical students, with some families incapable or unwilling to pay the cost of their daughter's tuition. In a patriarchal society, after graduation, male physicians could more easily get financial support from their families to start their medical business; for female physicians, even getting tuition to finish college study was not that easy. Starting a clinic required a substantial sum of money for leases and nurses' salaries, so new female physicians tended to see their best option as finding employment with a major hospital. Yet such employment meant greater pressure and less control over one's own schedule. Take Peking Union Medical College (PUMC) Hospital for example; if female physicians chose the big departments like internal medicine, surgery, or obstetrics and gynecology, they could expect not to marry. What's more, the hospital never sent married woman physicians to study abroad, because married woman physicians were supposed to allow their husbands to make decisions on their future career. In fact, very few women were ever admitted to study at PUMC. Those who had opportunities to study there at all wanted to realize their liberation as new women for themselves, so almost all these woman physicians remained single all their life. Ye Gongshao, who did marry, was an exceptional case in this respect. There were similar rules for nurses: they had to live and eat in their dormitories; if they wanted to get married, they first had to quit their job.[56] Working in the major hospitals, they faced the competition of their male peers, who had all the advantages of a patriarchal society. Remaining single or marrying late became the "natural" choices for women under such conditions.

Another factor affecting the rate at which female physicians married was the particular culture of learning and belief in which they found themselves.

It was Western missionaries who first started modern women's medical education in order to promote self-esteem and independence for women, and Christianity continued to be an important influence for many female physicians throughout the Republican period. Until the early decades of the twentieth century, while being trained to be a "dutiful wife and loving mother," women received education in order to serve society. It was in these Christian missionary schools, which were deeply influenced by contemporary Western cultural trends, that professional women unable to identify themselves with traditional notions of dutiful wife and mother were able to find a home.[57] Jinling Women's University and Huanan Women's University both trained a great number of professional women, most of whom remained single all their lives. These female physicians reflected the features characteristic of women in an era of drastic changes in gender roles. However, this does not mean that these women—whether Lin Qiaozhi and Yang Chongrui at PUMC hospital or Shi Meiyu and Zhang Zhujun in Shanghai—neglected families and children per se; all devoted their attention to the life and health of women and children in their medical practices.

When the issue of whether or not women who practiced medicine could marry arose, it led to heated public debate, although it was primarily of concern to female physicians themselves. It is worth comparing the experience of women entering the field of traditional medicine at the same time—a relatively new phenomenon. For example, *China's Female Physicians*, a magazine run by and for female doctors of traditional medicine, published an article titled "Should Women Who Practice Medicine Marry?"[58] In the following quote, we see the author providing multiple reasons to answer the question in the negative:

> A physician takes full responsibility for the life of the patient, so if you want to be a physician, you have to sacrifice your marriage; if you want marriage, then you are not qualified to be a physician. You cannot keep a balance between the two. A mother who has quite a few children cannot be at the same time a physician taking good care of the patients. If she is devoted to her profession and neglects her children, then she is not by any means a loving mother. Likewise, if she loves her children and neglects her duty as a physician, then where is her conscience? Both these situations are unsatisfactory. If this was the case, shouldn't all the girls who practiced medicine be unmarried?

Yet there is some room for ambiguity in the question, and the writer does not respond clearly for all readers, but instead makes her response specific to herself: "Now that I am a physician, I want to get some achievements in my career after all."[59] Apparently, she intends to forsake the desire to start her own family.

Restricted by the old conventions, women tended to shape themselves by the criteria of the male-dominant society. First of all, as a physician of traditional Chinese medicine, the author's negative attitude toward marriage is vividly expressed in the article. To be a responsible professional, the physician should "take full responsibility of the lives of her patients," and do whatever possible to help them. She should also be devoted to both her children and career; and because of her concern about marriage, she must be concerned with losing the balance between the two. This doctor's resolution to pursue her career is clear in her words, yet such attitudes were not exclusive to female physicians. Some female intellectuals thought being single was necessary to pursue their chosen career, if still abnormal. In a survey from the Republican era of sixty young women on marriage, some were in favor of being single just because they thought a life partner was hard to find, but they still thought remaining single was unusual.[60] Second, as a physician of Chinese medicine, the author thought it her duty to promote traditional medicine and compete with Western medicine. Yet her acceptance of the inferiority of the female physician is apparent. She considered men to have strong willpower and emotion and to be less affected by marriage, while professional women tended to be depressed after marriage, and often quit their jobs after getting married. Zhou Muying, a Western-trained medical doctor, once said that the responsibilities of being a wife and mother were incompatible with the responsibilities of being a doctor less because of any absolute gender roles than simply because the social structures didn't support doing so.[61]

Another article, "After Reading That Women Who Practice Medicine Cannot Marry," responded to the first and was also written by a female physician of Chinese medicine. This author approved of some female doctors not marrying.[62] She acknowledged that the choice to marry was a difficult decision for a medical woman to make: on the one hand, getting married fulfilled the expectation of one's parents and was the socially approved purpose of a woman's life. But for a modern woman, on the other hand, going to school, having one's own career *and* getting married and having children were all natural steps in life, and missing any of the three would leave one unfulfilled. The author argued that it was preferable for woman physicians to not marry, because evidence had proven that once a woman gets married, she becomes weak and depressed in spirit, temper, and body. Consequently, her attitude toward her profession would undergo a change compared with that before her marriage. Therefore, those woman physicians who refused marriage might be considered to be "martyring [their] individual freedom to fight for the freedom of the masses," and this sacrifice would be witnessed by the people and thus allow them to "achieve the highest moral standards." This kind of moralistic reasoning was common in the writings of female physicians wrestling with the conundrum of work-life balance.

Professional women thus experienced a paradox: at the same time their profession brought them both liberation and restriction. If getting married was "life's final destination," then giving it up must be painful. Among the well-educated of China at that time, there were many intellectual women who suffered from the pain caused by late or no marriage. Being single or marrying late each brought different challenges, so the average woman tended to conclude that being a professional was unpleasant. They returned to their traditional belief that being a housewife was their natural choice. In particular, those women who had to be professional under economic pressure pursued a career for a living only to find they had to sacrifice marriage as a result.

Whether or not to marry was a difficult enough question, but if a woman was to marry, she also faced the issue of what spouse to pick. Lu Tiying, a woman who studied Chinese medicine under her uncle, had gained much practical experience by watching him diagnosing and treating patients every day. When she was at an appropriate age for marriage, she was introduced to a clerk in a bank, and this experience made her "deeply afflicted as if a huge stone was pressing her heart." Her objections were three: that bankers were businessmen, and since businessmen succeeded only through scheming, they were not ideal husbands for a female physician; in addition, her mother was getting on in years, so she hoped that, in a year or two, she would be able to start her own medical business so as to live together with her younger brother and mother, and thereby "give her mother a better life in her declining years." Finally, according to her uncle's opinion (apparently she was happy to accept this opinion), she expected to marry another physician, because their goals would be compatible, their dispositions similar, and they would be able to learn from each other.[63] So her ideal husband should have similar interests and disposition, and they should have opportunities to learn from each other. For these reasons, she argued, a bank clerk would not make an ideal spouse.

Many professional women also shouldered the responsibility of financially supporting their families as the breadwinner, so the purpose of marriage was no longer simply to carry on the patrilineal family. In traditional patriarchal society, women had no economic status, and thus marriages were arranged by parents, who preferred a potential husband from a wealthy family, to ensure a secure life for their daughter after marriage. But women who were educated could decide to marry late or not at all. They had economic independence and did not need to depend on men, although getting married was not only for individual happiness but also to fulfill a sense of responsibility to one's family and society more generally. The dilemma that professional women faced in weighing family and career were not easily resolved.

Although women's liberation became a movement during the Republican period, the new-style woman still had to struggle to maintain proper roles in the public sphere, and this was also the case in regard to marriage. Men had always benefited from marriage, and they continued to benefit in the Republican era. Women physicians tended to marry late and, if they did marry, had fewer children. Their high professional and social status was a challenge to the self-confidence of men, and had the effect of making it difficult for these women to marry. A marriage survey conducted in the Republican period revealed that most male college graduates preferred to choose a spouse with only a high school education. Of the males surveyed, 85 percent would accept a spouse with less education, and 91 percent hoped to marry a woman younger than them. In other words, the majority of men expected their spouses to be less educated so as to put themselves in a dominant position in the marriage—that is, the apparent goal of many men was to gain a subservient wife.[64] Women, in contrast, preferred to marry a man with at least an equal or a higher social status, which greatly limited the choices of women who themselves had a high professional status. Many female physicians, for the sake of their careers, paid a price such as in late marriage, living alone, or divorce. This was the case for Dr. Ge Chenghui, who recalled that she had expected to marry; however, due to her professional status it was too difficult for her to find a suitable match, so she remained unmarried. The different criteria for finding a suitable spouse and the overloaded gender role expectations for all women in family life made it far more difficult to be a physician as a female than as a male.

A Feminist Perspective on Female Doctors

Female physicians argued that women's medical education was an integral part of the feminist movement in modern China. A large part of this was the role that obstetrics was to play in "saving the nation" from the scourge of high infant and maternal mortality, so advancing the health of mothers and infants became part of the discourse of modernization. An article in the *Guanghua Medical Journal* in 1934 made an impassioned plea to continue and expand the role of female medical education not just for future physicians, but for all women:

> If we want women to stand on their own feet, we must start with women's education. If women do not study and become self-sufficient, we are finished. And if we seek to study in order to stand on our own feet, we must begin with medical studies. . . . Without the development of women's education, there is no way to save women from ignorance! If women's medical studies do not develop, it will be impossible to keep women from sinking further into the cesspool of ignorance! If we are foolish and also sick, then what pretext can we use to apply ourselves to improve society? Therefore, if we want to improve society, then women all need common medical knowledge.[65]

Female doctors were arguably the most highly educated group of female professionals, and so they were more likely to appeal for equal rights for men and women. Furthermore, female doctors' acquaintance with their patients gave them insights into their private lives, enabling them to understand that the afflictions of their patients were not merely medical. Like their patients, female physicians also suffered from the constraints placed on them by a patriarchal society, so it should not be surprising why the ranks of advocates of women's rights were never short of female doctors.

In a patriarchal society such as that of Republican China, the position of professional women was very difficult, but compared to other females in the workforce, woman physicians who freely practiced their professions were more likely to enjoy independence, self-esteem, and pride. In comparison, companies recruiting female employees considered physical appearance first, rather than the knowledge and accomplishments of the applicants. Female employees also needed to defend their positions, sometimes suffering unwarranted verbal abuse from male superiors and coworkers.[66] Some female doctors like Qiu Yinwu were able to speak out about the discrepancy between woman physicians and other professional women: "The female professions in China in recent years have made considerable progress. However, the female employees in stores and companies have a purely ornamental function. In addition, the female employees in government offices are merely used by high officials and nobles as a "red vase" for decoration. In such a patriarchal society, the dignity of the professional women is negatively impacted by the social environment and depreciated by men."[67] In Qiu Yinwu's experience, some male physicians were addicted to opium and gambling with mah-jongg. According to Qiu, when these physicians of Chinese medicine were invited to make a house call to treat a patient, the patient's family members had to prepare an opium tray and mah-jongg table beforehand for the physicians. In contrast, Qiu wrote, self-employed female physicians had far greater respect and self-esteem than such men and than female shop clerks forced to please their male superiors: "We do not need to bear the exploitation of higher officials and bosses, and we do not need to lower ourselves to please others. This is the primary characteristic of female physicians. People should have self-respect, and self-respect should be the lofty distinction of the people. When we, as female physicians, are treating our patients, we must only focus on diagnosis and treatment, and not on meaningless sociality."[68]

The previously mentioned Police Bureau survey describes doctors as usually so busy that they rarely went out for relaxation, and thus many doctors were not able to be sociable. Yet some major hospitals stipulated that doctors socialize, and the people they would interact with the most were their patients. So if doctors desired, they could cast a wide social net since their patients came from diverse backgrounds. Doctors of Western medicine tended to offer an exclusive service just for wealthy elites due to there being a limited number of well-educated doctors, and the high cost and great reputation of Western medicine.[69] Doctors had their own specific social network related to their fame. This was true of female doctors of Western medicine as well.

Dr. Zhang Zhujun has attracted significant attention from historians. She played a great role in medical fields beyond just education, and she also was active in the feminist movement and in charities such as wartime medical aid and the establishment of Red Cross. She was revered as much for her personal style and courage as for her medical abilities. She dressed in a Western style and exhibited dauntless strength to the degree that she became almost a mythical figure, which can make it difficult to distinguish between fact and fiction in accounts of her life. Born in an official's family in Guangzhou in 1876, she studied medicine at the Nanhua Medical School affiliated with Boji Hospital. She became China's first female doctor to graduate from a domestic medical school. While still in Guangzhou, she established a school for girls, a hospital, and also a church that became the center of social gatherings. She hosted parties at which influential figures were brought together to exchange ideas. A typical gathering might include young military officers, newspaper editors, scholars, and other socially prominent individuals. Zhang felt strongly that women were the equals of men and should be treated as such in the social, political, and professional realms. She gave lectures expressing her ideas as well as conversing with them.

When cholera broke out in Guangzhou in 1902, and corpses littered the streets, Dr. Zhang raised significant funds for supplies, such as clean water, to be delivered to the city. When the Russo-Japanese War started, and Governor Cen Chunxuan of Guangdong and Guangxi made a public request for doctors' assistance at the battle zone, Dr. Zhang led a medical team thousands of miles north to Lüshun (Port Arthur) to treat the wounded. Then a few years later during the revolution of 1911, she formed the Chinese Red Cross in Shanghai. Working in association with the diplomat Wu Tingfang, in three days she was able to enlist between 123 and 300 members (depending on the source) and raise a large amount of money.[70] Remarkably, 54 of the 123 recruited to the original Red Cross were female. None of these volunteers were paid, and they were required to bring their own supplies as well, demonstrating their dedication to the cause and Zhang's leadership among them. Under her leadership, they regarded national service as their personal duty.[71]

In Shanghai, Dr. Zhang had wide social communication with influential individuals. Wealthy merchant Silas Aaron Hardoon's wife became her adopted mother, and the famous wealthy businessman Li Pingshu became her adopted father. She occupied a very different social sphere than those who were quietly dedicated to their own medical practices, and she was able to use her social connections to benefit her medical practice, as well as the public causes she supported. In collaboration with Li, Zhang opened Zhongxi Women's Medical School in 1904, where both Chinese and Western medicine were taught. It was the first women's school founded by Chinese. Zhang Zhujun was influential beyond the medical world, and was even compared to one of Republican China's most prominent intellectuals, Liang Qichao.

Women actually found it difficult to avoid taking the standards of the male-dominated society as their own. Independent women struggled for women's rights, even to the point of taking men as their model, in order to show their break from the traditional female temperament. Lu Lihua, a pioneer in promoting physical education for girls in Shanghai, commented that she herself possessed masculine characteristics and did not fear dealing with men. In her eyes, Zhang Zhujun's younger sister Zhang Xiangwen, also a physician, was a "manly type."[72] Zhang Zhujun, who liked to wear Western-style attire, was deemed to be a "rebellious" woman for her manner of speech and action. She was such an active advocate of gender equality that there were rumors that men with both a wife and many concubines were afraid of her; even bandits on the road did not dare to come close to her. Rather, a simple mention of her name would induce them all to bow to her and retreat. This legend of greatly exaggerated masculinity about Zhang Zhujun wasn't intended to be complimentary; rather, it was simply a socio-psychological prejudice: a public woman was not a woman at all.

Women who hoped to succeed as physicians needed to be talented, productive, strong, and ambitious, but these were not regarded as desirable feminine qualities. Such a woman would be criticized for her lack of attention to her proper role in the family. Lu Lihua described the challenges a woman faced in a patriarchal society this way: "If a woman wants to achieve something in this male-dominated world, she has to seek support from men of high standing. Yet, a woman, once successful, would invariably be defamed, as people may think that her success is only the result of her womanly charms rather than a result of her efforts."[73] Lu viewed Dr. Zhang Xiangwen as truly a woman worthy of respect, given her devotion to her career and long-suffering in the face of sexist gossip: "She was truly devoted to her career, and she also suffered the loss of her reputation. Many women gossiped about her, saying she was indecent and always meeting the head of some bureau." Zhang Zhujun also suffered this kind of social opprobrium as "everyone was constantly gossiping about her relationship with so-and-so." Lu remarked that this "was very ugly to hear" and an "abuse of women."

Women were caught in a conundrum: because most women did not dare challenge social propriety, only a few worked outside the home; and those who did work outside the home were considered women of loose morals, and the more a woman achieved, the worse she was regarded. This kind of social logic led to women being unwilling to work outside the home and to career women abandoning their careers.[74] Lu Lihua recalled some women's groups that consisted of female doctors, school principals, and teachers. They were not large groups, some having only twenty or so members, sometimes forty. All their efforts went toward constructing a new constitutional government in which women could have a voice. In the years before the Nationalist government nominally unified the country in 1928, their slogan was "Down with the warlords, Achieve gender equality."[75]

Yet as the overall number of Western-trained female physicians increased, so too did the number of female traditional physicians. One female Chinese doctor wrote that "it was like a dream" that "we just woke up from," observing that since the establishment of the Republic of China "women have a higher and higher social status" and that now "many women are well-educated."[76] As women gained a more respectable position in the public sphere, the signboards promoting their medical practices became more prominent.

Yet the impact on Chinese traditional medicine of the arrival of Western medicine was felt as deeply among the growing number of female doctors as among their more prominent male counterparts. Facing a great challenge in the success of Western medicine, some Chinese female doctors advocated that they should begin to participate in the public sphere alongside male traditional physicians to increase their standing in the medical field. This was particularly true of those female doctors who worked to help one another and take on the responsibility of developing traditional medicine and improving the social status of female doctors. Together these women founded the Chinese Women's Doctor Association and published the monthly medical magazine *China's Female Physicians* (*Zhongguo nüyi*). Those female doctors themselves provided financing for this endeavor and did not accept any support—even in 1940 in the midst of inflation—to show their determination to promote traditional medicine by their diligence and sacrifice. Zhang Zanchen, a prominent male practitioner of Chinese traditional medicine and the sponsor of the important journal *Annals of the Medical World* (*Yijie Chunqiu*), showed great respect to female practitioners when he said that in the ten years he had sponsored *Yijie Chunqiu*, he had rarely singled out any doctor for comment but nevertheless felt compelled to praise the efforts of these women. Dr. Zhang Jingxia and Qian Baohua wrote an article to answer why they formed the Chinese Women's Doctor Association, in which they primarily argued for equality with their male counterparts:

> To pursue women's equality with men, we have to attain equal status first; equal status is dependent on whether we have completed our education. A female doctor is self-employed, which can be the broad road of seeking equality. Medical education is a good way for us to seek freedom. We should be engaged in carrying forward the traditional essence of medicine like male doctors do, and to fight for equality. We propose an ideological doctrine of female doctors, to promote mutual spirit, and improve the status of female doctors.[77]

These prominent females who were in the Chinese Women's Doctor Association were generally from influential medical families, although some of them graduated from Chinese medical schools, a new trend in Chinese traditional medicine. Those doctors made contributions to the association and to the publication of its magazine. They managed all aspects of the operation without relying on men, building their friendship through their engagement with medical professionalization and equality for women.[78] Yet we see a particular pattern in the growth of the number of female practitioners of Chinese medicine. There was a significant increase in the number of women practicing even as traditional medicine declined and Western medicine expanded its influence in Chinese society. Stimulated by Western medicine and encouraged by a feminist movement, those female physicians shouldered the responsibilities to promote Chinese traditional medicine and to advance the cause of women's rights.

Although the voices of these women were drowned out in the rolling tide of the Western trend, female practitioners of Chinese medicine made significant contributions to modern Chinese feminism. Chinese and Western medical practitioners coexsited in competition and conflict and existed in an identifiable hierarchy based on some combination of education, social status, and income. At the top of the hierarchy were the Western-style physicians with their formal MD degrees and prominent reputations, while traditional medical practitioners generally took a lower place for a variety of reasons, including their less formal educational accomplishments and the cultural disparagement of Chinese medicine in some progressive circles because of the influence of scientism—a blind faith in science as a panacea for social problems. Nevertheless, modern Shanghai, given its vast population at all social levels, saw growth in the number of Chinese female medical practitioners because it provided the most suitable environment for their success.

As the number of female pracitioners of Chinese medicine as well as Western-style female physicians steadily increased, similar pressures applied to both groups because they were not accepted as the equals of men. Society had preset ideas about gender differences—namely, that women were by nature enthusiastic, genial, empathic, and patient, thus making them suited to fields such as obstetrics, gynecology, pediatrics, and nursing. Yet to compete in a male-dominated profession, female medical workers also needed to be as talented, productive, strong, and ambitious as any man. But although they made significant contributions in their "natural" field working with women and children, women's overall role as physicians was limited. As Li Shenglan describes in the following chapter, nursing increasingly became the medical career of choice for women, even though modern nursing, too, began as a male profession. There was a rapid growth of nursing schools oriented toward women, while male medical workers were expected to become physicians. Male physicians were regarded as representing rationality and authority in medicine, while females took on the work of assisting male physicians and caring for women and children. Men were experts representing the prominent medical associations, they were medical school professors, they were verifiers of medical qualifications, and makers of health policy. In the Republican period, merely to move into the public sphere to become a physician was a radical choice for a woman and involved many sacrifices. So rather than challenging men in most medical fields, women gravitated toward those areas of specialization that patriarchal Chinese society considered "natural"; they were careful not to be seen as impinging upon the field of male-centered medical sovereignty; women could become doctors for women, allowing men to be physicians for men. Suffering a variety of career obstacles while pursuing high occupational status, women fought to expand their role in medicine and struggled to gain equality in a male-dominated profession.

Notes

1. Xiaolian He, "The Social Status of Western Medical Doctors in Modern Shanghai," *Social Science* (Shanghai) 8 (August 2009): 137; see also Xiaoqun Xu, *Chinese Professionals and the Republican State: The Rise of Professional Associations in Shanghai, 1912–1937* (Cambridge: Cambridge University Press, 2001).

2. Judith Lorber, *Women Physicians: Careers, Status, and Power* (London: Tavistock Publications, 1984), 23; M. R. Walsh, *Doctors Wanted: No Women Need Apply: Sexual Barriers in the Medical Profession, 1835–1975* (New Haven, CT: Yale University Press, 1977), 213.

3. Charlotte Furth, *A Flourishing Yin: Gender in China's Medical History, 960–1665* (Berkeley: University of California Press, 1999): 266–300.

4. Yi-Li Wu, *Reproducing Women: Medicine, Metaphor, and Childbirth in Late Imperial China* (Berkeley: University of California Press, 2010): 181.

5. Sean Hsiang-lin Lei, *Neither Donkey nor Horse: Medicine in the Struggle over China's Modernity* (Chicago: University of Chicago Press, 2014), 121–40; Bridie Andrews, *The Making of Modern Chinese Medicine, 1850–1960* (Vancouver: University of British Columbia Press, 2014), 25–50.

6. According to the *Shanghai Business Directory*, in 1922 there were 21 female Western medical doctors, primarily specializing in obstetrics or pediatrics, concurrent with other fields. There were 4 Chinese medical physicians divided among specializations in acupuncture, pediatrics, ophthalmology, and obstetrics. In 1925, among nearly 200 Chinese medical doctors, there were only 3 women. There were 146 Western medical physicians, and of that number, 20 were women, excluding foreign physicians.

7. Shanghai shi zhengxie wenshi ziliao weiyuanhui (Shanghai Political Consultative Conference Oral Historical Committee), *An Orthopedic Specialist: Ni BaoChun* (Shanghai: Wenshi Ziliao Xuanji, 2007), 3.

8. Lorber, *Women Physicians*, 25.

9. Shanghai Medical Association, *Medical News*, no. 2 (1947): 20–22.

10. "Shanghai Medical Facilities Survey," *Shanghai Health* 4 (1947): 16. The survey shows that there were 685 physicians who opened practices, and among them 621 were men, 64 were female, predominantly forty-nine to fifty years old. The survey was conducted by the Ministry of Health Central Experimental Institute in conjunction with the Shanghai Municipal Health Bureau regarding Western medicine. At that time, Shanghai city was divided into thirty districts—of which nineteen urban districts, where medical institutions were concentrated, were investigated. The survey population of 3,142,661 accounted for a little less than 73 percent of the city's population, it was thus representative of most medical facilities in the city.

11. An analysis of Shanghai's Western medical practitioners shows there were 1,998 Western medical practitioners at the beginning of 1950, B 242-1-452-21, Shanghai Archives.

12. Annals of Shanghai Women Editorial Committee, *Shanghai funv zhi* [Annals of Shanghai women] (Shanghai: Shanghai Academy of Social Sciences Press, 2000). According to the statistics in 1951, 2,190 Chinese traditional medical practitioners operated in Shanghai, of which only 150 were female, less than 7 percent of the total.

13. Wang Hsiu-yun, "Refusing Male Physicians: The Gender and Body Politics of Missionary Medicine in China, 1870s–1920s," *Bulletin of the Institute of Modern History, Academia Sinica* 59 (2008): 46.

14. Ibid.

15. "Female Doctors," *Church News* 48 (1869): 10.

16. Qiu Yinwu, "Women Learning Medicine Promotes New Life Movement," *Guanghua Medical Journal* 1 (1939): 13–14.

17. Lorber, *Women Physicians*, 2.

18. Connie Shemo, *The Chinese Medical Ministries of Kang Cheng and Shi Meiyu, 1872–1937: On a Cross-Cultural Frontier of Gender, Race, and Nation* (Bethlehem, PA: Lehigh University Press, 2011).

19. *Women's Monthly* [funü yuebao] 7 (1936): 28.

20. In 1926, *LiangYou Pictorial* illustrated that Huang YuHua, who graduated from Obstetric School in Shanxi Province and whose obstetric clinic was located in Shanghai, was "the most famous obstetrician in Shanghai for years."

21. "Shanghai Medical Facilities Survey," 18.

22. Huang Yingdai, "Female Obstetricians: An Examination of Shanghai's Professional Women's Life," *Shanghai Life* 4 (1939): 22.

23. Huangsha, Mengyankun, ed., *Shanghai funü zhi* (Shanghai: Shanghai Academy of Social Sciences Press, 2000), 394.

24. Zhang Mingdao, ed., *Shanghai Weisheng Zhi* (Shanghai: Shanghai Academy of Social Sciences Press, 1998), 465.

25. Wang Yugang, *An Overview of New Medical Profession: An Analysis of the Profession* (Shanghai: Shanghai Vocational Education Society, 1927), 3–5.

26. Gu Shouchun, "The Dark Side of the Maternity Hospitals in Shanghai," *GuangHua Medical Journal* 4 (1934): 28–31.

27. Andrews, *Making of Modern Chinese Medicine*, 25–26.

28. Lei, *Neither Donkey nor Horse*, 125.

29. "The Library of Shanghai Women's Medical School," Y8-1-8-16, Shanghai Archives.

30. Wang, *Overview of New Medical Profession*, 17.

31. Lorber, *Women Physicians*, 2.

32. Because of inflation, the prestigious doctors were requiring payment in bullion and dollars.

33. Interview with Mei Tsu-Lin on April 23, 2013, Ithaca, NY.

34. "Shanghai Renji Hospital Overview," B242-1-146-1, Shanghai Archives.

35. Ibid.

36. Xu, *Chinese Professionals*, 59.

37. Police Bureau special household registration survey, 1948, Q133-3-26, Shanghai Archives.

38. *Assistance of Gongji Hospital's Benefits and Plans* (Shanghai: Gongji Hospital, 1945), 248.

39. "The Roster of Shanghai Renji Hospital physicians registered for more than three years, 1952," B242-1-377-54, Shanghai Archives.

40. "Songshan Branch of Shanghai Police Bureau special household registration surveys," Q136-4-67, Shanghai Archives.

41. An analysis of Shanghai's Western Medical Practitioners, 1951, B242-1-452-21, Shanghai Archives.

42. Zhang Mingdao, ed., *Shanghai weisheng zhi* [Annals of Shanghai public health] (Shanghai: Shanghai Academy of Social Sciences Press, 1998), 593.

43. Huang, "Female Obstetricians," 22.

44. Chen Mingyuan, *The Intellectuals' Economic Life* (Shanghai: Wenhui Press, 2007), 156–57.

45. Huang, "Female Obstetricians," 22.

46. Li Meili, "A Female Doctor's Personal Story," *Linglong* (1936): 50–54.

47. Ibid.

48. Ibid.

49. Qing (pseudonym), "He Saved the Lives of Countless Children: Dr. Su Zhenxiang," *Nü Sheng* [Female student] 7 (1947): 12.

50. Advertisement in *Shenbao*, August 3, 1915.

51. Advertisement in *Shenbao*, May 14, 1920.

52. Yun (pseudonym), "The Problems of Women's Careers," *Zhiye Funü* [Professional Women] 1 (November 20, 1944): 4.

53. Tianming (pseudonym), "Women's Occupation and Marriage—When Hearing That the Postal Bureau Dismissed a Married Female Staff Member," *Career and Life* 1 (1939): 366.

54. Wang Zheng, *Women in the Chinese Enlightenment: Oral and Textual Histories* (Berkeley: University of California Press, 1999), 263.

55. "Private Tong De Medical School's Historical Facts," 75, Q249-1-1, Shanghai Archives.

56. Ou Ge, *Xiehe yishi* [Medical Affairs at Peking Union Medical College] (Beijing: Sanlian Book Co., 2007), 261.

57. Cheng Yu, "The Ideological Trend of Encouraging Women to Obtain Jobs and Formation of the Creed of Being a Good Wife and Virtuous Mother in the 20th Century," *Shilin* 6 (2005): 66.

58. Guo Ruilin, "Should Women Who Practice Medicine Marry?" *China's Female Physicians* 1 (1941): 6.

59. Ibid., 9.

60. Liang Yisheng, "A Survey of Sixty Girls in Marriage," in Li Wenhai, ed., *The Corpus of the Republican Social Survey* (Fuzhou: Fujian Education Press, 2005), 68.

61. Huang Weizhi, "How She Became So Famous—Interview with Doctor Zhou Muying," *Jindai Funü* [Modern Woman] 5 (1947): 14.

62. Anonymous, "After Reading That Women Who Practice Medicine Cannot Marry," *China's Female Physicians* 2 (1941): 17.

63. Lu Tiying, "If I Should Marry," *GuangHua Medical Journal* 2 (1934): 53.

64. Lou Zhaokui, "Marriage Survey," in Li Wenhai, ed., *The Corpus of the Republican Social Survey* (Fuzhou: Fujian Education Press, 2005), 68.

65. "The Importance of Promoting the Cause of Female Doctors," *GuangHua Medical Journal* 5 (1934).

66. Yang Gonghuai, "Female Staff in Shanghai," *Shanghai Shenghuo* [Shanghai lifestyle] 4 (1939): 21.

67. Qiu Yinwu, "The Proper Accomplishment of Modern Female Doctors," *Guanghua Medical Journal* 5 (1934): 13.

68. Ibid.

69. Pang Jingzhou, *An Aerial View of the Past Decade of Medicine in Shanghai* (Shanghai: Chinese Science Company, 1933), 45.

70. "Doctor Zhang Zhujun," *Jindai Funü* [Modern woman] 2 (1928): 8.

71. "The Inauguration of the Chinese Red Cross," *Shenbao* 10 (1911): 24.

72. Wang, *Women in the Chinese Enlightenment*, 165.

73. Ibid.

74. Ibid., 169.

75. Ibid.

76. Editorial foreword for inaugural issue, *China's Female Physicians* 4, no. 1 (1941): 1–8.

77. Qian Baohua and Zhang Jingxia, "Why We Female Doctors Founded the Women's Doctor Association," *China's Female Physicians* 5 (1941): 1.

78. Wang Shuoru, "Doctor Gao Jianru," *China's Female Physicians* 5 (1941): 13.

Part Three

The Spread of Biomedicine to Southwest China, 1937–1945

Chapter Six

A Social History of Wartime Nursing Training in Hunan, 1937–1945

LI SHENGLAN

Metamorphosis, the patriotic play written by Cao Yu in 1940 after the outbreak of the Second Sino-Japanese War, depicts the wartime transformations of a decadent hospital in the context of Japanese aggression. While revealing the Chinese bureaucracy's inefficiency and corruption, Cao Yu portrays how the Chinese medical profession changed during wartime. In the play, a group of nurses work at gunpoint with a doctor to serve civilians, soldiers, and the national cause. The nursing staff, a man and two women, are dressed indistinguishably in white uniforms—"a gown of the bottom-up design, with the logo of a red cross embroidered on the left arm and a white cap on the head"—and working with "white gauze and white utensils."[1]

This dramatic portrait of medical workers was based on China's actual wartime realities, and it raises a series of historical questions about how gender and power relations affected the professionalization of wartime nursing.[2] Given that white is associated with death and funerals in Chinese culture, why would nursing pioneers in China insist that these agents of healing wear white uniforms? More importantly, how did the war shape the experience of nurses? The prominence of nurses in this play is remarkable given the fact that foreign missionary nurses had only introduced the profession into China a few decades earlier. Before the rise of nursing, relatives and servants within the family held the primary responsibility of caring for the sick; a trained person to take care of the sick would strike Chinese as an alien concept. Confucian ethics stressed that respectable women should remain in the home, so a profession of attending strangers including men other than their husbands was "a breath-taking innovation." During the 1910s, when the American nurse Nina Gage launched a pioneering nursing school in

Hunan, she found it necessary to coin a Chinese term for "nurse." Gage and her colleagues selected *hushi*, which might be translated as "guard scholars."[3] In contrast to nursing as a "women's profession" in the Anglo-American world during the early twentieth century, the enrollment of nursing students in China did not start as gender-exclusive.[4] In fact, for Gage, boys seemed to be more promising nursing students, as "too many problems complicated the lives of the girls."[5] By the 1920s, the Nurses' Association of China grew more influential and a number of prominent nursing schools were established across the country. Soon public health training became more important in nursing education, and thus was subjected to the Nationalist and Communist Parties' agendas during wartime.[6]

An examination of wartime nursing training in Hunan fleshes out our understanding of the transformations of medicine and gender roles during the war, and also illuminates some of the everyday realities of biomedicine. Seminal studies have accentuated the pioneering roles of missionaries and foreign philanthropy in the development of Western medicine in China, providing pertinent context regarding the missionaries that introduced modern nursing to China.[7] Scholars such as Sonya Grypma, Connie Shemo, David Kang, and Kaiyi Chen address the topic from perspectives either of missionaries or of Sino-US relations.[8] John Watt's pioneering overview of wartime medicine has shifted the focus to Chinese actors, and Chun-yen Chou's recent study on wartime first aid examines the development of modern nursing on the battlefield.[9] These studies offer important insights into changes in Chinese nursing, yet the implications of modern nursing in the daily lives of nurses themselves remain to be analyzed. Since Ruth Rogaski's groundbreaking work that highlights hygiene's essential role in modernity, others have expertly interrogated the interplay between medicine, public health, and modernity.[10] While these works provide the foundation for this study, its goal is to look deeper than their focus on the discourse of elite reformers, which limits our understanding of how these ideas affected the lives of ordinary people.

This study also builds on emerging trends in women's history and war studies that have showcased everyday realities as a critical approach to dissect social changes. By centralizing everyday lives, scholars such as Danke Li, Gail Hershatter, Chien-Ming Yu, and Joan Judge illuminate women's agency at different stages of Chinese social history.[11] Similarly, research on professional women by scholars such as Emily Honig, Ling-ling Lien, Hui-chi Hsu, and Helen Schneider collectively address the shifting gendered social norms in Republican China.[12] Other recent studies on war history have extended the scope of inquiry with more attention to social and cultural dimensions to examine wartime medicine and public health, or to focus on certain social groups, such as refugees, workers, students, or soldiers. They have greatly enriched our understanding of wartime society, and several other authors in this volume are contributing to expanding this knowledge.[13] This chapter further advances the field by exploring the significance of nursing in relation to wartime gendered social dynamics.

Placing local nursing training in the context of the Second Sino-Japanese War, this study investigates the ways in which historical contingencies relocated resources and reshaped lives at transitional moments. By analyzing nursing training as a gendered practice, I hope to illuminate the agency of nursing students and Chinese women—the active yet largely neglected actors in the history of medicine during the World War II period. While existing scholarship reveals that cultural imperialism tainted the processes of transplanting biomedicine into China, I focus on critical transformations uncovered by the experiences of nurses.[14] By examining this history primarily from the perspective of nurses themselves, this study moves beyond the framework of cultural imperialism and focuses instead on the gender dynamics and daily politics inherent in biomedical development in China.

The Hunan-Yale Nursing School, known as Hsiangya (Xiangya) for short, offers a case study to interrogate the significance of nurses' wartime professional experiences in modern China.[15] Established in 1913 by Nina Gage and the Yale-in-China Association, the wartime Hsiangya, located in central-south China, remained functional and trained a number of female students despite circumstances of war. Similar to the Nursing School of the Peking Union Medical College, also known as Xiehe, supported by the Rockefeller Foundation, Hsiangya represented a prominent nursing program that adapted an American model. Keeping English as its instructional language, the wartime Xiehe maintained an elite approach through maintaining the highest admission standards in the country and offering training that sought to measure up to international criteria and cultivate Chinese nursing leaders.[16] In comparison, wartime Hsiangya exemplified a more common pattern of negotiating and compromising with local conditions, such as adopting translated textbooks and using Chinese language in both classrooms and wards. Hsiangya accommodated a diverse student body, unlike the majority of students at Xiehe who came from affluent or intellectual backgrounds. Some Hsiangya students were from wealthy families, drawn into nursing by their parents' expectations or their own interests, but a large portion of students endured poverty and relied on the professional training to make a living. Some grew up in missionary orphanages, and several escaped from war zones or transferred from suspended programs.[17] In this sense, wartime Hsiangya provides a crucial microcosm to probe into quotidian experiences of adapting and practicing nursing and biomedical knowledge driven by the war. Through this account of Hsiangya's tenacity under wartime pressure, we see how the atrocities of war brought trauma to the land and the people, but also induced a redefining moment for nursing. The contingencies of war contributed to the mobilization of nursing students, the formation of a nursing consciousness, the reshaping of gender dynamics in the medical sphere—all under the influence of surging patriotic propaganda. Subject to wartime nationalism, nursing students also gained further legitimation by fulfilling the government's agenda in public health and midwifery.

Nursing Refugees and Services

The circumstances of the Second Sino-Japanese War imposed critical tests for institutions of higher education to survive, relocate, and operate. Considering educational institutions to be centers of cultural movements and political resistance, the Japanese army launched extensive attacks against Chinese campuses, in particular institutes of higher education. Threatened by the flames of war, one-fifth of colleges and universities consolidated or closed within one year. The schools in Japanese-occupied areas either chose to close temporarily, or moved to "Free China."[18] By 1937, nationwide at least 143 nursing schools were running and facing increasing challenges to survive.[19] While nursing programs of smaller scale had to close or merge with others, more resourceful ones joined refugees in retreating to interior regions. For example, the National Central Nursing School of Nanjing evacuated to Guizhou and reopened in 1938; Xiehe evacuated to Sichuan in 1943.[20] In the case of Hunan, while several missionary nursing programs struggled to function during the early stage of the war, Hsiangya was the only school in the province that managed to systematically evacuate and continue operating throughout wartime. The period of turmoil was disastrous for nursing training; however, Hsiangya's survival exemplified the ways in which the experience of war brought nursing to the fore.

Supported by the Yale-in-China Association, Hsiangya managed to maintain regular recruitment and training for a year after the outbreak of war with Japan in 1937. Hsiangya continued its training programs because of the belief that China was undefeatable and the hope that the Japanese army would consider the school neutral because of its American connections.[21] The curriculum continued to be as strict as it had been before the war under wartime conditions. Huang Junyuan, a student nurse who enrolled in 1934, recalled that the nursing curriculum took three and a half years to finish with both theoretical and practical courses. Since most students entered the program after graduating from middle school, they had to continue studying basic subjects, including Chinese, anatomy, biology, chemistry, arithmetic, and practical nursing for the first year. During the second year, students started learning more specialized subjects, such as materia medica, dietetics, ethics for nurses, and introductions to caring for patients with various diseases and specific medical cases. For juniors, the school offered courses on public health and lectures on medicine, surgery, and ethics. Students received a half-year's training in midwifery after the third year. For technical training, nursing students interned in the wards from eight to nine hours a day starting in the second year. The school provided students with accommodations, stipends, and three weeks of vacation each year. However, any additional absences were not permitted except for extreme cases. If sick, pupils needed to catch up with studies and complete work after they recovered. According to Huang Junyuan, her graduation was delayed a few days to make up for her sick leave during the course of study.[22]

Besides the professional training, air-raid drills became a daily routine for nurses. Nursing students and almost everyone had to be ready for *Pao jingbao* (running for safety when the air-raid siren rang) at any minute during the war years. For some students, such experiences, though nerve-racking, were somewhat entertaining at first. One student recounted that the basement of the Hsiangya Hospital was the safest place in the area. The *Jingbao* (air-raid siren) sometimes went off in the middle of the night and caused chaos. Some students ran to the basement without their glasses on and could only guess peers by their accents; some realized that they were wearing someone else's pants when they tried to reach into a pocket for a handkerchief; some sprained their ankles because they put their shoes on the wrong feet. As the war dragged on, the siren and the accompanying desperation turned into real nightmares for students and faculty. Nurses, doctors, patients, and nearby residents who were all packed underground could barely breathe; many wept out of fear and uncertainty.[23]

A more disheartening moment came when the city of Changsha was abandoned and largely destroyed by the Nationalist government. In November 1938, falsely believing that the Japanese army was approaching, panicked government officials informed citizens to leave and ordered soldiers to set fire to Changsha so as to leave "an empty city [and a] piece of scorched earth" for the arriving Japanese troops, rather than attempt to defend the city. After the fall of Hankou, Chiang Kai-shek (Jiang Jieshi) quoted the Chinese proverb that it was "better to be broken jade than a whole tile," to explain the rationale of the Nationalists' "scorched earth" policy.[24] In addition, as historians Keith Schoppa and Paul Russell suggest, ill-informed rumors tended to be "the *lingua franca* of the war" expressing the overall anxiety and uncertainty caused by the psychological terror of bombings and invasion.[25] Yet wartime also forced people to be resourceful when pressed. Aware of the scorched-earth policy, administrators of smaller nursing schools in Hunan dissolved their programs or merged with others. With support from the Yale-in-China Association, Hsiangya merged with the Changsha Union Hospital's nursing school and evacuated the new joint program to safe ground.

After the Nationalist government's self-inflicted fire in Changsha in the face of the arrival of Japanese troops, Hsiangya was broken into various parts. The nursing program was divided in far-flung locations, yet nevertheless played a significant role in the war effort. The Hsiangya Hospital was left to function in Changsha on a much reduced scale, while the majority of the nursing school moved to Yuanling in western Hunan by 1940. A group of junior nursing students mobilized to Guiyang in the neighboring province along with the medical school. Meanwhile, most senior students were scattered in the hospitals in Changsha, various towns of Hunan, and the war-time capital of Chongqing for internships. After students, faculty and their families, equipment, and baggage arrived in Guiyang, the people of Hsiangya sheltered in an old temple hidden on a wooded mountain slope. There they found conditions to be difficult; they "slept on the floor and the rats raced over them in the darkness and the fleas didn't wait for the darkness." In Yuanling, students and faculty helped build a primitive classroom building with an auditorium, combined with wards and operating rooms, a library with a study hall, and dormitories. In these simple facilities there was a dearth of sanitary necessities, and unidentified insects could be seen scampering across the floors. Despite the distress about living and working conditions, the very fact of the survival of the nursing school boosted students' morale, according to a faculty member. A nursing student supported this interpretation saying, "It would be easy to go on recounting the miseries of the early months after evacuation, yet that is changed now. We still have many hardships, but we have our own campus."[26] While accommodating its own students and faculty, Hsiangya also accepted and quartered refugees from other nursing programs that had to suspend operations due to warfare.[27]

As a group, Hsiangya students performed a key role in addressing war-time needs. A few senior nursing students joined relief units after the school dissolved.[28] Later on, the remaining nursing branch in Changsha served as a camp for civilians desperate when the Japanese army reached the city. Refugees quickly crowded the hospital, assuming American property to be a sanctuary from the onslaught of the Japanese attack. For overwhelmed nurses and doctors, an average day consisted of caring for fifty inpatients, a hundred outpatients, and conducting five or six operations. Medical staff of the Hsiangya Hospital attempted to conduct as many operations as possible, but still could not meet the demand as more cases arrived every day.[29] Frustration prevailed among hospital staff, and the situation worsened after the Japanese attack on Pearl Harbor. After the United States entered the war, Hsiangya lost its neutrality, making senior nursing internships in occupied Changsha impossible; consequently, unoccupied Yuanling became the center of the nursing program.

Relatively free from threats of invasion, yet nonetheless under the fear of bombings, Hsiangya in Yuanling became an appealing choice for female students in central-south China seeking to receive nursing education. Nursing leaders and reformers in China had attempted to feminize nursing since the 1920s.[30] Responding to the trend, from 1928 onward, Hsiangya restricted its admission to women only.[31] Although particular fields, such as military and public health nursing, continued to train male nurses, nursing's womanly connotations were reinforced during wartime. As of 1942, ninety-three female students enrolled in Hsiangya Nursing School in Yuanling, while eight graduate nurses and ten doctors taught at the school and kept the locally established Hsiangya Hospital running. While the majority of students came from Hunan, some transferred from other nursing schools in provinces across the country, such as Shandong and Hubei to the north and Fujian to the southeast.[32] The exclusive enrollment of females during wartime seems to have been the effect of both supply and demand. On the one hand, there was a shortage of potential young male students during wartime when the Nationalists press-ganged large numbers into their armies. On the other hand, nursing became a more attractive profession for Chinese women, as seen by the considerable number of enrolling students and their extensive geographic origins. One reason for the attraction to the profession for women was likely the relatively safe environment of the school given its American affiliation. Another was the financial aid provided by the program, which refugees from the Japanese-occupied areas in particular might have found appealing. The ideological construction of nursing as a respectable occupation and the formation of an identifiable nursing consciousness were also influenced by another attractive feature: the transfer of the mystique of Florence Nightingale to China.

"Nightingale-ism" in China

In *The Development of the Japanese Nursing Profession*, Aya Takahashi argues that Red Cross nurses contributed to constructing the model of modern nursing in Japan. By selectively adapting aspects of Florence Nightingale's teachings, nursing ideals in Japan emphasized moral training based on Japanese Confucianism and the feminine virtues summarized by the phrase "good wives and wise mothers."[33] Overall, there were striking similarities between "Nightingale-ism" in Japan and China in terms of the emphasis on character training, the elevation of Nightingale as a "sage" for nurses, and the construction of nursing as a noble career. However, in the case of the wartime Hsiangya Nursing School, Nightingale-ism stood for the professionalization of nursing and wartime service, unrelated to the Confucian dogma of female virtue.

Although Florence Nightingale neither participated in any Chinese nursing activities nor ever visited China (she died three years before Hsiangya was founded), the iconic image of her holding a lamp while attending to the needs of wounded soldiers during the Crimean War became emblematic in the early twentieth century and continued to influence the wartime Chinese nursing profession. In 1943, a senior nursing student interning in Guiyang wrote a letter to her professor in which she made the connection explicit: "at 9 p.m. every night, I come up to the second floor with a tiny oil lamp to check on every patient, make the bed, and ask the *coolie* to bring boiled water and pills. I then go through the general wards, the special care units, obstetric wards, and baby room. Every time like this reminds me of the fact that Ms. Nightingale inspecting patients with a lamp during wartime. But I am of course not as great as she was!" Nor was this student alone in seeing Nightingale as her role model. In 1944, another Hsiangya nursing student wrote, "I am on the night shift from 9 p.m. to 7 a.m.," where there was "a single floor lamp in the ward for fifty patients." The lamp simultaneously took on an implication at once both heroic and desolate when interpreted through the lens of Nightingale-ism: "The dim light looks so sad and lonely. Looking at such a scene, I could not help but to think of our predecessor, Ms. Nightingale, who held a lamp and walked 12 miles at night alone to take care of patients. Her spirit indeed encourages me!"[34] The iconic image of Nightingale was further ingrained into students through yearly celebration of her birthday. On this day, Hsiangya kept the tradition of paying tribute to Nightingale by performing student plays, publishing articles or special issues, and so forth.[35] In 1944, a Hsiangya nurse published an article to introduce their nursing school to nationwide students in honor of Nightingale's birthday. Addressing Nightingale as the "goddess," the article highlighted the fact that her "light of philanthropy" continued to inspire programs like Hsiangya and their students.[36]

One might ask why the image of Nightingale, a woman of the Victorian era, would be so influential among Chinese nursing students. Through these records we see that for Hsiangya students, Nightingale with her lamp symbolized a heroic and positive force that sustained hope while also imbuing a sense of professionalism that was deeply attractive to women seeking an increased role in society. Like the Nightingale of nursing mythology, Hsiangya nursing students and graduates were working in a wartime situation under extreme difficulties, and Chinese nurses easily found a resonance with her despite cultural differences. Yet turning Nightingale into a professional icon was by no means a given; instead, nursing pioneers carefully constructed this image and incorporated it into wartime nursing training in China.

In contrast to the image of Nightingale in nursing reforms in the Anglo-American world, which included Christian values, her celebrity in China, similarly in Japan, concentrated on her secular ethics and professional spirit.[37] In the Hsiangya school journal's special issue in celebration of its tenth anniversary, a featured column introduced Nightingale as the ultimate ancestor of nursing. The biographical sketch highlighted Nightingale's determination and devotion to becoming a nurse despite her parents' opposition. The author applauded her exceptional courage as a nurse, for taking care of various strangers, particularly male patients, which was not considered virtuous in Victorian Britain.[38] By depicting Nightingale rebelling against restrictive gendered social norms, the author implicitly criticized similar social and cultural obstacles for women pursuing a nursing career in China. When Gage, the founder of the Hsiangya school, remarked that "too many problems complicated the lives of the girls," she was aware that traditional Chinese values treasured female domesticity, which expected respectful women to be confined to the "inner quarters"—obedient to parents, respecting husbands, raising children, and dealing with domestic work.[39] By constructing the arc of the story of Florence Nightingale as a woman who rebelled against traditional values but who eventually gained respect and success, the biography presented her image as a role model with whom Chinese female nursing students could identify. Thus the students could correspondingly form their new identities free from the restraints of Confucian moral judgments regarding female virtues.

The biography also amplified the gender-neutral qualities of attentiveness, integrity, diligence, and benevolence through the epic tale of Nightingale bringing light and care to patients during wartime.[40] Nightingale's lamp became a symbol for noble and kind-hearted nurses who endeavored to serve under difficult circumstances. Through the implication that a woman could actively participate in the "masculine" sphere of war and attend "dangerous" patients with professionalism, the author employed Nightingale's image to represent the new set of womanly virtues based on individual professional discipline, instead of Confucian filial norms that revolved around obeying the patriarchal order.

Nightingale's portrayal served the purpose of ethical training of nurses, which Hsiangya's credo reinforced and nursing students internalized. In reminiscing about nursing training after seventy years, the very first memory that Huang, a graduate of the wartime class, articulated was the school motto of "diligence, sincerity, rigorousness, and determination." According to Huang, these words emphasized the professional, moral, technical, and personal aspects of nursing, which distinguished nurses from other occupations.[41]

Wartime ethics training, with Nightingale as a symbol, was particularly important in the Chinese nursing world. For administrators of Hsiangya Nursing School, student ethics was pertinent to their professional identities and nursing consciousness, while also reflecting the quality of the institution. The school made nursing ethics courses mandatory for both the second and third year, and kept strict rules and high standards to keep students disciplined.[42] Regardless of the frequent war-related disruptions, Hsiangya seized the yearly special occasion of commemorating Nightingale's birthday to "enhance students' morale and improve their nursing professional ethics."[43]

The focus on the cultivation of ethics and Nightingale-ism in wartime China could be properly seen as part of the growth of nursing consciousness and professionalism, evident in the activism of the Nurses' Association of China (NAC). To promote professional development nationwide, the NAC strove to gain support from the Nationalist government by underscoring the moral traits of loyalty and patriotism of Nightingale to its members. In February 1942, the first national conference of the NAC since the outbreak of the war commenced in Chengdu with about 150 representatives from across the country in attendance. In the opening speech, Aizhu Xu, the president of the association, called the attendees' attention to the "essence" of Nightingale's work—"assisting the government and serving the country." Xu highlighted the indispensability of nurses in developing public health in China, and the urgent wartime need of expanding nursing training. Reflecting on Nightingale's concerns for public health and the spirit of serving the nation, Xu further emphasized the cultivation of social responsibility for Chinese nurses, so as to form a professional consciousness in cooperation with the Nationalist government.[44]

Nightingale in China, as an adaptable symbol, therefore, enabled Chinese women to transcend restraints of conventional gendered values and come to dominate a modern profession when such domination was not a foregone conclusion. The strategy of selectively promoting Nightingale's tale further feminized nursing. The next stage of Nightingale-ism in China was the adoption of the white uniforms despite the ominous cultural association of the color.

Warriors in White Uniforms

While Chinese Nightingale-ism and ethics training shaped a nursing consciousness, we must also look to the influence of material culture in constructing the wartime roles of nurses—in particular, the adoption of white uniforms in accordance with the Anglo-American nursing custom. However, the Hunan nursing students did not merely accept this foreign uniform; they embraced the austere color, and combined it with the Chinese term for nursing to emphasize their contribution to the national interest during wartime. Their wartime nickname thus became the "warriors in white uniforms,"[45] demonstrating the significance of the uniform in framing the perception of the profession, while also spotlighting the inextricable link between nursing and national defense.

Despite the fact that Chinese considered white as a sensitive color in cloth-ing, following an Anglo-American model, wearing white uniforms became the emblem for both nursing students and nurses in China. Adopting white nursing uniforms for Chinese denoted the process of acculturation, as Deborah Washington has suggested. Seeing nursing as culturally competent care, Washington suggests that in a transcultural environment, accultura-tion demonstrates the newcomers' capability to manage the cultural shock and navigate the health system. As a mode of medical cultural encounters, it also asks for the natives' ability to "adapt to the rules and conventions" of a society different from their origins.[46] The case of adopting white uniforms for Chinese nurses illustrates the dynamics of navigation and adaption. As Hsiangya was modeled on the US training system, it required Chinese stu-dent nurses to wear white on duty as US nurses did—aprons on colored or white uniforms.[47] However, traditional Chinese culture treated white clothing, nearly synonymous with mourning apparel, as ominous, thus its acceptance required a strategic approach.[48] The offer of free uniforms for students was probably the key tactic to resolve this obstacle, as the free cloth-ing could be quite an allure for students. Another important step was the reconstruction of the meanings of white in hygienic and moral terms. The color of white designated the meaning of neatness and orderliness, as white was applied in almost all possible hygienic occasions. Through the title of "warrior in white uniform," the color white also began to carry the symbolic meanings of nobility for its devotion to the wartime national cause, which further popularized the image of trained nurses wearing white apparel. The success of acculturating the white uniforms is also evident in the illustra-tion of the nursing staff in white and their white equipment in Cao Yu's *Metamorphosis*.[49]

Originally the nursing uniform in the Chinese case was gender-neutral, despite its gendered meaning in the case of American nurses.[50] Although Hsiangya allowed only women to enroll during wartime, the uniform was not much different from that of the male medical staff. One reason for the similarity is that the plain-colored gown-style uniform actually resembled the common style of dress for men before 1949, so Chinese did not associate a gender-specific connotation to the attire. It is difficult to infer, with current available sources, whether the similarity between the Western-style nursing uniform and the Chinese male gown made students feel more feminine by imitating Nightingale and her sister nurses, or more masculine by wearing clothes close to men's. But what we see is that the nature of the nursing uni-form in the Chinese context might at the same time demonstrate accultura-tion by expanding the cultural meanings of white attire from mourning to hygiene while also, at least initially, avoiding any gender particularity.

A gendered wartime agenda may have contributed to this ambiguity. In the ancient folk tale of Hua Mulan, a young woman takes the place of her father during wartime, winning accolades for her martial prowess even while cross-dressing as a male and covering her great beauty. The tale, told in several famous versions in the Ming and the Qing dynasties, continued to have purchase in narratives of the 1930s to encourage women to make contributions to the war effort. The tale of Mulan regained popularity in the press and *Mulan Joins the Army* became a feature film in 1939.[51] By promoting Mulan as a heroine cross-dressing as a man to participate in the male-exclusive military, propaganda like the 1939 film directed by Bu Wancang advocated that the anti-Japanese national cause prioritized conventional gender norms. Louise Edwards's study on Mulan suggests that Bu's film delivered a "thinly disguised tale of resistance to foreign invasion" metaphoric to the war against Japan. In the film, Mulan's transgressions of womanly expectations, as Edwards contends, from growing up as a "mischievous tomboy," to disguising herself in the army as a man, to undergoing hetero- and homosexual tensions, were subordinate to service to the state.[52] Similar to the Rosie the Riveter campaign to recruit American women to factory work to replace males after the US entry in World War II, wartime Chinese authorities also mobilized women into the "masculine sphere" of national defense.[53] Official organizations and institutions such as the Red Cross Society of China and the Nationalist Ministry of War urged female volunteers and trainees to join battlefield service and military medical care.[54] Despite the fact that Hsiangya remained a private institution, the National Health Administration (NHA) monitored and intervened in nursing training from the beginning of the war.[55] It was no surprise that nursing uniforms would be regulated under the national regime, while the gender-neutral term "warriors in white uniforms" coincided with the official interest in national defense. Yet despite any gender neutrality of the uniform, gender-specific values were increasingly evident in everyday practices of nurses and wartime medical culture.

Sisters and Guards

As a female-dominant profession that aligned with the interests of authorities, nursing provides a crucial microcosm to interrogate the gendered politics of wartime China. There were two types of gendered relationships for nurses that were key in transforming their identity during the war: the sisterhood among nurses as well as among nursing and medical students themselves; and the nurse-physician relationship. These gender dynamics in particular, along with a larger medical culture, shaped the group identity of nurses. Subject to wartime agendas, nursing students were also cast as a safeguard of the nation's hygienic modernity.

The sense of sisterhood conditioned nurses' experiences and choices. For nursing students interning in remote hospitals, they often found alumni nurses to be helpful "sisters," and easily bonded through their shared professional identity.[56] Despite frustrations over local inadequate facilities and uncooperative patients, one intern was "relieved" that the "sisterlike" care from a Hsiangya senior colleague helped her and two other classmates navigate and "establish patients' trust."[57] Similar rapport was weighed into nurses' professional choices. When choosing job offers at the end of her internship in Guiyang, a Hsiangya senior rejected a more prestigious position in Sichuan, deciding to stay and assist the fledgling military nursing program. Her "friendship with Ms. Zhou Meiyu," who was in charge of the program, swayed her to join Zhou's efforts to gain ground for military nursing training.[58] The camaraderie among female students was also extended across specializations. Yuanxiu Lao, one of the few female medical students, described the "widespread" cordiality among fellows at their Hsiangya compound in Guiyang "as if siblings" to "overcome hardships." Female medical and nursing students often played sports and performed plays together.[59]

In contrast to these peer relationships, workplace relations between doctors and nurses, or between administrators and nurses, were hierarchical as they were in Europe or the United States. As the Chinese nursing profession became increasingly feminized during the war, the subordination of nurses to authoritative physicians also became gendered. These asymmetrical power relations were pervasive in the medical professional environment and could even be operative in other areas of nurses' lives, as they were forced to take responsibility for physicians' errors during long working hours, and yet were still on call at a moment's notice during their leisure time. An excerpt from a popular poem among students depicted the situation:

> Taking the blame for the doctor's mistakes,
> Oh dear, what a lot of patience it takes.
> Going off duty at seven o'clock,
> Tired, discouraged, and ready to drop,
> But called back on special at seven fifteen,
> With woe in her heart that must not be seen.
> Morning and evening, noon and night,
> Just doing it over and hoping it's right.[60]

Letters to the Hsiangya Nursing School from female senior students similarly reflected their inferior position and lack of protection within and beyond hospital wards. One nursing student, Tianwen Pan, inquired for help regarding the harassment she encountered as an intern at a county hospital where the hospital's director attempted to set her up with his divorced friend. Taking her refusal personally, the director constantly found fault with her and made the work environment "unbearable."[61] Similar hierarchical tensions and unfair treatment were common complaints from nursing interns. One Hsiangya intern, Jingwen Guan, was disturbed by her vulnerability to "unexpected nitpickings" from various personages acquainted with her supervisors, which "severely hindered" her work. Another intern, Dong Xiuying, underwent "unreasonable humiliations" from her hospital's director when she asked him for a two-week leave to take care of her sickly and only parent. Showing "no empathy," the director "strictly scolded" her for the request and even threatened to fire her. In a following letter to the school, Dong stated that as "a frail woman in a foreign town" she had "no one to seek assistance" from when subject to the director's frequent bullying. Dong further petitioned Hsiangya to reassign her internship and report her case to the provincial health administration to "establish protection" for herself and other nurses in like situations.[62] Although there is no evidence whether assistance from Hsiangya was forthcoming, these cases nevertheless illustrate the deficiency of legal standing for nurses regarding their asymmetrical relations with male physicians. Given the inadequate rights for nurses, sisterhood became their shield against both professional and wartime distress. As Dong expressed her desire for comradeship in her working environment, students like Fu Xizhen also addressed the importance of peer relations in wartime. In her plea to the school, Fu reported that her daily routines were overwhelmed given that she was the only nurse at her clinic and that she was constantly dealing with floods, soaring inflation, or banditry on top of the threat of Japanese bombings. Fu requested a fellow Hsiangya nurse to provide not only "mutual help at work" but also "moral support."[63]

The concept of sisterhood was also appropriated to engage nursing students to think transnationally about their contributions to the war effort. For example, during the Battle of Changsha, the Young Women's Christian Association (YWCA) circulated printed material among nursing students calling for volunteers to join a first aid team that was part of an international movement. One pamphlet addressed students as "sisters" while prompting them to join in the international battle against fascism with the slogan, "Let's unite to fight!"[64] By highlighting the first aid group organized by the YWCA during the Battle of Changsha, the pamphlet employed the bonds of sisterhood to recruit volunteers based on shared war-relief experiences. Another example comes from an influential 1942 speech by Madame Chiang Kai-Shek that was broadcast and circulated widely on the Hsiangya campus, in which she reflected on her recent visit to India and implored women everywhere to unite on their faith and works. Students at Hsiangya were deeply inspired by the speech, and one Hsiangya faculty member later wrote that the nurses saw themselves as being responsible to "safeguard" the new freedom Chinese women had achieved during this time.[65]

Vague internationalist movements like that of Madame Chiang were acceptable, unlike the many movements gripping students in "Free China" who protested the corruption of the Nationalists. Student nurses were seen by the authorities, along with others, as potential threats, and were also subject to disciplinary wartime propaganda. For the Chinese Nationalist authorities, the major concern centered on students' potential role in uprisings against the government, and the Nationalist administration issued a series of regulations and preventative policies that were implemented in all schools. These included the delivery of patriotic speeches to enhance students' loyalty to the government, requiring regular reports of student activities, and the immediate cessation of any radical movements among students. At the same time, the government attempted to improve student living conditions to ensure their emotional stability.[66] Meanwhile, the Chinese Communist Party (CCP) seized the opportunity to mobilize students, considering them a major revolutionary force. In December 1937, Xu Teli, the CCP director of the Changsha Eighth Route Army Office, spread propaganda emphasizing the determination of the Communists to defeat the enemy, an attempt to encourage students to leave the Nationalist-controlled region and make the long and arduous journey to the Communist base in Yan'an. Xu's propaganda received a strong response, and it altered a number of students' negative impressions of the CCP. After his talks, two medical students and four nursing students came to Xu and volunteered to serve wounded soldiers in Yan'an.[67] Although no records suggest that Hsiangya officially responded to Xu, these four nursing students were publicly expelled from the school for their choice to go to Yan'an.[68]

Public health training for nursing students became another primary concern for the Nationalist government. Given the potential for epidemics because of mass migration from war zones, the NHA established a chain of highway health stations and mobile antiepidemic units along the main routes of transportation. The pressing need for nurses to participate in epidemic control and medical care led to an intensification of efforts to train nursing staff with public health knowledge. In particular, the Japanese use of germ warfare in Hunan Province in 1941 made public health nursing training critically urgent; therefore, a public health campaign was initiated with the aid of international forces.[69] In December 1943, the Hunan Provincial Health Administration convened the province-wide mission hospitals and medical training institutions to reinforce public health education. For nursing training, the Provincial Health Administration developed and regulated a curriculum that emphasized the need to combine training in public health theory with real-world experience. The curriculum placed nursing graduates under governmental control since the recognition of their graduation certificates became contingent on an official seal by the provincial government.[70] To increase the reach of its campaign, the government expected the school to instill nationalism with slogans such as "healthy citizen, healthy nation" while educating civilians about common sense in public health. Nursing students were considered the front line of hygienic safeguard against epidemics and were asked to participate in the public health campaign. Students learned public health knowledge combined with the ideology of building a healthy and strong nation, as one student's notes highlighted: their work in the campaign was tied to "the destiny of China."[71]

In addition, the provincial government required the Hsiangya Nursing School to plaster propaganda posters on campus that combined public health rhetoric with the language of patriotism and anti-imperialism. In one particular poster issued by the Department of Health in Yuanling, a bayonet is seen punctuating the heart of an epidemic-ridden rat wearing a Japanese flag. If the graphic was too subtle, certainly the ominous title spoke volumes, "Kill the enemy as if [you would] kill a rat."[72] Such posters employed vivid metaphors accusing Japan of being a public health menace, while also conjuring up images of China's foe as a perpetrator of germ warfare. In this way, the posters imbued public health consciousness with a nationalistic anti-Japanese ideology that nursing students were expected to communicate to citizens through their routine work.

While nurses acted as a bulwark for the preservation of national health and imparted daily sanitary knowledge to civilians, both the provincial government and Hsiangya Nursing School supplemented all students' education with training in reproductive hygiene. They thus joined midwives, who had a long history in China, as another group of female professionals through whom the government sought to influence childbearing and maternity. Tina Johnson's study on childbirth in Republican China suggests that the popular discussions regarding the significance of maternal health drew on Western theories of reproduction and were part of a larger emphasis on urban sanitation and hygiene.[73] These trends can be seen in nursing training in Republican China more generally, even as the case of Hsiangya illustrates the complexities of carrying out midwifery hygiene plans in wartime China.

After completing the three-year coursework, Hsiangya nursing students had the option to receive additional training in midwifery before their internships.[74] With wartime needs leading to surging demands for credentialed midwives, in 1941 the provincial government commanded the nursing school to open specialized midwifery classes. For Hsiangya, the new obligations magnified both physical and spiritual difficulties: despite monthly stipends from government coffers to support the wartime midwifery program, soaring inflation and material shortages meant the stipends were often inadequate. The government's overly ambitious plan worsened the conditions at the school. The official goal of enrolling fifty students per year proved unrealistic, since Hsiangya neither received enough qualified applications nor possessed sufficient faculty to accommodate so many students. Consequent problems arose when the Hsiangya-trained nurses or midwives started interning for obstetrical care. Since the provincial government failed to provide adequate support for obstetrical departments, these students found it frustrating to work in hospitals that lacked even the most basic equipment. More discouraging to them was the fact that local pregnant women were often skeptical about their services. As a Hsiangya intern wrote, her job was "quite idle," for only four cases of delivery happened within twelve months. Women from well-off families, as she explained, lived in secluded places that she and her colleagues had difficulty reaching. Most other pregnant women had little previous exposure to biomedical knowledge or Western-style hospitals; this student found it "helpless and futile" that these expectant mothers "refused to trust" their advice on maternal care.[75]

The gap between official goals and everyday reality in Hsiangya nursing students' practice speaks to the general deficiency of state resources. While the idea of sisterhood empowered women to bond and establish their professional footing in the face of wartime hardships, it provided only a mild challenge to the gendered hierarchy of the medical field in demanding rights for nurses. Despite nurses' extensive outreach, without adequate supporting measures, their ability to practice public health and maternal care was restrained. However, the limitations and strengths of nurses' work exposed under wartime circumstances rendered nursing as both target and device for postwar rehabilitation.

With Japan's surrender in 1945, the Hsiangya Nursing School returned to the Hunan provincial capital. The former campus was in a state of almost complete destruction or neglect, as was much of the city. While vigorously helping restore the school buildings and clean the equipment, Hsiangya nursing students were also sent to the Provincial Relief Committee Refugee Camp to tend those infected during a cholera pandemic that had broken out after the war.[76] By the summer of 1946, all Hsiangya students and branches had settled in Changsha and begun the work of rehabilitation.[77]

The tumultuous period of the Second Sino-Japanese War was devastating to individuals and society at various levels, yet out of the destruction, wartime circumstances catalyzed a new chapter for nursing in China, as the case of the Hsiangya Nursing School illustrates. The institution provided shelter and a purpose for refugees from all over China, and maintained a base for professional training. The war years saw nurses empowered through a growing professional identity drawing selectively from systems and uniforms in Anglo-American models, even as the feminizing of the profession created new sets of gendered restraints and frustrations for nurses. Gaining particular momentum from patriotic service for the wounded and the sick, nursing training became highly pertinent to governmental concerns regarding public health and midwifery.

Recognizing the importance of the "warriors in white uniforms" to the nation, governmental authorities strove to seize the administrative power of the Hsiangya compound. In 1940, the Nationalist government took over the Hsiangya medical sector; but owing to both domestic and international efforts, the nursing school staff and the committee board of the Yale-in-China Association managed to keep the nursing school operating independently through the Chinese Civil War era until the establishment of the Communist regime when the state system absorbed Hsiangya. The CCP's ideology in the 1950s sought to purge Hsiangya's foreign ties and subsume nursing under the slogan of "serving the people." Practices and ideas such as wearing the white uniform, the bond of sisterhood, and the metaphor of guards were appropriated and repackaged to indoctrinate nursing students' commitment to the "unity" and "the people's health" under "the banner of Mao Zedong."[78] This episode of nursing training at Hsiangya reassesses the gender dynamics and legacy of wartime society and accentuates the heterogeneous nature of health care as biomedical knowledge and care were transformed from theoretical training into everyday practice.

Notes

1. Yu Cao, *Cao Yu Xiju Ji: Tuibian* [Yu Cao's Plays: Metamorphosis], (Chengdu: Sichuan Renmin Press, 1984). The quote is my translation.

2. According to Cao, the storyline was developed while he fled to Hunan in 1937, witnessing and experiencing the sufferings of war, the upsurge of patriotism, the wartime social evils, and the good deeds by Western-style medical staff. See Cao, "Cao Yu Tan Tuibian" [Cao Yu on Tuibian] (originally published in *Chongqing Daily*, October 18, 1985), in *Cao Yu Quanji* [Complete Works of Cao Yu] (Shijiazhuang: Hua shan we yi Publishers, 1996), vol 2, 357–58.

3. Edward H. Hume, *Doctors East Doctors West: An American Physician's Life in China* (New York: Norton, 1946), 167–70.

4. See Kimberly Jensen, *Mobilizing Minerva: American Women in the First World War* (Urbana: University of Illinois Press, 2008); Jean Quataert, "Gendered Medical Services in Red Cross Field Hospitals during the First Balkan War and World War I," in *Peace, War and Gender from Antiquity to the Present: Cross-Cultural Perspectives*, ed. Jost Dulffer and Robert Frank (Essen: Klartext Verlag, 2009), 219–33.

5. Hume, *Doctors East Doctors West*, 167–70.

6. The schools of nurses were attached to either hospitals or medical schools, such as Hsiangya Hospital in Changsha, Margaret Williamson Hospital in Shanghai, Sleeper Davis Hospital in Beijing, and the Peiping Union Medical College in Beijing. See Evelyn Lin, "Nursing in China," *American Journal of Nursing* 38, no. 1 (1938): 1–8.

7. See Mary Brown Bullock, *The Oil Prince's Legacy: Rockefeller Philanthropy in China* (Washington, DC, and Stanford, CA: Woodrow Wilson Center Press and Stanford University Press, 2011); Jane Hunt, *Gospel of Gentility: American Women Missionaries in Turn-of-the-Century China* (New Haven, CT: Yale University Press, 1984); Motoe Sasaki-Gayle, "Entangled with Empire: American Women and the Creation of the 'New Woman' in China, 1898–1937" (PhD diss., Johns Hopkins University, 2008).

8. Sonya Grypma, *Healing Henan: Canadian Nurses at the North China Mission, 1888–1947* (Vancouver: University of British Columbia Press, 2008); Connie Shemo, *The*

Chinese Medical Ministries of Kang Cheng and Shi Meiyu, 1872–1937: On a Cross-cultural Frontier of Gender, Race, and Nation (Bethlehem, PA: Lehigh University Press, 2011); David Kang, "Missionaries, Women, and Health Care History of Nursing in Colonial Hong Kong (1887–1942)" (PhD diss., Chinese University of Hong Kong, 2013); Kaiyi Chen, "Quality versus Quantity: The Rockefeller Foundation and Nurses' Training in China," *Journal of American–East Asian Relations* 5, no. 1 (2003): 77–104.

9. John Watt, "Breaking into Public Service: The Development of Nursing in Modern China, 1870–1949," *Nursing History Review: Official Journal of the American Association for the History of Nursing* 12 (2004): 67–96; Chun-Yen Chou, "Funv yu Kangzhan Shiqi de Zhandi Jiuhu" [Women and battlefield first aid during the Second Sino-Japanese War], *Jindai Zhongguo Funvshi Yanjiu* [Research on women in modern Chinese history], no. 24 (2014): 133–220.

10. Ruth Rogaski, *Hygienic Modernity: Meanings of Health and Disease in Treatyport China* (Berkeley: University of California Press, 2004); Yang Nianqun, *Zaizao "Bingren": Zhong Xiyi Chongtu xia de Kongjian Zhengzhi, 1832–1985* [Remaking "Patients": Spatial politics under the conflicts between Chinese and Western medicine] (Beijing: China Renmin University Press, 2006); Sean Hsiang-lin Lei, *Neither Donkey nor Horse: Medicine in the Struggle over China's Modernity* (Chicago: University of Chicago Press, 2014); John R. Watt, *Saving Lives in Wartime China: How Medical Reformers Built Modern Healthcare Systems amid War and Epidemics, 1928–1945* (Leiden: Brill, 2014); Nicole E. Barnes, "Protecting the National Body: Gender and Public Health in Southwest China during the War with Japan, 1937–1945" (PhD diss., University of California–Irvine, 2012); Tina Phillips-Johnson, *Childbirth in Republican China: Delivering Modernity* (Lanham, MD: Lexington Books, 2011); Ming-cheng M. Lo, *Doctors within Borders: Profession, Ethnicity, and Modernity in Colonial Taiwan* (Berkeley: University of California Press, 2002).

11. Danke Li, *Echoes of Chongqing: Women in Wartime China* (Champaign: University of Illinois Press, 2009); Gail Hershatter, *The Gender of Memory: Rural Women and China's Collective Past* (Berkeley: University of California Press, 2014); Chien-Ming Yu, "Chuchu Wujia Chuchu Jia: Zhongguo Zhishi Nvxing de Fenghuo Suiyue" [Home is nowhere, home is everywhere: A female intellectual's life in Sino-Japanese wartime], *Jindai Zhongguo Funüshi Yanjiu*, no. 23 (2014): 1–63; Joan Judge, *Republican Lens: Gender, Visuality, and Experience in the Early Chinese Periodical Press* (Oakland: University of California Press, 2015).

12. Emily Honig, *Sisters and Strangers: Women in the Shanghai Cotton Mills, 1919–1949* (Stanford, CA: Stanford University Press, 1986); Ling-ling Lien, "Searching for the 'New Womanhood': Career Women in Shanghai, 1912–1945" (PhD diss., University of California–Irvine, 2001); Hui-chi Hsu, "Guanyu Dushi Xiaofei yu Nüxing Zhiye de Tantao [Female waitresses of Republican China] (1928–1937)—on Urban Consumerism and Female Profession," *Jindai Shi Yanjiusuo Jikan* [Bulletin of the Institute of Modern History, Academia Sinica], no. 48 (2005): 47–93; Helen M. Schneider, *Keeping the Nation's House: Domestic Management and the Making of Modern China* (Vancouver: University of British Columbia Press, 2011).

13. Keith Schoppa, *In a Sea of Bitterness: Refugees during the Sino-Japanese War* (Cambridge, MA: Harvard University Press, 2010); Diana Lary, *The Chinese People at War: Human Suffering and Social Transformation, 1937–1945* (Cambridge, MA: Harvard University Press, 2010); Joshua H. Howard, *Workers at War: Labor in China's*

Arsenals, 1937–1953 (Stanford, CA: Stanford University Press, 2004); Guotai Hu, *Yu Huo Chong Sheng: Kangzhan Shiqi de Gaodeng Jiaoyu* [Reborn of fire: Higher education during the Second Sino-Japanese War] (Taipei: Daoxiang Press, 2004); Aaron W. Moore, *Writing War: Soldiers Record the Japanese Empire* (Cambridge, MA: Harvard University Press, 2013); Barnes, "Protecting the National Body"; Watt, *Saving Lives in Wartime China.*

14. Cultural imperialism in China's medical development has been discussed in such works as Iris Borowy, ed., *Uneasy Encounters: The Politics of Medicine and Health in China, 1900–1937* (Frankfurt: Peter Lang, 2009); Shemo, *Chinese Medical Ministries.*

15. The Hunan-Yale (pinyin: Xiangya) Nursing School, which was used during wartime, has been referred to by many different names. For convenience, in this chapter the name of the nursing school will be given as Hsiangya (as it was at that time).

16. Chen, "Quality versus Quantity," 77–104; Watt, "Breaking into Public Service," 67–96; Zhengxie Beijing Shi Weiyuanhui Wenshi Ziliao Yanjiu Weiyuanhui [CPPCC Beijing Committee for Oral Historical Records], ed., *Huashuo Lao Xiehe* [Stories of the PUMC] (Beijing: Chinese Literature and History Press, 1989), 205–11; Li Shenglan, "Refashioning Care: Nursing, Intimacy, and Citizenship in Wartime China, 1930–1950" (PhD diss., Binghamton University, 2017), chap. 2.

17. Xiangya Di, "40 ban Xuesheng Jiating Kaikuang Biao, Huxiao Xuesheng Jiating Qingkuang Diaocha, Ruxue Zhengjian, Sujia Zheng Ji Gexiang Jianbiao Deng Wengao" [Students' family background charts, surveys, admission paperwork, leave permits, and other documents of the Hunan-Yale Class of 1940], 1939–45, box 67-2-501, Collection of the Hunan-Yale Medical College, Hunan Provincial Archives, Changsha [hereafter cited as HPA]; Li, "Refashioning Care," chap. 2.

18. Hu, *Yu Huo Chong Sheng*, 20–30.

19. "Wartime Christian Mission in China," 1937, box 10, file 167, Edward H. Hume: Writings, Edward H. and Lotta C. Hume Papers (MS787), Manuscripts and Archives, Yale University Library, New Haven, CT [hereafter cited as YUL].

20. Zhu Bihui, "Guiyang Hushi Jiaoyu Gaikuang ji Shicha Yijian" [Survey of nursing education in Guiyang and recommendations], 1940, Chuan Gui Dian Sansheng Zhuchan Jiaoyu ji Chengdu Guiyang Hushi Xuexiao Shicha Baogao Deng Youguan Wenshu [Midwifery education in Sichuang, Guizhou, and Yunan: Reports on nursing schools in Chengdu and Yunan . . .], box 5-14899, Second Historical Archives of China, Nanjing; Nie Yuchan, "Xiehe Yixueyuan Hushi Xuexiao de Bianqian" [A history of the PUMC Nursing School], in Zhengxie Beijing Shi Weiyuanhui Wenshi Ziliao Yanjiu Weiyuanhui, ed., *Huashuo Lao Xiehe*, 195–204; Li, "Refashioning Care," chap. 2.

21. The American faculty actually laid out their country's flag to be visible from the sky during Japanese bombings in order to avoid attacks.

22. "Bainian yaolan tianshi qugao wanren tideng renjian nuanhe: Jinian Xiangya huli jiaoyu 100 zhounian" [Special issue on the 100th anniversary of the Xiangya Nursing School], *Zhongnan daxue xuebao* [Journal of the Central South University] 21 (October 8, 2011): 1; "National League of Nursing Education, 1923–1946," National League of Nursing Education, 1923–46, box 10, file 419, Yale-China Association Records (RU 232), YUL.

23. Hunan Yixueyuan Yuanshi Zhengjizu, *Hunan Yixueyuan Yuanshi Ziliao Diyi Ji: Xiangya Chunqiu* [Historical sources of the Hunan Medical College, vol. 1: Xiangya's past], 1984, Central South University Archives, Changsha.

24. "Broken Jade," box 6, file 178, Subject Files, Writings, Photographs, Phillips F. and Ruth A. Greene papers (MS 797), YUL; Nancy E. Chapman and Jessica C. Plumb, *The Yale-China Association: A Centennial History* (Hong Kong: Chinese University Press, 2001), 52.

25. Schoppa, *Sea of Bitterness*, 106–10.

26. Xiaoqian Zhang to Dwight Rugh, April 25, 1940; Dwight Rugh to Xiaoqian Zhang, February 17, 1941, box 67-2-90, 1939–1942 Zhang Xiaoqian yu Guoji Jiujihui Yu Daocun deng Xinjian [1939–1942 correspondence between Zhang Xiaoqian and Dwight Rugh from the International Relief Committee], HPA; "Yale-in-China Report of the 34th year—1940, Dec.," 1940, box 67-2-569, *Xiangya Journal*, Meiguo Yali Ge Danwei jiqi zai Zhongguo Jianli de Jige Qinlue Jigou [US Yale-in-China branches and its imperialist institution], HPA.

27. "A Summary Report of the Hsiangya Medical College," 1939, box 67-2-88, Xiangqian Zhang the Acting Director, Shenqing Keyan Shiyanshi ji Zhang Xiaoqian Guanyu Benyuan de Nianzhong Baogao [The application for the laboratory and Xiangqian Zhang's annual reports], HPA; "The Hsiang Ya Medical College: A Brief Report for 1939–1940," 1940, *Xiangya Journal*, HPA.

28. "A Summary Report of the Hsiangya Medical College," 1939.

29. "Air Raids in Changsha," 1941, box 3, file 76, William Winston Pettus, Writings, the William Winston Pettus Papers (MS 786), YUL; "Reports on the Changsha International Relief Committee—Refugee Camp at Yale-in-China 1941," 1941, box 2, file 34, Pettus, Correspondence of the Pettus Family and Others.

30. "Report of the School of Nursing of the Hunan-Yale Hospital, June 1924–June 1925," 1925, box 66, Yale-China Association Records (RU 232), YUL; Li, "Refashioning Care," chap. 1.

31. Hunan Sili Xiangya Yixueyuan Fushe Gaoji Hushi Zhiye Xuexiao Zhangcheng [Constitution of the Hunan Private Hsiangya Nursing School], 1937, MW 0256, Central South University Archives.

32. "China's Wartime Nursing," *American Journal of Nursing* 42, no. 5 (1942): 519–20; "1941 nian Sili Xiangya Gaoji Hushi Zhiye Xuexiao Gaikuang" [Survey of the Hunan-Yale Nursing School in 1941], 1941, box 67-2-503, Hunan-Yale Nursing School, Huxiao Yuansheng Tongji Baogao [Statistics of the staff and students of the nursing school], HPA.

33. Aya Takahashi, *The Development of the Japanese Nursing Profession: Adopting and Adapting Western Influences* (London: Routledge Curzon, 2004), 36–54. I borrow the term "Nightingale-ism" from Takahashi's study of Japanese nurses. My comparison between nursing in China and Japan mostly relied on this work.

34. Huxiao Xuesheng gei Xuexiao Xinjian [Correspondence from the nursing students], 1943–44, box 67-2-512, HPA.

35. "Nandinggeer Danchen Benxiao Te Juban Zhuankan" [A special issue in honor of Nightingale's birthday], n.d., Huxiao Jiaowu ji Qita Xingzheng Fangmian Wenjian 1930–1946 [Nursing school's documents on teaching and administration], 67-2-537, HPA; Dwight Rugh to Xiaoqian Zhang, February 17, 1941, HPA.

36. Fengzi, "Xiangya Gaoji Hushi Xuexiao" [Hsiangya Nursing School], Xuesheng Zhi You [Students' Friends] 1944, 41–42.

37. For Nightingale, see Takahashi, *Japanese Nursing Profession*; Linda C. Andrist, Patrice K. Nicholas, and Karen A. Wolf, eds., *A History of Nursing Ideas* (Sudbury: Jones and Bartlett Publishers, 2006).

38. Hunan-Yale-in-China, *Xiangya: Xiaoqing Shi Zhounian Jinian Hao* [Xiangya: Ten-year anniversary issue], 1925, Archive Reading Room, Central South University Archives.

39. Hume, *Doctors East Doctors West*, 167–74.

40. Hunan-Yale-in-China, *Xiangya*, 7–10.

41. "Bainian Yaolan Tianshi Qugao Wanren Tideng Renjian Nuanhe."

42. "Hunan-Yale School for Nurses (Student Manual)," 1924, Accession 2009-A-198, box 10, Hunan-Yale School of Nursing: School Records, 1923–24, Yale-China Association Records (RU 232), YUL.

43. "Nandinggeer Danchen Benxiao Te Juban Zhuankan."

44. China Nursing Association, *Hushi Jibao: Zhongguo Hushi Xuehui Diyijie Daibiao Dahui Zhuanhao* [Nursing Quarterly: The first Nursing Association Conference issue], 1942, box 67-2-153, Hushi Yiyao Ziliao [Nursing and Medical Materials], HPA.

45. Hunan Yixueyuan Yuanshi Zhengjizu, *Hunan Yixueyuan Yuanshi Ziliao Diyi Ji*, Central South University Archives.

46. According to Deborah Washington, nursing is a multicultural professional that provides culturally competent care. She identifies three modes of medical cultural encounter: cultural autonomy, acculturation, and cultural imposition. See "Moving towards a Culturally Competent Profession," in *A History of Nursing Ideas*, ed. Linda C. Andrist, Patrice K. Nicholas, and Karen A. Wolf (Sudbury: Jones and Bartlett Publishers, 2006), 45–55.

47. "Hunan-Yale School for Nurses."

48. Yang, *Zaizao "Bingren*," 176–77.

49. See Cao, "Cao Yu Tan Tuibian."

50. Kara Dixon Vuic, *Officer, Nurse, Women: The Army Nurse Corps in the Vietnam War* (Baltimore: Johns Hopkins University Press, 2010), 95–98.

51. Antonia Finnane, *Changing Clothes in China: Fashion, History, Nation* (New York: Columbia University Press, 2008), 188–99.

52. Louise Edwards, *Women Warriors and Wartime Spies of China* (Cambridge: Cambridge University Press, 2016): 28–29.

53. D'Ann Campbell, *Women at War with America: Private Lives in a Patriotic Era* (Cambridge, MA: Harvard University Press, 1984).

54. Zhou Meiyu, *Development of Army Nursing School in China*, trans. Wang Shijun (Taipei: National Defense Medical Center, 1985), 25–35, 57–62. The original English version of the book was Zhou's master's thesis submitted to the Massachusetts Institutes of Technology in 1944. Li, "Refashioning Care," chap. 4.

55. The National Health Administration is also known as Weishengshu. The Nationalist government nationalized the Xiangya Medical School in 1940, but the nursing school remained private under the Yale-in-China management until the 1950s.

56. See Huxiao Xuesheng gei Xuexiao Xinjian, 1943–44, HPA.

57. Duoli Li to Teachers, January 17, 1943, Xuesheng Gei Xuexiao Xinjian [Students' letters to the school], 67-2-512, HPA.

58. Debiao to Taiyuan Wang, n.d., Xuesheng Gei Xuexiao Xinjian, 67-2-512, HPA.

59. Hunan Yixueyuan Yuanshi Zhengjizu, *Hunan Yixueyuan Yuanshi Ziliao Diyi Ji,* Central South University Archives.

60. Author unknown, "The Nurse," n.d., in "Poems collected by Nina Gage," Accession 2004-A-006, box 1, Letters and photographs of Nina Gage concerning the Yale-China Program circa 1924–1938, Yale-China Association Records (RU 232), YUL.

61. Tianwen Pan to teachers, n.d., Huxiao Xuesheng gei Xuexiao Xinjian 1943–44, HPA.

62. Jingwen Guan to teachers, July 28, 1944; Xiuying Dong to Director Liu, July 15 and 26, 1945, Xuesheng Gei Xuexiao Xinjian, HPA.

63. Xizhen Fu to Taiyuan Wang, June 1 (n.d.), Xuesheng Gei Xuexiao Xinjian, HPA.

64. See "Miscellaneous notes and printed matter," n.d., box 5, file 170, Young Women's Christian Association in Changsha, Subject Files, Writings, Photographs, Phillips F. and Ruth A. Greene Papers (MS 797), YUL.

65. Ruth A. Greene, "Chinese Women and War" and "Wartime Hsiang-Ya," 1944, box 6, file 177, Phillips F. and Ruth A. Greene Papers (MS 797), YUL.

66. "Hunan Shengjiaoyuting Fangzhi Jianwei Youhuo Xuesheng zhi Duice" [Hunan Provincial Education Department's policies to prevent abduction of students by spies], 1944, box 67-2-57, Hunan Provincial Education Department, HPA.

67. Hunan Yixueyuan Yuanshi Zhengjizu, *Hunan Yixueyuan Yuanshi Ziliao Diyi Ji,* Central South University Archives; "Xiangya 90-year Anniversary Exhibition," Exhibition room, Central South University Archives.

68. Jin Xin, *Qinli Yan'an Suiyue: Yan'an Zhongyang Yiyuan de Wangshi* [Experiencing Yan'an: Memories of the Yan'an Central Hospital] (Beijing: Renmin University Press, 2014), 268.

69. In November 1941, the Japanese dropped grain infected with plague bacteria in Changde, Hunan, in an attempt to accelerate the occupation process. A number of civilians died of the plague within a few days, although this attempt at germ warfare was far less successful than the Japanese had hoped. See "Changde Guangde Yiyuan Baogao" [Changde Guangde Hospital Reports], 1942, 77, vol. 1, box 54, Changde Presbyterian Mission Hospital, Hunan Shengweishengchu Zhaoji ge Jiaohui Yiyuan Huiyi Jilu ji Changde Guangde Yiyuan Baogao [Conference of mission hospitals in Hunan and the Changde Guangde Hospital reports], HPA.

70. "Conference of Mission Hospitals in Hunan and Health Organizations Called by the Hunan Provincial Health Department in Leiyang," 1943, Hunan Provincial Health Department, HPA.

71. "Xiangya Huxiao Jianban Shehui Jiaoyu Gongzuo Baogaobiao" [Reports on the social educational activities of the Xiangya Nursing School], 1944, HYNS, and "Hunan sheng Sasi niandu geji Xuexiao Jianban Shehui Jiaoyu Jihua Bingbaobiao" [Plans and reports on Hunan schools' joint-education for the public in 1944], 1944, box 67-2-502, Hunan Provincial Education Department, Huxiao Tianbao Xuexiao Qingkuang Diaochabiao he Jianban Minzhong Jiaoyu Baogaobiao [Survey on the nursing school and report on its education to the public], HPA.

72. "Shadi Ru Shashu" [Killing enemy as if killing mouse], n.d., box 7A, Yuanling Health Department, Drawings, Paintings, and Cartoons with Primarily Anti-Japanese Themes, 1930s–1940s, Yale-China Association Records (RU 232), YUL.

73. Phillips-Johnson, *Childbirth in Republican China*, 35–72.

74. "Zhaosheng Jianzhang" [Admission information], July 1940, box 67-2-513, Huxiao Kaoshi he Ruxue de Wenjian [Nursing school's documents on exams and admissions], HPA.

75. Wu to Teachers Wang, Liu, and Chen, January 10, 1944, Xuesheng Gei Xuexiao Xinjian; Zhang to Rugh, January 15, 1942, 1939–1942 Zhang Xiaoqian Yu Guoji Jiujihui Yu Daocun deng Xinjian; Zhang to Balfour, April 10, 1942, and Rugh to Zhang, August 26, 1942, Zhang Xiaoqian Yu Luokefeilei Jijinhui Baerfu dengde Xin [Correspondence between Xiaoqian Zhang and Balfour from the Rockefeller Foundation . . .]—all in box 67-2-91, HPA; Huxiao Xuesheng gei Xuexiao Xinjian, 1943–44, HPA.

76. "Hsiang-Ya Hospital and College Reports," 1946, Phillips F. and Ruth A. Greene Papers (MS 797, 5/167), YUL; Shanqi Huang, *Xiangya lao gushi* [Old stories of Xiangya] (Changsha: Central South University Press, 2012), 245–60.

77. "A Life for China," n.d., box 3, file 80, China Council in California, Writings, William Winston Pettus Papers (MS 786), YUL; Shanqi Huang, *Xiangya lao gushi* [Old stories of Xiangya] (Changsha: Central South University Press, 2012), 245–60.

78. Xingshu Zhu, "Huxiao Sannian Shenghuo Duanji" [On the three years at the nursing school]; Taiyuan Wang, "Fayang Gaodu de Fuwu Jingshen [Developing a high level of spirit of service]; Erfa Ma and Zhitian Qi, "Yihu Tuanjie Jinxingqu" [The march of the unity between doctors and nurses], in *Xiangya Biye Jinian Kan* [The commemorative issue for the Hsiangya graduates], July 1950, MW 0257, Central South University Archives.

Chapter Seven

Frontiers of Immunology

Medical Migrations to Yunnan, Vaccine Research, and Public Health during the War with Japan, 1937–1945

MARY AUGUSTA BRAZELTON

In September 1938, a man named Tang Feifan drove into the southwestern Chinese city of Kunming. He was at the head of a convoy of six trucks that carried rabbits, glass bottleware, and a variety of scientific instruments. Tang's curious cargo was a consequence of his position as the new chief of the National Epidemic Prevention Bureau (NEPB), a Chinese government agency that developed, manufactured, and distributed vaccines. Originally stationed in Beijing and Nanjing, Tang and his staff had been forced to flee these cities as the Japanese army expanded its occupation of China during World War II. When China's Nationalist government fled to Chongqing in 1937 and established its wartime base of operations there, a variety of official bureaus, private companies, and institutions of higher learning also moved their personnel and offices to China's far southwest. Tang and his staff had joined this exodus. The NEPB set up temporary facilities in Changsha in 1937 but moved again the next year to Kunming, capital of Yunnan Province. Here, Tang faced the formidable challenge of reestablishing an institute that could provide wartime China with vaccines and sera while withstanding bombings, supply shortages, and epidemic outbreaks.

The road to Kunming was not lonely. Between 1937 and 1945, Kunming became a temporary home to a large population of biomedical experts, both Chinese and foreign. Yunnan's capital had quickly become a center

184 * MARY AUGUSTA BRAZELTON

of education and intellectual inquiry in the wartime Republic. In 1938, faculty and students at three of China's most prominent universities—Peking, Tsinghua, and Nankai—had established the Southwest National United University, or Lianda, in Kunming. Their precedent attracted other refugee institutions of higher education, and as a result, a number of prominent medical schools like the National Tongji University Medical College and the National Shanghai Medical College moved their wartime instruction to Yunnan. Biomedical experts streamed into Kunming from the west as well, joining the community of medical research and education that these schools and governmental institutes, like the National Epidemic Prevention Bureau, were building. As the eastern terminus of the wartime Burma Road, a strategic supply route crossing the Allied China-Burma-India military theater, Yunnan's capital also became a base of operations for international aid organizations. These groups, including the Rockefeller Foundation and the League of Nations Health Organization, contributed to the Nationalist cause via public health initiatives and research. A common endeavor soon bound together many of these institutes: the making of vaccines.

Vaccination demonstrates the increasingly extensive influence that Western medical science had on public health in twentieth-century China. Although provincial immunization rates remained generally low until after 1949, the development, production, and distribution of vaccines for smallpox, cholera, and other diseases became a common goal that united the variety of biomedical groups in Yunnan. In this chapter, I explore the identities of refugee scientists who found themselves in wartime Kunming, the development of a scientific community there that focused on vaccine development and distribution, and the impact of this group's work on the growing field of immunology worldwide. Although China's southwest had heretofore been a borderland at the fringes of modern public health and medical intervention, during the war the region became a laboratory space for biomedical research that shaped the rise of modern immunology in China. In the process, vaccines integrated Nationalist China into a global network of biomedical material circulation, providing grounds for transnational collaborations in which Chinese scholars actively participated in leading immunological studies.

Medical Migrations to Kunming

The universities and institutes that built temporary bases in Kunming included many of China's leading scientific organizations, and the biomedical researchers and physicians who came with these institutions stood among China's scientific elite. Their migrations indicated a reconfiguration of medical networks that united physicians, students, and researchers in one small city. In order to understand the impact of the wartime move to the southwest on these medical professionals and their work, it is critical to understand the careers that people like Tang Feifan and his colleagues spent their lives building before the Japanese invasion.

One of the most prominent medical organizations in wartime Kunming, the National Epidemic Prevention Bureau had been founded at Beijing's Temple of Heaven in 1919 in response to a 1917 plague outbreak in north China. Its work quickly grew over the next years to include manufacturing of sera and vaccines, biomedical research on communicable diseases, epidemiological data collection, and the development of vaccination campaigns.[1] When the Nationalist Party consolidated control over the Republic in 1927, the NEPB became part of efforts by policymakers to develop a national health infrastructure.[2] By the mid-1930s, it was "the primary agent" in efforts to control and eradicate communicable diseases in China. The bureau also grew physically, adding a new branch and moving its headquarters to Nanjing in 1935. By this time, its offices manufactured over forty different types of sera, vaccines, and antitoxins against human and animal diseases (notably cholera, plague, typhus, tuberculosis, and diphtheria in addition to smallpox) and exported products to Taiwan, Korea, and other sites in East Asia.[3]

When the NEPB was forced to transfer to Kunming, it brought established biomedical researchers to southwest China. Tang Feifan had supervised the move of bureau headquarters from Nanjing to Changsha and then to Kunming in 1938. Born in 1897 in Hunan, Tang was at the top of the first class to graduate from Xiangya Medical College. After postdoctoral training at Peking Union Medical College, he traveled to Harvard Medical School to work under a leading bacteriologist of the day, Hans Zinsser.[4] In 1936, Tang was also a visiting scientist in virology at London's National Institute for Medical Research, where he collaborated with Sir Henry Dale, winner of the 1936 Nobel Prize in medicine and renowned for his studies of ergot alkaloids, acetylcholine, and histamines.[5] Before taking up the leadership of the NEPB in 1937, Tang had served as head of the Department of Bacteriology at the Henry Lester Institute of Medical Research and as a faculty member of the Medical College at National Central University in Shanghai.[6]

Tang Feifan was a pioneering expert on bacteriology in China. In the early 1930s, he had won both respect and notoriety for his work attempting to isolate the agents that caused trachoma, reportedly going so far as to perform a series of inoculation experiments on his own eyes.[7] While he was stationed in the southwest, Dr. Robert Kesheng Lim—wartime head of the Chinese Red Cross Medical Relief Corps, Guiyang's Emergency Medical Service Training School, and the joint US-China Blood Bank in Kunming—described Tang as "the local authority on bacteriology and a good friend to all of us."[8] When the blood bank that Lim's Chinese Red Cross ran in

Kunming encountered problems of contamination, Lim requested that Tang personally check the quality of its samples. When in 1944 Joseph Needham visited wartime Kunming as the representative for the newly established Sino-British Science Cooperation Office, he described Tang as "well known to bacteriologists, immunologists and tropical disease specialists in England and America."[9]

Once head of the NEPB, Tang Feifan found himself in charge of an organization that had virtually bankrupted itself and for which safety was an ever-present concern. Wartime refugees brought skyrocketing inflation with them to southwest China. This caused severe shortages in the operating funds of wartime medical institutes. By 1945, Tang had to request US$12 million in emergency funds from the American Bureau for Medical Aid to China (ABMAC) to help cover a budget shortfall at the bureau. P. Z. King (Jin Baoshan), head of the Weishengshu, or National Health Administration (NHA), in Chongqing, added a note in support saying, "The price of biologicals cannot be increased to a level comparable with the increasing cost of manufacturing and transportation. This makes it especially difficult to produce enough to meet the wartime needs and to distribute to distant areas."[10] The NEPB faced a constant struggle to keep these prices artificially lowered. Moreover, the threat of Japanese invasion loomed large. In a 1947 speech at the postwar reopening of the bureau's original offices in Beijing, Tang reflected on his wartime days in Kunming saying, "During this time we underwent some of the most terrible experiences of our lives, when we had to prepare plague vaccine or to perform animal experiments with plague bacilli, without any protection from the enemy raiders." The rats that infested the Western Hills of Kunming, where the NEPB was given territory to build laboratories, and frequent Japanese air raids made Tang's work especially dangerous in light of western Yunnan's historical role as a disease well for bubonic plague.[11] Tang shared that responsibility with several close colleagues, particularly Wei Hsi, a senior specialist at the NEPB who also hailed from Hunan and Xiangya Medical College. Like Tang, Wei had also studied at the Lester Institute and Harvard with Zinsser.[12]

The medical schools that moved to Kunming also contributed new members to the city's growing community of biomedical experts. The nascent Yunnan University Medical College was joined in 1938 by the National Tongji University Medical College and National Shanghai Medical College. Both transplants from Shanghai, during the Nanjing Decade these medical schools had been involved in rural health demonstrations at Gaoqiao and Wusong, projects that sought to establish a small-scale model of modern public health administration that could eventually be applied across the nation.[13] In October 1938, the National Zhongshan Medical College, a medical school and research university in Guangzhou, came to Chengjiang County, Yunnan.[14] The National Zhongzheng Medical College, formerly of

Nanchang in Jiangxi Province and founded under the auspices of Robert Kesheng Lim, also moved to Kunming in autumn 1938. It had entered into a joint agreement with the Shanghai Medical College to form a conglomerated medical school there, making Yunnan a unique center for Chinese medical students and faculty.[15]

Very few of the scientists and doctors who came to Kunming would have seen themselves as "immunologists," even though since the early 1910s, Chinese experts had translated (mostly Japanese) texts and written their own treatises on the subject. By the 1930s, immunology in China was an emerging subfield of the biological sciences.[16] A 1933 volume, *Mianyixue yuanli* (Principles of immunology), published in Shanghai, gives an overview of knowledge about immunology in China before the war. The book distinguished between congenital and acquired immunity, describing the causes of antibacterial and antitoxin immunity and outlining debates between theories of humoral and cellular immunity that had evolved in Germany in the late nineteenth century.[17] In discussing these competing theories, *Mianyixue yuanli* demonstrated its authors' awareness of contemporary debates in the field of immunology.

The 1930s saw a proliferation of Chinese research, writing, and translation on immunology, bacteriology, microbiology, and related fields.[18] A dictionary of immunology and bacteriology published in 1937, *Xijunxue mianyixue mingci*, includes the German, English, French, and Japanese translations of key terms and lists the term that a committee of experts had chosen as the Chinese version for each.[19] Comparison with a similar dictionary published in 1918 provides an illustrative contrast: by 1937 "immunology" had its own section comprised of forty-nine terms. The newer dictionary dropped words for "immune agglutinin," "immune opsonin," and "inoculation" via lungs, stomach, muscles, and pleural cavity in favor of a focus on types and principles of immunity.[20] Terms that fell under the domain of "immunology" comprised just one section alongside the vocabularies of many other new subdivisions in the life sciences, such as toxicology, serology, bacteriology, and microbiology.

Translations and dictionaries were not the only forms in which knowledge about immunology was transmitted to medical spheres in Republican China. Magazines for medical and popular audiences offered Chinese-language introductions to the field at varying levels of specialized knowledge. For example, a 1931 article in the medical journal *Yiyao pinglun* (Medical review), outlined Ehrlich's "side-chain" theory. The theory suggested that all cells have special receptors or "side-chains" that have unique structures that permit the introduction of external nutrients to the nucleus. Ehrlich had argued that when these receptors combined with nonnutritious foreign matter or "antigens," the cell would overproduce the receptors, or "antibodies," and secrete them into tissue fluids.[21] The piece in *Yiyao pinglun* devoted

188 ♠ MARY AUGUSTA BRAZELTON

space to discussing the practical implications of the side-chain theory for individual adverse reactions to vaccination. It also detailed how, according to Ehrlich, vaccination produced immunity by creating antibodies that circulated in the blood.[22] These were by no means cutting-edge theories—Ehrlich had first published on the side-chain theory in 1897 in German—but their discussion in Chinese medical journals indicated that physicians of the early 1930s might find these principles of immunology relevant to clinical practice.[23]

Immunology was also a topic of interest for more casual Chinese readers in the 1930s. For instance, a 1931 article in the *Jisheng Yiyuan Yuebao* (Aid-life hospital monthly magazine) gave a basic overview of immunity and immunology using a question-and-answer format. Author Liang Guifang explained the three different kinds of immunity then accepted in medical literature: natural, inherited, and acquired. Liang devoted special attention to acquired immunity, explaining that it could develop in an individual either by contracting a contagious disease or by receiving vaccination, using cholera as an example.[24] Liang's use of simpler language indicated an attempt to communicate the basic concepts of immunity to a nonscientific audience that was less familiar with the specialized terminology of microbiology.

It was just as immunological research and discussion in China began to gain momentum that war forced the evacuation of many researchers to the southwest. Transferring to Kunming would not have been the first long-distance move for many of the Chinese scholars and professionals who fled there in the late 1930s. Most of them had undertaken advanced training at universities in the United States and Europe. But whereas previous journeys of these scholars and administrators to the West had generally kept them within elite intellectual circles, the move to remote Kunming was in character quite different.[25] It was born of exigency, not ambition. To the students and staff newly arriving there, Yunnan and its environs posed new medical, logistical, and social issues that evoked considerable trepidation and created logistical barriers to the establishment of research and manufacturing facilities.

Disease, a lack of equipment, shortages of funds, reduced living standards, inflation—all of these hardships connected medical personnel and researchers in Kunming and forced them to reach out across disciplines, regions, and national borders. The story of one team struggling to establish a medical school in nearby Guizhou Province aptly illustrates the wartime straits in which professors and scientists in southwest China found themselves. A 1940 article in the American *Science News Letter* gives a report by a "Tang Pei-sung" at "Tsing Hua University, Kunming, Yunnan Province [in a] remote corner of China": Following Nanjing's fall, Tang undertook "an arduous trip . . . during the coldest part of the year plus motoring over difficult robber-infested highways to Kweiyang to help start a medical school from nothing, absolutely nothing, except a 'hospital' of four beds and a group of determined men."[26] The article was adapted from a letter written by Tang Peisong, a plant physiologist at Lianda. His role in helping to build a medical school suggests the degree to which medical work in wartime China drew in anyone with remotely useful skills, even if their specific expertise lay well outside the clinical realm. "Six months later," the report continued, there was "a 'hospital' of over 100 beds, laboratories which compare well with any school in China in equipment, most of the apparatus improvised, such as the hand-made pneumothorax machine rigged up from junk shop parts."[27] While its hyperbolic tone underscored the hardships of working in the southwest, the report also suggested ways in which the move reconfigured professional networks for those working in medicine and the life sciences. That Lianda staff traveled to Guiyang to establish a new medical school indicates the growing role not only of Kunming, where many medical schools and research institutes were temporarily based, but also of other cities in China's southwest like Guiyang that were growing the capacity to house new medical infrastructure.[28] Although this chapter focuses on the role of Kunming, Nicole Barnes and John Watt have considered the growth of this new medical network across the wartime southwest more broadly.[29]

Kunming was not the only site of medical education, manufacturing, and research that formed in southwest China during the war. A new biomedical network emerged across China's hinterland, and the research and production of vaccines was a common endeavor that linked many nodes in this network. Chongqing became the center of Guomindang public health administration as home to the NHA, which provided financing and administrative oversight to vaccine production and distribution. Guiyang, capital of Guizhou Province, hosted a rich variety of military medical organizations: notably the Chinese Red Cross Medical Relief Corps and the Emergency Medical Service Training School, which included a pharmaceutical factory and laboratory to supply Guomindang troops with vaccines.[30] Along the northern front, Lanzhou was home to the Northwest branch of the NEPB, supplying the unoccupied northwestern hinterland with vaccines, drugs, and sera, as well as the National Northwest Medical School, Personnel Training Institute, and Hospital.[31] Vaccine work in Lanzhou focused on livestock as much as, if not more than, on humans, and the Lanzhou center oversaw substations in Qinghai, Gansu, and Ningxia.[32] The medical network that emerged during the war thus covered much of Guomindang-occupied territory.

Vaccination in the Wartime Southwest

As a critical part of wartime public health services, vaccination became a central focus for research, manufacturing, and clinical testing in Nationalist-occupied China. Consequently, researchers and physicians in wartime

Kunming began to see themselves as participants in the developing field of modern immunology—a field that was itself becoming critical to the changing relationship between public health and medical science in China's wartime southwest. Because vaccination at this time typically involved professional administration in a clinical setting, its implementation in local health programs required new, extensive cooperation with researchers and manufacturers. These collaborative efforts both formed new connections between Chinese organizations involved at the various stages of vaccine production and required new interactions with the wider Allied biomedical community.

The development, manufacture, and dissemination of vaccines took on new importance during the war because epidemics threatened so many zones of conflict. American scholar Dorothy Borg noted that the "primary wartime function" of the entire National Health Administration soon became the prevention of epidemics.[33] By 1938, cholera had ravaged Hubei, Hunan, and Jiangxi Provinces, and relapsing fever had spread across northwest China. Dysentery, plague, and malaria also troubled several critical regions.[34] Southwest China's legendarily unhealthy environment made vaccines a particularly critical instrument in fighting disease among military and civilian populations there. The malarial diseases associated with Yunnan's geography had made this region an enduring borderland, famously inhospitable to Chinese settlement and governance since the Qing era.[35] With good reason, wartime migrants to Kunming feared disease. Many students at Lianda, for example, contracted trachoma, typhoid fever, scarlet fever, and malaria after their arrival.[36] In 1939, the plague struck western Yunnan, and in 1942 a cholera outbreak ravaged the province. In addition to incurring the dangers of endemic illness, wartime migrations themselves changed the epidemiological map of China. The movements of soldiers and refugees into China's interior allowed contagious diseases such as cholera, typhoid, and plague to spread farther and faster.[37] In a 1943 article for the *Chinese Medical Journal*, P. Z. King noted that plague and cholera were the most serious epidemic threats facing the nation. At the same time, more mundane illnesses struck relentlessly, as he observed, "Under war conditions there have been serious outbreaks of typhus fever and relapsing fever among the soldiers and refugees."[38] The threat of epidemic outbreak was particularly serious in Yunnan, since it had become a key transport hub for communications between Nationalist China and the West.[39] King remarked that in the case of a 1942 cholera outbreak, the disease "rapidly spread along the main routes of communication" and followed the Yunnan-Burma Highway from Xiaguan to Kunming.[40]

As the threat of epidemic disease spread, vaccines became an important component of Nationalist resistance to Japan in the southwest. The need for both military and civilian populations to receive vaccinations against several key diseases was publicized in the media as well as through official channels. One 1941 radio broadcast in Chengdu, published in the wartime medical magazine *Zhanshi yizheng*, proclaimed, "The officers and men on the front, and fellow citizens at the rear, should have every man receive the cholera, dysentery, and typhoid vaccines' preventive injection."[41] King, as director general of the NHA, wrote in a *Xinyun daobao* article that one of the primary tenets of wartime public health was "to hold large-scale dissemination of smallpox inoculation and to inject vaccines for cholera, typhoid fever, etc," as well as to focus on public health education and environmental health.[42] King specifically stated in a discussion of recent wartime public health work that "the National Epidemic Prevention Bureau and Northwest Epidemic Bureaus are the NHA's two organs of vaccine and serum production," underscoring that vaccine production in Kunming was a key component of Nationalist antiepidemic strategy.[43]

Several epidemics in wartime Yunnan demonstrated just how important vaccine production had become by the early 1940s. When cholera broke out in 1942, vaccines were a first line of defense, and local authorities quickly turned to the wartime groups in Kunming for help. As soon as the first signs of the disease began to show up in rural towns like Zhongdian, the Yunnan Provincial Health Administration asked the NEPB to mail cholera vaccines to the Burma Road region. They also turned over stool samples from the local population to the NEPB to request that they confirm that the epidemic spreading across Yunnan was cholera, which the bureau did. Consequently, local government formed the Kunming Temporary Medical Treatment and Disease Prevention Committee, which met with local medical groups and organized free vaccinations through the Public Health Experimental Station.[44]

The NEPB eventually also supplied cholera vaccines to Yunnan's beleaguered public health authorities. The Yunnan Provincial Health Administration originally provided the immunizations—a total of 78,000 ml—and mailed them out to every county for use starting May 12. Within six days, all these supplies were exhausted. "Alternately, we continued to buy instead from the National Epidemic Prevention Bureau," one report noted, "purchasing a total of 120,000 mL, which lasted until June, but then we again bought 100,000 mL." The same report goes on to note that in Kunming, the vaccines were distributed to fourteen public and private hospitals for free immunizations. The Yunnan University Medical School, the Central No. 2 Military Medical School, Kunhua Advanced Medicine Occupational School, Tenth Disease Prevention Brigade, Provincial Instruction Group for Protecting Childbirth, and all organizations directly under the city public health bureau sent students or workers to organize thirty-three vaccination teams.[45] Aside from supplementing official stocks, the NEPB also published advertisements in the local medical journal *Yunnan yikan* (Yunnan medical journal), a publication intended for local physicians. The bureau sold vaccines for smallpox, cholera, rabies, typhoid combined vaccine, dysentery, meningitis, pertussis, plague, and others through a sales office at Jinbi Park, where Kunhua Hospital was also located.[46]

By August 1942, cholera vaccines made by the NEPB had been distributed by the Yunnan Experimental Public Health Department to almost every corner of the province, either directly or via subsidiary health organizations. The cholera vaccines that the NEPB supplied to local public health bureaus were also used in new, sometimes coercive ways. For instance, when people tried to enter or exit Yunnan, they had to supply a certificate showing proof of inoculation—or else be forcibly vaccinated.[47] Vaccine certificates became necessary to buy tickets for travel. One local public health magazine notes, "On May 5 it was announced to every communications organization: for ordinary people entering or leaving [the province], those without vaccination certificates are not allowed to buy train tickets and airplane tickets."[48] A detailed order explaining vaccine restrictions on travel was reprinted in the magazine in a later issue, underscoring its importance.[49] The requirement posed particular difficulties for laborers who came to work in new factories set up in Kunming, so factories assumed the responsibility of helping new workers get the necessary vaccine certificates, along with passports and visas.[50]

As part of antiepidemic work, vaccination in wartime China was much closer to medical treatment than other forms of public health, or *gonggong weisheng*. Vaccines were usually discussed as part of *fangyi* (disease prevention) or *fangzhi* (disease prevention and treatment). Following contemporaneous work in the West on "serotherapy" and "immunotherapy," scientists in China sought new ways of using vaccines not only as a means of preventing disease, but also as a way to cure it.[51] The perceived therapeutic value of vaccines affected the way that they fit into local public health measures. For instance, in one discussion of the effectiveness of NEPB vaccines, public health officials in Yunnan made a detailed analysis of the efficacy of vaccines in ameliorating the symptoms of cholera (see table 7.1). They observed that people who were vaccinated could still get sick, but at much lower rates than those who had not been immunized, and those who received more injections of the vaccine got sick at proportionally lower rates.[52] Officials thus noted the vaccines' efficacy in clinical terms of medical *treatment* and not just prevention, speaking to the murky area between treatment and prevention of disease that vaccines occupied.

In wartime China, vaccines served both therapeutic and preventive aims, but the protection against cholera that they provided was likely limited to a year or two. The type of cholera vaccine then used worldwide had been developed by German researcher Wilhelm Kolle; in 1902, Kolle had claimed that large-scale use of his vaccine in Japan was 80 percent effective, but his study lacked a control.[53] It was only in 1963 that controlled studies in

Table 7.1. Biological products of National Epidemic Prevention Bureau, 1937–41

Item	July 1937–June 1938	July–Dec. 1938	Jan.–June 1939	July–Dec. 1939	Jan.–June 1940	July–Dec. 1940	Jan.–June 1941	July–Dec. 1941
Cholera vaccine	2,973,000	1,075,410	381,820	1,070,089	4,170,000	359,500	2,174,320	423,960
Typhoid-paratyphoid combined vaccine			227,240	46,482	48,000	110,000	22,150	8,600
Cholera-typhoid combined vaccine (TABC)	3,680,000	759,400	2,750,880	5,021,569	1,530,000	160,000	6,339,480	1,380,900
Cholera-typhoid-paratyphoid combined vaccine	1,340,000	140,480	233,160	189,160	180,240	250,000		110,080
Dysentery vaccine	60,000		8,120	14,169			33,790	
Gonococcus vaccine	35,540		1,180	2,820	1,920	5,100	9,485	
Meningococcus vaccine	94,400				32,090	6,340	13,341	70,359
Pertussis vaccine	7,650		2,520	340	2,100	1,500	547,850	11,558
Plague vaccine	80,000		4,750	10,289			5,250	1,011,440
Staphylococcus vaccine	18,900		2,260	249				
Streptococcus vaccine	9,720		1,740		12,000	1,300	14,094	1,781
Rabies vaccine (for human)	11,270	2,156	3,628	7,904	12,680	6,940		14,760
Rabies vaccine (for dog)	1,820	182	511		480	190		180
Smallpox vaccine	142,885.333	34,420	1,296,172	614,676	1,062,168	591,870	734,160	830,011
Normal horse serum	23,200				4,000	18,800	27,000	
Anti-meningococcus serum	182,000	7,360	43,700	36,760	91,500	97,100	61,500	36,400
Anti-dysentery serum	70,250	42,310	18,040	11,810	17,045	84,600	37,500	24,000
Anti-streptococcus serum	58,159		9,280	5,000	17,660			

Table 7.1. (*continued*)

Item	July 1937–June 1938	July–Dec. 1938	Jan.–June 1939	July–Dec. 1939	Jan.–June 1940	July–Dec. 1940	Jan.–June 1941	July–Dec. 1941
Anti-scarlatina serum	27,950			2,369	10,000	18,700	8,800	
Anti-plague serum				3,469			41,000	18,000
Anti-tetanus serum					3,038,200			
Concentrated diphtheria antitoxin	29,950		15,002,000	8,769,000	29,772	4,108,000	9,500,000	
Diphtheria antitoxin	146,070	5,187,000	4,986,500	498,000	1,904,440	16,125,400		17,937,500
Concentrated tetanus antitoxin	9,000			5,684,000	17,710	2,211,000	16,100,000	
Tetanus antitoxin	611,440	20,179,500		1,763,000	7,620	6,119,000	15,560,000	7,500,000
Diagnostic suspension, B Typhosus, "H" Antigen	25,370		3,760	9,560	7,500	5,960	9,640	20,289
Diagnostic suspension, B Typhosus, "O" Antigen	24,850	80		9,680	5,000	9,560		10,160
Diagnostic suspension, B Paratyphosus, "A"	23,900	40	4,760	9,360	7,590		7,690	10,140
Diagnostic suspension, B Paratyphosus, "B"	30,000		3,520	9,440	5,000		5,320	10,160
Diagnostic suspension, B Proteus X2 for Weil-Felix Test	13,000		4,680	9,640		9,560		20,208
Diagnostic suspension, B Proteus X19 for Weil-Felix Test	15,000		4,600	9,480		9,720		26,200
Diagnostic suspension for Typhus				4,440		10,280		
Diagnostic serum, V. Cholera	293	27	10	5	26	26	24	
Diagnostic serum, B. Dysenteriae	103	39	10	89		213		

Table 7.1. (*continued*)

Item	July 1937–June 1938	July–Dec. 1938	Jan.–June 1939	July–Dec. 1939	Jan.–June 1940	July–Dec. 1940	Jan.–June 1941	July–Dec. 1941
Diagnostic suspension, B. Meningococcus			15					
Diagnostic suspension, B. Typhosus	349	40	10	20	58	80	25	34
Diagnostic suspension, B Paratyphosus, "A"	183	36	5	8	22	76	39	12
Diagnostic suspension, B Paratyphosus, "B"	129	28	5	2	27	128	57	19
Antigen for Kahn Precipitation Test	11,880	3,700	3,380	2,310	5,250	4,500	6,940	3,510
Antigen for Wassermann Test			4,080					
Antigen for Dick Test			147	165		1,000	3,305	
Antigen for Schick Test			78	184	2,545	1,970	700	1,590
diphtheria precipitate toxoid					16,330		29,000	155,000
Distilled water	3,850						40,400	80,000
Diagnostic serum, Pneumococcus, Type III	34	55						
Tetanus toxin						89,780		
Tetanus toxoid						17,650		
Scarlatina toxin						16,400		
Scarlatina toxoid	7,500					9,500		
Diphtheria toxin						142,950		
Diphtheria toxoid	10,000			850		61,500		
Alum toxoid for diphtheria						11,700		

Table 7.1. (continued)

Item	July 1937–June 1938	July–Dec. 1938	Jan.–June 1939	July–Dec. 1939	Jan.–June 1940	July–Dec. 1940	Jan.–June 1941	July–Dec. 1941
Sheep amboceptor	76			2				
Sterile physiological salt solution	7,920			1,289,000				
Cholera vaccine (containing 2 bil. bacteria @cc)	555,000							
Cholera vaccine (containing 6 bil. bactera @cc)	2,418,000							
TABC (3 bil. bacteria @cc)	2,689,000							
TABC (4 bil. bacteria @cc)	1,000,000							
Triple typhoid vaccine	560,000							
Diagnostic serum, B. Dysenteriae Polyvalent	360							
Diagnostic serum, B. Dysenteriae Shiga	95							
Diagnostic serum, B. Dysenteriae Y	120							
Diagnostic serum, Meningococcus, Polyvalent	40							
Diagnostic serum, Pneumococcus, Type I	87							
Diagnostic serum, Pneumococcus, Type II	65							
Tuberculin	520							

Source: Tongji yuebao 1939 (38, 39), 1940 (41, 42, 48), 1941 (55), 1942 (73–74), Shanghai Library, Shanghai.
Note: Quantities are in milliliters. Units for smallpox are in dozens; units for Schick and Dick Tests are in portions.

Pakistan and Manila found that Kolle's vaccine was effective for approximately one year in areas where cholera was endemic, and about 30 percent effective during outbreaks of cholera in nonendemic regions.[54] Information on the combined cholera-typhoid TABC (or CTAB) vaccine that the NEPB also distributed is less clear on questions of efficacy.[55] However, given that killed whole bacterial cell vaccines such as TABC are generally seen today as "associated with high toxicity and limited duration of immunity," the combined vaccine—and other immunizations produced using similar methods, including many antiplague vaccines—likely also had limited effectiveness.[56]

Cholera was not the only epidemic that evoked a massive coordinated response, centered around vaccination, from the many refugee medical organizations based in Kunming. When plague struck western Yunnan in 1939, efforts quickly arose to subdue the epidemic since it affected the strategically critical Burma Road. A Western Yunnan Plague Prevention and Treatment Committee quickly formed, and drew members from the Medical Supervisory Division and Headquarters Supply Office of the US Military Base in China, the Chinese Red Cross, the American Red Cross Public Friendship First Aid Brigade, the Chinese Army Headquarters Office of Public Health, the NEPB, the China-India Public Road–Eastern Part Guard Headquarters, the Sixth Administrative Division Experts, the Tengchong County Government, and the Yunnan Department of Public Health.[57] In Baoshan, where the plague struck hard, local public health authorities purchased over 300,000 cc of plague vaccine, which between June and August 1946 the Yunnan Public Health Department Disease Prevention Brigades, county public health clinics, and "every doctor in business" distributed to the masses for free. "The effectiveness of these preventive injections is clear not only in terms of the clinical statistics," reported Chen Shiguang, "but also in that afterwards, the masses also had a much better understanding of it. When I went to inspect the area, the commoners mostly urgently wished that they could get the fresh vaccine injected."[58] Yunnanese thus not only received vaccines from wartime institutes in Kunming, but also apparently learned at least some information about their immunity-producing roles in the science and clinical application of immunology.

The Rise of New Alliances and Methods
in Immunological Research

As the NEPB and other institutions developed vaccine research and production endeavors in Kunming, they attempted to adhere to models of standardization, efficiency, and innovation. In 1937, NEPB staff had hauled six trucks' worth of rabbits and guinea pigs all the way from Nanjing in order to standardize vaccines and sera in the new Kunming facility.[59] Standardization also required strict sterilization, and the NEPB invested substantial time and resources into maintaining sterile conditions. Needham said of the NEPB: "[It] maintains high standards of cleanliness in the stables and animal houses in spite of the lack of any running water supply."[60] To prevent impurities in the manufacturing process, the bureau went so far as to build its own makeshift glass factory.[61] It also tried to make its vaccines efficient to produce, a difficult task given that wartime inflation made medical manufacturing a business with high overhead. "One of our main problems," one staff member wrote, "is to find a source of supply of the commonly used products such as tetanus antitoxin, T. A. B. vaccine, diphtheria vaccine . . . that does not result in their being, when delivered here, four or five times the price of the former N. E. P. B. supplies."[62] And another noted, "It was found during a temporary shortage of unvaccinated rabbits that guinea pigs are also a suitable animal for the titration of smallpox vaccine."[63] Efficiency in wartime thus faltered, or required innovation with scarce resources.

The bureau's wartime accomplishments were significant for a perpetually underfunded ad hoc laboratory—although vaccination rates in Yunnan Province remained far below 100 percent of the population. For instance, by June 1942, Yunnan provincial authorities had overseen 335,986 anticholera vaccinations, a number that represented less than 3 percent of the provincial population of 12 million.[64] Yet vaccine production figures for Yunnan suggested a substantial increase in immunization rates there, as compared to conditions before the war. According to *Statistics Monthly*, from July 1937 to December 1941, the bureau produced approximately 1.2 million ml of cholera vaccine, almost 500,000 ml of typhoid-paratyphoid combined vaccine, 2.2 million ml of TABC, more than 1 million ml of plague vaccine, and almost 64 million doses of smallpox vaccine (see table 7.1).[65] For the years 1942 and the first half of 1943, the NEPB reported new production figures to ABMAC, which included 6.6 million cc of cholera vaccine, 4.2 million cc of TABC, and 1.4 million capsules of smallpox vaccine (see table 7.2).[66] For comparison, in 1931 the provincial government of Yunnan had reported that just twenty thousand citizens had received the smallpox vaccine; in 1942 the NEPB produced almost fifty times that many, or 960,622 capsules of the vaccine.[67] Medical journals in Yunnan reported steadily on the work of the NEPB and other medical organizations in Kunming. "Since the NEPB moved to Yunnan, it has worked hard to carry out all work," wrote one local physician in *Yunnan yikan*, "and as every place needs large quantities of every kind of vaccine and smallpox inoculation, they have really worked overtime to hasten production. Now they have already produced smallpox vaccine, and distributed it to every medical service site. Furthermore, their prices are relatively inexpensive."[68] For Yunnan—a place that had heretofore remained on the fringes of central public health measures—the work of the NEPB and other wartime medical institutes in Kunming signaled a significant change.

Table 7.2. Biological products of National Epidemic Prevention Bureau, 1942–43

Item	Unit	1942	Jan.–June 1943
Cholera vaccine	cc	4,055,000	2,520,000
Typhoid vaccine	"	3,725,000	0
cholera-typhoid combined vaccine	"	3,810,000	375,000
Typhoid and paratyphoid vaccine	"	110,000	170,000
Typhoid, paratyphoid and cholera vaccine	"	260,000	150,000
Plague vaccine	"	5,099,500	0
Smallpox vaccine	capsule	960,622	421,752
Anti-streptococcus serum	cc	2,680	0
Anti-meningococcus serum	cc	40,000	50,000
Anti-dysentery serum	"	40,000	30,000
Anti-plague serum	"	111,500	10,000
Tetanus antitoxin	IU	25,453,900	3,100,000
Diphtheria antitoxin	"	37,979,200	4,395,000
Tetanus alum toxoid	cc	6,000	2,500
Diphtheria toxoid	"	4,000	0
Diphtheria alum	"	4,000	0
Rinderpest vaccine	"	0	0

Source: "Report of Anti-Epidemic Activities for 1942–43, National Health Administration, January 1, 1942, to June 30, 1943," box 20, American Bureau for Medical Aid to China Records, Columbia University Rare Book & Manuscript Library, New York.

In addition to ensuring continued mass production, bureau staff and collaborators developed new immunizations and novel methods of making vaccines. For instance, Wei Hsi collaborated with the American Anti-Typhus Commission in Burma and military medical researchers at Guiyang on projects to develop a vaccine against typhoid fever.[69] The NHA wrote of progress in developing a new smallpox vaccine by using penicillin, streptomycin, and phenol-glycerine to reduce the original NEPB vaccine's virus content.[70] Wei Hsi published a paper in 1947 explaining his work with Tang Feifan in developing a new, faster method to prepare smallpox vaccine using gum acacia. He noted that the exigencies of war had demanded their development of the new method, saying, "During the war (1937–1945) there was such a constant, urgent and heavy demand by both the military and civilian medical services for this vaccine, that [the prior preparatory] method was considered too slow to cope with the requirements."[71] The bureau also became the first unit to domestically produce penicillin in China. In September 1944, Tang and collaborators at the NEPB manufactured the drug using mold samples from "clothes, boots, bean curd, meat broth, and shoe polish," as well as strains imported from India.[72]

Other wartime refugee organizations in Kunming contributed to biomedical research there, and vaccines were an important component of this work. The National Tongji University Medical College sent students to serve on the Yunnan Provincial Public Health Department's disease prevention teams, injecting vaccines that the NEPB had created.[73] Some Lianda students set up local public health stations.[74] The Zhongzheng Medical College and the National Shanghai Medical College cooperated in opening a local clinic in Kunming, as well as an experimental public health station in the eastern Yunnan town of Qujing.[75] The Nationalist government's Epizootic Epidemic Prevention Station at Kunming also manufactured and sold vaccines for livestock, seeking in part to prevent the transmission of animal-borne diseases like rabies and diphtheria to humans.[76] The Central Drug Research Institute, Nationalist China's official pharmacological research group, set up shop near the NEPB in Xishan and began researching drugs that could be produced from local plants and that might be of use for emergency medicine.[77]

Cooperation between civilian and military medical institutes in Kunming was a major aspect of vaccine work (and, indeed, of all biomedical research) there. After the war, Tang praised the "very cordial relationships" that had grown between the US armed forces in Yunnan and Chinese laboratories there, saying, "Besides supplying them with our biological products, we also performed various laboratory tests for them, while they in turn helped to solve many of our transportation difficulties by getting us supplies over the 'Hump' . . . and in flying vaccines and sera to different parts of China, Burma, and India." Cooperation with Chinese military forces was intrinsic to research and development in Kunming. Tang described the NEPB's priorities in distributing vaccines as "first to supply the needs of our own fighting forces, then the allied armed personnel and finally to our civilians."[78] When the military-organized joint US-China Blood Bank in Kunming experienced troubles over a case of contaminated plasma in 1944, Robert Lim turned to Tang as a resident expert. In a report to ABMAC, Lim wrote, "We felt it was imperative that every sample of plasma should be checked by Tang in order to protect the Bank and ABMAC, as well as to restore confidence on the part of the Army and public. . . . Dr. Tang has promised that he will carry out checks and thus in a measure clear you of all responsibility should samples be contaminated after they leave your hands."[79] Lim thus relied on Tang to take on accountability for the integrity of the blood bank, although it is not clear that Tang himself saw the situation in precisely the same light.

The NEPB also benefited from cooperation between Tang and Lim, particularly in terms of its work with penicillin production. Although ABMAC had originally planned to develop a penicillin plant of its own in China, the work that Tang had already done with strains from India was encouraging enough that the NEPB and the US-China Blood Bank pooled their resources and set up a joint project to foster further work.[80] Lim advocated for ABMAC to divert funding and supplies for its penicillin plant to the NEPB, saying, "If . . . we might get enough equipment, we might use the Epidemic Prevention Bureau and set up a real plant."[81] ABMAC members agreed, recording in a 1944 report that rather than developing its own pilot plant, they would "support Dr. F. F. Tang, who is producing penicillin in China, by buying equipment for him and sending Dr. Tsun Tung back to China as soon as possible to help in the production of penicillin there."[82] The penicillin project thus strengthened the NEPB's funding situation, as well as its ties with military medical programs.

International aid organizations that were based in Kunming or that involved Kunming-based researchers helped shape vaccine production into a research endeavor that fell squarely within immunology. Tang sent staff abroad to gain more knowledge and research experience in the production of vaccines; international agencies in Kunming facilitated such foreign exchanges for Chinese scholars. For instance, the Rockefeller Foundation sponsored Wei Hsi's travel to the United States Typhus Commission in Mytikyna, Burma, to study scrub typhus with US military medical researchers, and Huang Youwei's journey to Bombay's Haffkine Institute to study plague vaccine manufacture.[83] These international exchanges sought to rectify specific problems that the NEPB faced in its vaccine research and development, but also allowed bureau staff to form new connections to global networks of immunology and bacteriology.[84]

While Chinese scholars traveled widely in search of relevant experience and information, world organizations also came to their doorstep to provide medical aid and collaboration. On October 5, 1937, a special subcommittee of the League of Nations Health Committee meeting in Geneva decided to pursue "anti-epidemic action" in wartime China. A rare project undertaken in the twilight years of the League, the scheme placed three public health teams, led by experts, or "Epidemic Commissioners," and equipped with sufficient medical matériel, at the disposal of the Nationalist government to send wherever it saw fit.[85] As part of its support of these medical teams, the League of Nations committee also provided cholera vaccines to China from all over the world after the 1938 outbreak of the disease. The Secretariat of the League of Nations advertised the need for 6 million doses of the vaccine in China and soon collected donations from a variety of national bacteriological institutes, ranging from Australia to the State Serum Institute of Copenhagen, the Cantacuzene Institute of Bucharest, and the Egyptian Ministry of Health. In accepting donations of vaccine from such a wide variety of global partners, the NHA demonstrated that vaccines in wartime China were part of a global circulation of medical resources.[86]

The public health aid from the League of Nations was subsidiary to China's National Health Administration, and thus was part of the larger medical network that had developed across China's southwest with nodes at Guiyang, Chongqing, Lanzhou, and other cities. The NHA in Chongqing directly supervised the NEPB, monitoring its funding and the travels of its employees. The NHA sent its own staff to Kunming to buy vaccine for local rabies outbreaks in Chongqing.[87] Outside Chongqing, the Lanzhou Northwest Epidemic Prevention Bureau (NWEPB) fell under the directorship of Yang Yung-nien, who like Tang had worked with Sir Henry Dale in London.[88] The NWEPB, although semiautonomous vis-à-vis financing and day-to-day activities, remained subsidiary to the NEPB and sent reports on the state of its facilities to Kunming.[89] Tang also sent Wei Hsi from Kunming to Guiyang to work on studies of scrub typhus.[90] Tang also personally visited army camps outside Kunming, underscoring the bureau's attention to military medical work.[91]

Researchers based in Kunming traveled widely outside Yunnan's capital, but many Chinese biomedical experts also came to visit them. Between April 2 and 5, 1940, the Chinese Medical Association held its Fifth General Conference in Kunming.[92] Underscoring Kunming as a critical hub in China's wartime medical networks, this conference served as an exposition of medical research, education, and practice in the city. "An attractive programme of sight-seeing and entertainments were arranged. Medical colleges, hospitals, and other institutions in Kunming acted as hosts to the delegates," noted one report.[93] Attendees visited the medical colleges that had moved to Yunnan, local public health organizations, hospitals, and the NEPB headquarters at Xishan. They also presented papers on wartime medical relief, education, public health, clinical medicine, pathology, and pharmacology. Epidemic prevention was a major focus of the meeting, and many staff from the NEPB presented their recent work. Tang gave a paper on his work accelerating the development of smallpox lymph in order to hasten vaccine production, and Wei Hsi spoke about "the so-called two weeks fever in Kunming in relation to typhus." Senior bureau researchers Wang Youwei and Chen Dinghong discussed the reuse of agar-agar for cultures in emergency conditions, a procedure they had adopted as a result of wartime supply shortages.[94] Over four hundred delegates, students, and guests attended the conference, including consular officials from Britain, France, and the United States; representatives from the Yunnan provincial civil administration, Department of Education, Vice Minister of Health Jin Baoshan; and

Department of Military Medicine president Lu Zhide.[95] The next meeting of the Chinese Medical Association would not occur until 1943, in Chongqing. The Kunming conference in 1940 was thus one of the major opportunities for China's national medical community to convene and exchange news and findings. It also emphasized the importance of wartime organizations in Kunming as hosts of the meeting—as well as wartime Yunnan as an important laboratory space for medical research.

The *Gongyi* Ideal: Implications of Wartime Vaccine Work for Health Policy

The collaboration that marked Kunming's wartime biomedical institutes— between civilian and military, elites and ordinary locals, researchers and physicians, Chinese and foreigners—suggest that Yunnan had become a space for extensive biomedical exploration and experimentation. That space had also given rise to a new model of public health policymaking in China, one that entailed sustained and extensive involvement of biomedical research and development in routine public health measures. Vaccination research and implementation exemplified this dynamic, but it was also evident in other projects like Tang Feifan's development of penicillin, the NEPB's collaboration with Robert Lim's blood bank, and the roles that refugee medical students played in local public health stations.

Writing a few days after the 1940 meeting of the Chinese Medical Association, physician M. C. Balfour noted this shift in southwest China and placed it in the context of *gongyi zhidu*, or "the system of state medicine." Balfour wrote, "Though [*gongyi*] is not the official policy of the government, the question has already been decided in the South-west, and there is no doubt that every doctor is engaged in some sort of public service there. . . . This explains in a way the great importance being attached to Public Health and Preventive Medicine in medical education."[96] *Gongyi* represented a new system of state-run, socialized health administration that stirred considerable debate on the part of physicians and health officials in wartime China. Its central tenet was that the government should provide free, equitable health care to all citizens.[97] In terms of policy, discussions over *gongyi* provided a signal that even in their southwestern exile, health experts in China were growing ever more engaged with the global medical community, as they reckoned with questions of the government's role in health care that nations across the world were grappling with.[98]

Medical work and collaboration in Yunnan suggested a different way to approach the *gongyi* ideal than previous models. Ka-che Yip has discussed the early development of *gongyi* in China during the 1920s, when medical elites in Beijing and Shanghai developed rural county health models at Dingxian,

Gaoqiao, and Wusong. From 1929, the NHA sought to institute similar county-based health programs that would provide basic health services to residents.[99] But the *xian* health system had quickly run into numerous problems, chiefly due to a persistent lack of funds that prevented it from reaching its goals. In his study of medical education in wartime China, John R. Watt argues that the exigencies of war made *gongyi* a "much more immediate challenge" for medical students and professors, and that although these few could only continue to provide basic services and prophylactic measures, they did preserve *gongyi* as an active ideal.[100] Balfour suggested that biomedical work in wartime southwest China indicated a significant step toward establishing *gongyi* insofar as it integrated private interests with public needs. Kunming—where private medical students, physicians, and academic research scientists contributed time and labor to help provide the local population with medicines, health services, and vaccines—provided an example of such a dynamic.

The lasting effects of biomedical research and development in wartime Kunming are difficult to gauge given the subsequent upheavals of civil war and Communist revolution, but vaccination did remain a critical aspect of epidemic prevention throughout the postwar era. Many of the scientists and students who had sought temporary refuge in Yunnan returned to their prewar homes in Beijing, Nanjing, and Shanghai, where they reassumed positions of prominence. After the war and establishment of the People's Republic of China (PRC) in 1949, the National Epidemic Prevention Bureau changed its name to become the National Vaccine and Serum Institute in Beijing (Beijing shengwu zhipin yanjiu suo), which survives today as a research group specializing in immunology and serology. Tang Feifan retained his leadership there until his death in 1958.[101] Health policy in the early PRC certainly stressed vaccines as part of preventive health, making the practice of inoculation a goal in its own right. Republican authors had tended to include vaccination in discussions of individual diseases, usually as one of many preventive strategies. In contrast, in the 1950s, public health guides—several penned by scientists who had worked in Kunming during the war—discussed vaccines and immunology independently of specific disease etiologies, encouraging the use of vaccines as a necessary tool to prevent epidemics.[102]

The Effects of Wartime Vaccination on Immunology in China

The work of the NEPB and other organizations during the war brought new methods, concepts, and resources to the field of immunology in China. It also brought Chinese professionals in the field into more extensive working relationships with immunological experts across the world. In Yunnan, wartime science popularized the practices and concepts that comprised immunology. As "immunology" rose as a distinct field, the concepts that constituted it became more prevalent in local medical discourse. The terms for "immunity," *mianyixing* and *mianyili*, began to appear more often in medical writing during and after the war. Discussions of the etiology, treatment, and prevention of specific diseases often dedicated entire sections to "immunity," discussing whether vaccines were available for a particular illness and other means by which immunity might be attained. For instance, one article on smallpox notes, "After one instance of inoculation . . . immunity against smallpox will be supported for about five years."[103] As in the case of the Baoshan plague, the actual practice of vaccination also served to disseminate popular knowledge about immunity and vaccines' roles in producing it.

Wartime vaccine development in Kunming also changed the way that those who made the vaccines saw their work and presented it to others. At this time, vaccine production was generally described as the production of "biological products," alongside production of drugs, cultures, and other organic materials used for research. A 1940 advertisement for the NEPB in the local medical journal *Yunnan yikan* touts the bureau as a developer of biological products that is also active in "researching bacteriology and immunology." The ad goes on to claim that the bureau "takes the utmost care to do research, and has expertly produced every kind of biological product, and consults and follows the newest international methods."[104] Comparison with a 1935 advertisement for the NEPB, which merely describes the bureau as a maker of sera, vaccines, and medical equipment, demonstrates that it was in Kunming that NEPB staff first presented themselves to potential buyers as an institute specializing in immunology and bacteriology.[105] That the NEPB changed its name to the National Vaccine and Serum Institute seems to underscore the increasing importance it attributed to its work in immunology and serology.

The war also marked a turning point when Chinese immunologists began increasingly translating from English-language (as opposed to Japanese) works and a period in which they worked more extensively with US colleagues. In the 1930s and 1940s, Chinese medical journals were filled with translations from the *New England Journal of Medicine* and *American Journal of Public Health*. Although Chinese scientists had long been making journeys to the United States for study, the arrival of US military and philanthropic medical experts in southwest China provided new avenues for exchange. As discussed above, Wei Hsi's work in Mytikyna at the United States Typhus Commission, his and Chen Dinghong's Rockefeller Foundation–funded journeys to India to study vaccine manufacture, and support offered by ABMAC all provided new venues for exchange between American and

Chinese scholars of immunology. And this dynamic was one of exchange, not simple technology or knowledge transfer. The war also marked the point at which Chinese scientists made increasingly important contributions to experimental immunology. The hardships of war encouraged innovation to the point that researchers at the NEPB published a considerable amount of work during this era in domestic and foreign journals, most notably Wei Hsi's progress developing smallpox and typhus vaccines.[106]

Vaccine research and development in wartime Kunming produced new knowledge about immunology, especially the means to produce vaccines and sera under less than ideal conditions that provided immunity against the particular diseases that affected Yunnan. This was only possible through extensive cooperation that stretched from Kunming across Guomindang-occupied territory, among research scientists, medical students and physicians, military and philanthropic medical organizations, and local public health groups. As a laboratory space where a variety of domestic and international teams carried out exploration and research, China's wartime southwest played a critical role in the nation's growing immunological community, as well as the interactions of that community with a global network of experts in the life sciences. Immunological R & D in this Chinese space contributed to the globalization of biomedicine because it not only contributed new knowledge about how to make vaccines under severe constraints of matériel and money, but also because it provided justification for collaboration between a variety of actors, Chinese and foreign, who would become postwar players in a global immunological community.

Notes

1. Ka-che Yip, *Health and National Reconstruction in Nationalist China: The Development of Modern Health Services, 1928–1937* (Ann Arbor, MI: Association for Asian Studies, 1995), 16.

2. Ibid., 5.

3. Ibid., 109.

4. Guangsheng Cheng, Ming Li, and George F. Gao, "Recollection: 'A Friend to Man,' Dr. Feifang Tang: A Story of Causative Agent of Trachoma, from 'Tang's Virus' to Chlamydia Trachomatis, to 'Phylum Chlamydiae,'" *Protein Cell* 2, no. 5 (2011): 349–50.

5. Wu Anran and Xie Shaowen, "In Memory of Professor Tang Fei-fan," *Chinese Medical Journal* 100, no. 6 (1987): 512; Joseph Needham Photographs—Wartime China, 1942–1946, photo SWEST/8 caption: "Scientists and technical staff of the NEPB/National Epidemics Prevention Bureau (Zhong yang fang yi chu) at Hsishan (Xishan) near Kunming," January 1, 1945, accessed February 22, 2013, http://www.nri.org.uk/JN_wartime_photos/all.htm. See also "Obituary Notices: Sir Henry Dale, O.M., G.B.E., D.Sc., LL.D., M.D., F.R.C.P., F.R.S.," *British Medical Journal* 3, no. 5613 (August 3, 1968): 318–21.

6. Cheng, Li, and Tao, "Recollection," 349. Tang would go on to discover, in 1955, the virus strain that causes trachoma.

7. Ibid.

8. Letter from Dr. Robert Lim to Dr. Yi Chien-Lung, Kunming, December 5, 1944, American Bureau for Medical Aid to China Records, 1937–1979, box 2, Columbia University Rare Book & Manuscript Library, New York [hereafter cited as ABMAC Records].

9. Joseph Needham, "Article II: Science in South-west China," in *Science Outpost* (London: Pilot Press, 1948), 88–89.

10. F. F. Tang and P. Z. King, "A Request for Subsidies for Increased Production of Vaccines and Sera and Their Distribution," January 25, 1945, box 2, ABMAC Records.

11. Carol Benedict, *Bubonic Plague in Nineteenth-Century China* (Stanford, CA: Stanford University Press, 1996).

12. "Wei Xi," *Zhonghua renmin gongheguo renwu cidian 1949–1989* [Dictionary of persons in the People's Republic of China], ed. Wang Naizhuang and Wang Deshu (Beijing: Zhongguo jingji chubanshe, 1989), 580. See also Joseph Needham, "Manuscript Notes on Visits to Institutions," Papers and Correspondence of Joseph Needham, CH FRS, Record Group (RG) C.63, Cambridge University Archives, Cambridge, UK.

13. Ka-che Yip, "Health and Nationalist Reconstruction: Rural Health in Nationalist China, 1928–1937," *Modern Asian Studies* 26, no 2 (May 1992): 402.

14. Wang Yuanchen, "Chuxi Zhonghua yixuehui di wu jie da hui ji canguan dian zhu yiyao weisheng" [Attending the Chinese Medical Association's Fifth General Conference and taking a look at medicine and public health in Yunnan and Guiyang], *Yiyu* [Medical education] 4, no. 2 (1940): 5.

15. Sun Daixing and Wu Baozhang, eds., *Yunnan kangri zhanzheng shi: A History of Anti-Japanese War in Yunnan* (Kunming, China: Yunnan daxue chubanshe, 2005), 274.

16. The few Chinese who were actively researching in the field included Liu Sizhi and Xie Shaowen at the Peking Union Medical College and Yu He and Lin Feiqing, both in Shanghai. Cao Xuetao, "Immunology in China: The Past, Present, and Future," *Nature Immunology* 9, no. 4 (April 2008): 329–43.

17. The cellular theory of immunity, advocated by Elie Metchnikoff of the Paris Pasteur Institute, claimed that immunity resulted from macrophages and microphages, now known as polymorphonuclear leukocytes. The humoral theory, in contrast, argued that "only the soluble substances of the blood and other body fluids" caused immunity. It was endorsed by Robert Koch and most researchers at the Koch Institute in Berlin. Arthur Silverstein, "History of Immunology: Cellular versus Humoral Immunity; Determinants and Consequences of an Epic 19th-Century Battle," *Cellular Immunology* 48 (1979): 208–21. See also Arthur Silverstein, *History of Immunology* (London: Elsevier, 1989). Similar Chinese volumes include *Xijunxue zonglun ji mianyixue—Allgemeine Bakteriologie und Immunologie* [A general introduction to bacteriology and immunology] (Cheng Muyi: Tongde Yixueyuan, 1937).

18. For an overview of this subject, see Laurence Schneider, *Biology and Revolution in Twentieth-Century China* (New York: Rowman and Littlefield, 2005).

19. *Xijunxue mianyixue mingci* [Dictionary of bacteriology and immunology], ed. Guoli bianyi guan (Shanghai: Shangwu yinshuguan, 1937). Tang Feifan was on the

committee that translated these terms, along with Wu Liande and Jin Baoshan. For a full account of the translation of bacteriological and immunological terms into Chinese before the Second Sino-Japanese War, see "Xijunxue mianyixue mingci" [Dictionary of bacteriology and immunology], ed. Guoli bianyi guan, *Tushu jikan* (Books quarterly) 1 (1939): 47–48.

20. *Xijunxuezonglun, mianyixue, xijun mingcheng, xijun fenlei: Kexue mingci shencha hui yixue mingci shencha ben* [Report of the General Committee on Scientific Terminology: Terms in general bacteriology, immunology, names of bacteria, classification of bacteria] 1918, Modern Historical Materials Reading Room, Shanghai Library, Shanghai, file R37-62.

21. Ernest Witebsky, "Ehrlich's Side-chain Theory in the Light of Present Immunology," *Annals of the New York Academy of Sciences* 59 (September 1954): 168–81.

22. Ji Jilin, Vaccin, "Yufang jiezhong zhi mianyixue shang jianjie" [Gaining an understanding of the immunology of vaccinations], *Yiyao pinglun* 55 (1931): 18–20.

23. According to Witebsky, the citation is P. Ehrlich, *Klin. Jahr.* 6 (1897): 299.

24. Liang Guifang, "Mianyixing" [Immunity], *Jisheng yiyuan yuebao* 9, no. 9 (1932): 1–2.

25. See Ye Weili, *Seeking Modernity in China's Name* (Stanford, CA: Stanford University Press, 2001); and Paula Harrell, *Sowing the Seeds of Change: Chinese Students, Japanese Teachers, 1895–1905* (Stanford, CA: Stanford University Press, 1992).

26. "Medical Science Goes on in War-Torn Remote China," adapted from letter of Dr. Pei-sung Tang to William S. Cooper, *Science News Letter*, March 23, 1940, 184.

27. Ibid.

28. Guiyang is the capital of Guizhou, the other province that has historically constituted "southwest China" as defined by the Skinnerian Yun-Gui macroregion.

29. Nicole E. Barnes and John R. Watt, "The Influence of War on China's Modern Health Systems," in *Medical Transitions in 20th-Century China*, ed. Bridie Andrews and Mary Brown Bullock (Bloomington: Indiana University, 2014); Nicole E. Barnes, "Protecting the National Body: Gender and Public Health in Southwest China during the War with Japan, 1937–1945" (PhD diss., University of California–Irvine, 2012); John R. Watt, *Saving Lives in Wartime China: How Medical Reformers Built Modern Healthcare Systems amid War and Epidemics, 1928–1945* (Leiden: Brill, 2014), 227–43.

30. Joseph Needham and Dorothy M. Needham, "Report on a Journey in the South-West of China, Occupying August, September and October, 1944," in *Chinese Papers 1942–1946*, 1:18–28, Needham Research Institute, Cambridge, UK.

31. It is worth mentioning that serious public health work was being done in the Yan'an base camps on the Communist northwest front, although no substantive research was carried out as in Lanzhou, Guiyang, and Kunming. See I. Epstein, "Scientific Research and Education in the Border Region," in *Science Outpost* (London: Pilot Press, 1948), 199–205.

32. "A Brief Report of the Northwest Epidemic Prevention Bureau, Lanchow, Kansu, from January 1939 to December 1942," box 20, ABMAC Records.

33. Dorothy Borg, "Chinese Health Work Progressing Despite War," *Far Eastern Survey* 9, no. 11 (May 22, 1940): 132–34.

34. Ka-che Yip, "Disease and the Fighting Men," 174, cited in Diana Lary, *The Chinese People at War: Human Suffering and Social Transformation, 1937–1945* (Cambridge: Cambridge University Press, 2010), 120.

35. See David A. Bello, "To Go Where No Han Could Go for Long: Malaria and the Qing Construction of Ethnic Administrative Space in Frontier Yunnan," *Modern China* 31, no. 3 (July 2005): 283–317.

36. John Israel, *Lianda: A Chinese University in War and Revolution* (Stanford, CA: Stanford University Press, 1998), 319.

37. Yip, "Disease and the Fighting Men," 174.

38. P. Z. King, "Epidemic Prevention and Control in China," *Chinese Medical Journal* 61 (1943): 51.

39. One discussion of antimalaria efforts in southern Yunnan notes, "The situation has been aggravated by the construction of the Yunnan-Burma Road which greatly increases the opportunities for spreading the disease." Borg, "Chinese Health Work Progressing," 132–34. The fact that western Yunnan is a "disease well" for endemic plague only exacerbated the situation; see Benedict, *Bubonic Plague in China.*

40. King, "Epidemic Control and Prevention," 49.

41. Guo Keda, "Dijun shiyong xijun zhan de kenengxing he women ying you de zhunbei" [The possibility for the enemy army's use of biological warfare and the preparations we should have], *Zhanshi yizheng* [Wartime medical administration] 3, nos. 8–9 (October 1941): 11. The article speaks to broader issues around Japanese biological warfare and concerns over protecting racial health, which also may have contributed to health officials' focus on vaccines to prevent disease. Guo discusses the nature of biological warfare, suspicions of its past and future use by Japanese forces, and methods by which China could resist biological weapons.

42. Jin Baoshan, "Chang qi kang zhan yu fangyi" [The long war of resistance and preventing disease), *Xinyun daobao* 14 (1938).

43. Jin Baoshan, "Zuijin de weisheng jianshe" [Recent public health establish-ments], *Zhandou zhongguo* [China in combat] 1, no. 5 (1945): 14–19.

44. "Yunnan sheng san shi yi nian huoluan liuxing ji qi fangzhi gongzuo chu (zi wu yue shier ri zhi liu yue san shi ri zhi)" [Cholera's spread in Yunnan in Minguo year 31 and work to prevent and cure it], *Yunnan weisheng* [Yunnan public health] 2, no. 7 (September 30, 1942): 1–19.

45. Ibid.

46. "Zhongyang fangyi chu" [National Epidemic Prevention Bureau], *Yunnan Yikan* [Yunnan medical journal] 2, no. 2 (April 1940).

47. "Yiqing: Yunnan quansheng weisheng shiyan chu sa yi niandu ba, qi liang yue huoluan fangzhi gongzuo jianbao" [Epidemic situation: Brief report of the work of the Yunnan Provincial Experimental Health Station to control cholera during July and August 1931], *Yunnan weisheng* 2, no. 8 (November 1942): 13–15. The coercive nature of some immunization programs raises the question of the extent to which the attitudes of Chinese vaccinators in the Southwest were colonial in nature—that is, the extent to which they believed they were enforcing a modern hygienic regime on a population they considered ignorant and lacking in modern methods of public health. For detailed explorations of this theme, see Ruth Rogaski, *Hygienic Modernity: Health and Disease in Treaty-Port China* (Berkeley: University of California Press, 2004); and Sean Hsiang-lin Lei, "Habituating Individuality: The Framing of Tuberculosis and Its Material Solutions in Republican China," *Bulletin for the History of Medicine* 84 (2010): 248–79.

48. "Yunnan sheng sanshiyi nian huoluan liuxing ji qi fangzhi gongzuo chu," *Yunnan weisheng* 2, no. 7 (Sept 1942).

49. "Yiqing: Yunnan quansheng weisheng shiyan chu sa yi niandu ba, qi liang yue huoluan fangzhi gongzuo jianbao" (November 1942).

50. Shih Kuo-heng, *China Enters the Machine Age: A Study of Labor in Chinese War Industry*, ed. and trans. Fei Hsiao-tung and Francis L. K. Hsu (Cambridge, MA: Harvard University Press, 1944): 20.

51. See "Mianyi zhiliao fa: Therapeutic Immunisation," *Guangji yikan* 1, no. 9 (1924): 5–7. See also "Yimiao liaoxue: Vaccinotherapie," *Guangji yikan*, 11, no. 10 (1934): 11–15.

52. Miao Ancheng and Chen Shiguang, "Yunnan yi xi qu xian shu yi" [Bubonic plague in western Yunnan], *Yunnan weisheng* 4, no. 3 (May 15, 1947): 6–7.

53. Wilhelm Kolle, "Zur aktive immunisierung des Menschen gegen Cholera," *Zbl Bakt I Abt Orig* 19 (1896): 97–104. See also Charles C. J. Carpenter and Richard B. Hornick, "Killed Vaccines: Cholera, Typhoid, and Plague," *Vaccines: A Biography*, ed. Andrew W. Artenstein (New York: Springer, 2010), 92–93.

54. Carpenter and Hornick, "Killed Vaccines," 93. In East Pakistan, where cholera was endemic, researchers found that the vaccine provided over 70 percent protection against cholera in adults for the first year and declining efficacy over the next two years. In the Philippines, where cholera is usually not present, the vaccine provided about 26 percent effective protection during a 1968 outbreak there.

55. NEPB labs started producing this vaccine in 1930. They used three different strains of typhoid obtained from the United States Army Medical School in Washington, DC (Rawlings strain of B. typhosus, Kessel strain of B. paratyphosus "A," and Rowland strain of B. paratyphosus "B"). Between 1932 and 1934, they produced a total of 3,693,292 cc of the vaccine; in 1933–34 it was their most-produced vaccine, at approximately 3 million ccs. National Health Administration and Central Field Health Station, *National Epidemic Prevention Bureau: A Report, Being a Review of Its Activities from Its Foundation in March 1919 to June 1934* (Beijing, 1934), 37–42. In 1967, two Dutch scientists investigated the optimal time and delivery system of the combined cholera-typhoid vaccine. They described it as a suspension of heat-killed bacteria preserved in phenol and containing "8000 × 10⁶ *Vibrio cholera* bacteria, 1000 × 10⁶ *Salmonella typhi*, 750 × 10⁶ *Salmonella paratyphi A* and 750 × 10⁶ *Salmonella paratyphi B* bacteria." They did not describe the effectiveness of the vaccine, but did note that only 9 out of 1,100 test subjects, or approximately 1 percent, reported reactions to the vaccine. H. A. L. Clasener and B. J. W. Beunders, "Immunization of Man with Typhoid and Cholera Vaccine: Agglutinating Antibodies after Intracutaneous and Subcutaneous Injection," *Journal of Hygiene* 65, no. 4 (December 1967): 449–56.

56. Gerald B. Pier, "Vaccines and Vaccination," in *Immunology, Infection, and Immunity*, ed. Gerald B. Pier, Jeffrey B. Lyczak, and Lee M. Wetzler (Washington, DC: ASM Press, 2004), 515; Stephen T. Smiley, "Current Challenges in the Development of Vaccines for Pneumonic Plague," *Expert Rev. Vaccines* 7, no. 2 (March 2008): 209–21.

57. "Gongzuo baogao yu gongzuo yijian" [Work report and work recommendations], *Yunnan weisheng* 3, nos. 9–10 (October 1946): 6.

58. Chen Shiguang, "Baoshan shuyi shicha baogao" [Report of a survey of the plague in Baoshan], *Yunnan weisheng* 4, no. 1 (March 1947): 6. See also Miao and Chen, "Yunnan yi xi qu xian shu yi: yu fang zhu she zhi xiao yong."

59. John Cameron, "Pharmacy in China in 1938," *Chemist and Druggist* 130 (February 1939): 147–48.

60. Needham, "Article II," 88–89.

61. Ibid.

62. Cameron, "Pharmacy in China," 148.

63. "Progress Report on ABMAC Projects: III. Standardization of Biological Products," box 20, ABMAC Records.

64. According to Kuo, a 1932 census listed the population at 2,338,272 households, with 6,095,549 men and 5,699,937 women for a total population of 11,795,486. Yunnan's population was 2 percent of China's total population. The population of Kunming was 143,700. Kuo Yuan, *Yün-nan sheng ching-chi wen-t'i* [Economic problems of Yunnan Province] (Chongqing: Cheng-chung shu-chü, 1940), 3–4, 14 (reprinted by Center for Chinese Research Materials, Association of Research Libraries, Washington, DC, 1945).

65. *Tongji yuebao* 1939 (38, 39), 1940 (41, 42, 48), 1941 (55), 1942 (73–74), Shanghai Library, Shanghai.

66. "Report of Anti-Epidemic Activities for 1942–43, National Health Administration, January 1, 1942, to June 30, 1943," box 20, ABMAC Records.

67. Yunnan sheng difang zhi bianji weiyuanhui, ed., *Yunnan shengzhi, juan liu shi jiu: Weisheng zhi* [Yunnan provincial gazetteer: vol. 69, Public Health] (Kunming: Yunnan renmin chubanshe, 2002), 333; "Report of Anti-Epidemic Activities for 1942–43," ABMAC Records.

68. "Zhongyang fangyi chu zhizao xueqing" [The National Epidemic Prevention Bureau is producing serum], *Yunnan Yikan* 1, no. 6 (March 1939): 45.

69. Letter from Wei Hsi, Guiyang, to Dr. George W. Bachman, Chungking, July 6, 1943, box 20, ABMAC Records.

70. "Progress Report on ABMAC Projects," ABMAC Records.

71. Wei Hsi, "Preparation of Simple and Dried Smallpox Vaccine in Gum Acacia," *Chinese Medical Journal* 65 (May–June 1947), 163–66.

72. Robert Bud, *Penicillin: Triumph and Tragedy* (Oxford: Oxford University Press, 2007), 80.

73. "Kunming Shi Huoluan Yufang Zhushe Gongzuo Baogao" [Report on preventive injection work for cholera in Kunming city], *Tongji yixue jikan* [Tongji medical journal] 7, no. 3 (March 1940): 146.

74. Israel, *Lianda*, 198.

75. Wang, "Chuxi Zhonghua yixuehui di wu jie da hui ji canguan dian zhu yiyao weisheng," 6.

76. Nonglin bu [Ministry of Agriculture and Forestry], "Fangzhi shouyi zhi xingzheng sheshi" [Administrative structure of work in preventing epizootic diseases], 1946, RG 20-25-11-19, Institute of Modern History Archives, Academia Sinica, Taipei.

77. Wang, "Chuxi Zhonghua yixuehui di wu jie da hui ji canguan dian zhu yiyao weisheng," 4.

78. Tang Feifan, "The National Vaccine and Serum Institute: Retrospect and Prospect," *Chinese Medical Journal* 65 (May–June 1947): 177–81.

79. Letter from Dr. Robert Lim to Dr. Yi Chien-Lung, Kunming, December 5, 1944, box 2, ABMAC Records.

80. "Report on Penicillin Work," letter from C. S. Fan to Dr. Donald Van Slyke and Dr. Co Tui, September 4, 1944, box 2, ABMAC Records.

81. "Minutes of the Meeting of the Special Advisory Committee on Penicillin for China Project of ABMAC and Indusco, held at the office of ABMAC," New York City, June 23, 1944, 8 p.m., box 24, ABMAC Records.

82. American Bureau for Medical Aid to China, "Report on Penicillin Meeting," September 22, 1944, box 24, ABMAC Records.

83. National Health Administration to Dr. F. F. Tang, Kunming, August 15, 1941, Zhongyang fangyi chu [NEPB], RG 1029.1.51, Yunnan Provincial Archives, Kunming [hereafter cited as YPA]; Paxton Davis, *A Boy's War* (Winston-Salem, NC: J. F. Blair, 1990), 222–23; Hsi Wei, Kunming, to Dr. Yieh Tien Hsin, Chinese Red Cross Society Medical Relief Corp, Guiyang, April 3, 1942, Zhongyang fangyi chu [NEPB], RG 1029.1.51, YPA.

84. Wang Youwei to Dr. Marshall Balfour, November 10, 1943, Zhongyang fangyi chu [NEPB], RG 1029.1.51, YPA.

85. "League of Nations Technical Collaboration with China: Scheme of Anti-Epidemic Action, Report by the Supervisory Committee," October 22, 1937, document C.524.M.363.1937.X, Archives of the League of Nations, Geneva.

86. "League of Nations Health Organization: Collaboration of the League of Nations in the Control of Epidemics in China," July 26, 1938, document C.H.1353, Archives of the League of Nations.

87. "Related to the Weishengbu Anesthesia Medicine Manager's Station at Chongqing Office Sending Staff to the NEPB to buy rabies vaccine," RG 0030-0001-00183, Chongqing Municipal Archives, Chongqing, China.

88. Needham, *Science Outpost*, 134.

89. "Zhongyang fangyi chu: Zhongyang fangyichu Lanzhou zhizao suo caichan qingce" [National Epidemic Prevention Bureau: Detailed list of the property of NEPB Lanzhou Branch], April 19, 1938, Zhongyang fangyi chu [NEPB], RG 1029.2.43.3, YPA.

90. Needham, *Science Outpost*, 209.

91. Letter from Yan Wai, Xishan, Kunming, to Dr. Tang Feifan, October 28, 1941, Zhongyang fangyi chu [NEPB], RG 1029.2.51, YPA.

92. The Chinese Medical Association seems to have moved at least part of its organizational leadership to Kunming after 1937. The *Chinese Medical Journal*, which it published, moved its offices to Kunming, and the editor of the association's bimonthly public health magazine, *Zhonghua jiankang zazhi*, directed all his correspondence to a new address at the Kunhua Hospital.

93. "Fifth General Conference of C.M.A.," *Shanghai yishi zhoukan* [Shanghai medical news] 6, no. 15 (April 8, 1940): 4.

94. "Di wu jie da hui lun wen ti mu" [Fifth General Conference Paper Titles], *Zhong hua yi xue za zhi* [Chinese medical journal] 26, no. 7 (July 1940): 603–11.

95. Wang, "Chuxi Zhonghua yixuehui di wu jie da hui ji canguan dian zhu yiyao weisheng," 1.

96. M. C. Balfour, "Travels in South-west China: Summary of an Address Given by Dr. M. C. Balfour to the Shanghai Public Health Club at the YMCA, Blvd. de Montigny, on April 8, 1940," *Shanghai yishi zhoukan* [Shanghai medical news] 6, no. 16 (April 15, 1940): 2.

97. Jin Baoshan (P. Z. King), "'Gong yi' zhi shi ming" [The mission of "state medicine"], *Gong yi* [State medicine] 1, no. 1 (January 1945): 1–2. For wartime discussion and debates on *gongyi*, see "Gongyi lunzhu: Gongyi zhidu yu xin zhongguo" [A treatise on state medicine: The system of state medicine and the New China], *Yiyu* 4, no. 4 (1940). See also "Taolun gongyi zhidu" [Discussing the system of state medicine], *Yiyao pinglun* 149 (1937): 1–2; "Kangzhan jianguo yu gongyi zhidu" [The War of Resistance and the system of state medicine], *Yiyu* 4, no. 4 (1940): 8–14; Huang Mingzhou, "Gongyi zhidu yu quanmin jiankang" [The system of state medicine and the health of the whole people], *Xuesheng zhi you* 1, nos. 2–3 (1940): 221–33; "Wo guo ying shixing gongyi zhidu" [Our nation ought to implement the system of state medicine], *Yiyu* 3, no. 4 (1939): 1–2; and *Gongyi* [State medicine], a periodical dedicated to discussing and furthering the cause of state medicine that ran from January to November 1945.

98. Chinese authors who wrote about *gongyi zhidu* often invoked the example of Western nations like the United States in arguing for a greater state role in Chinese public health. P. Z. King (Jin Baoshan) discussed the examples set by post–World War I "new and strongly recovering nations" in Europe, such as Yugoslavia, Czechoslovakia, and Poland, in medical reform. See Jin Baoshan, "Gong yi zhi du: Yi yue er ri zai zhongyang diantai bojiang" [State medicine: January 2 broadcast on Central Radio], *Guangbo zhoubao* 124 (1937).

99. Yip, "Health and Nationalist Reconstruction," 399–402.

100. John R. Watt, "Public Medicine in Wartime China: Biomedicine, State Medicine, and the Rise of China's National Medical Colleges, 1931–1945," Rosenberg Institute Occasional Paper No. 1 (Boston: Rosenberg Institute for East Asian Studies, Suffolk University, 2012), 70–71.

101. Cheng et al., "Recollection." Tang committed suicide during the Anti-Rightist campaigns of 1957 and 1958.

102. See Tang Feifan, *Yufang jiezhong* [Preventive inoculation] (Beijing: Kexue puji chubanshe, 1956); *Xijunxue ji mianyixue shiyan zhidao* [An experimental guide to bacteriology and immunology], ed. Luo Haibo and Guo Maofu (Hangzhou: Xin yi shu ju, 1951); *Weisheng changshi* [Practical knowledge about public health], ed. Wu Yundong (Fuzhou: Fujian renmin chubanshe, 1960).

103. "Niudou bixu" [Smallpox inoculation requirements], *Yunnan Yikan* 1, no. 5 (January 1939): 7. See also "Chuanranbing guanli fangfa: Control of Communicable Diseases—a Manual of the American Public Health Association," trans. Wang Baoshu, *Yunnan weisheng* 5, nos. 1–2 (January 1948): 4; and "Xiao'er ke zhong chang jian zhi chuanranbing de yufang" [The prevention of diseases that small children often encounter in the classroom], ed. Xu Duanqing, *Yunnan yikan* 1, no. 6 (January 1939): 1.

104. "Zhongyang fangyichu" [NEPB], *Yunnan Yikan* 2, no. 2 (April 1940).

105. "Zhongyang fangyi chu" [NEPB], *Gonggong weisheng yuekan* 1, no. 6 (December 1935).

106. Wei Hsi and Wen Pin Wei, "Experimental Infection of Silkworm Pupa with Typhus Rickettsia: A Preliminary Report," *Chinese Medical Journal* 65 (May–June 1947): 171–75. See also "Tang Feifan and Wei Hsi, "Morphological Studies on Vaccinia Virus Cultivated in the Developing Egg," *Journal of Pathology and Bacteriology* 45, no. 2 (1937): 317–23; Wei Hsi, "Preparation of Simple and Dried Smallpox Vaccine in

Gum Acacia"—both in *Chinese Medical Journal* 65 (May–June 1947): 163–66; Wei Hsi, "Wo guo zhi huigui rebing" [Our nation's relapsing fever], *Yiwu shenghuo* 3, no. 11 (1946): 14–21. Wei Hsi was also listed as a coauthor in Colonel Thomas T. Mackie, M. C., A. U. S., et al., "Observations on Tsutsugamushi Disease (Scrub Typhus) in Assam and Burma: Preliminary Report," *American Journal of Hygiene* 43, no. 3 (May 1946): 195–218.

Chapter Eight

Serving the People

Chen Zhiqian and the Sichuan Provincial Health Administration, 1939–1945

Nicole Elizabeth Barnes

Dr. Chen Zhiqian, China's "father of public health," is consistently celebrated for the five and a half years he spent as director of the Department of Health in north China's model county in Hebei, Dingxian Province. Dr. Chen (also known by the Anglicized name of C. C. Chen) directed public health work in this chief site of the Rural Reconstruction Movement from January 1932 to July 1937.[1] However, he left another important and lasting legacy in his home province of Sichuan during the Second Sino-Japanese War (1937–45), work for which he is seldom recognized. For six years during the war, from May 1939 to November 1945, Chen Zhiqian served as director of the Sichuan Provincial Health Administration (Sichuan sheng weishengchu), or SPHA, in the southwestern province that boasted the wartime capital of Chongqing. Founded in spring 1939 and headquartered in Chen's hometown of Chengdu, the provincial capital, the SPHA established county health centers (*xian weishengyuan*), or CHCs, in 131 of the province's 139 counties before the war ended in 1945, and continued to operate through 1948.[2] The bulk of this work built on and greatly expanded the Dingxian legacy. Taken as a whole, Chen's Rural Reconstruction work in prewar northern China and his wartime work in Sichuan laid the foundations for the expansion of public health services into rural China in the Communist period.

The work of the SPHA also played a key role in two wartime processes of enormous importance to the nation. First, the establishment of a county health center in all but eight of Sichuan's counties was a chief means by which the once independently ruled province was incorporated into the nation. Doctors, nurses, midwives, and public health personnel who had worked to establish state-administered public health services in other parts of China prior to the war transferred their talents to Sichuan during the war, building a health infrastructure in the once remote province that mirrored that of communities in northern and eastern China. Since public health administration constituted an important part of state formation and nation building, this work did more than treat individual bodies; it constructed Sichuan as part of the national body. Second, CHC staff actively promoted scientific biomedicine in semiurban and rural towns throughout Sichuan. Far from being a foreign import, by this time in Chinese history biomedicine was quickly becoming an indigenized and fully integrated part of medical care in China, and many people living in rural areas received their first introduction to biomedicine through public health work. Recent scholarship has shown that the barefoot doctors who worked under the Communist state brought biomedicine to the countryside; this chapter contends that this process began in wartime Sichuan under the leadership of Dr. Chen Zhiqian. By paving the way for medical professionals with biomedical training to enter rural Chinese villages, the SPHA furthered the indigenization of scientific biomedicine and eroded the status of Chinese traditional medicine in the same way that barefoot doctors did in the 1960s and 1970s.[3]

Curiously, all of this activity occurred not in spite of the war but because of it. The war did bring seemingly insurmountable troubles to health workers: bombs dropped in air raids destroyed offices and equipment, wartime hardships eroded employee morale, inflation threatened staff retention, and severe supply shortages occasionally rendered even the most basic treatments impossible. However, the war also created all the right conditions for the establishment and operation of the SPHA. The Japanese occupation of northern China forced the closure of operations in Ding County in summer 1937. Soon thereafter, Dr. Chen returned to his home province in unoccupied China, where he employed well-trained medical professionals who also sought work in the Nationalist Party–controlled interior. With the Japanese invasion threatening its very survival, the Nationalist government gained new interest in promoting public health, and while it continued to commit meager resources to the project, its financial contribution compared favorably with prewar numbers.[4] China's solitary battle against the Japanese Imperial Army also appeared in the international press, spurring charitable groups around the world to provide additional support that augmented that of the government, particularly in the later war years when runaway inflation threatened nearly all state ministries. Organizations such as the Rockefeller Foundation's China Medical Board, United China Relief, the International Red Cross, and the American Bureau for Medical Aid to China donated millions of dollars' worth of funding and equipment. Meanwhile, within China the rhetoric of resisting the Japanese encouraged members of the public to strengthen their bodies so as to strengthen the nation for the war effort, and the dire conditions invited individuals to compromise with state reforms that they might have resisted in times of peace. For all of these reasons, the War of Resistance marked a period of unforeseen opportunity. Chen Zhiqian and his colleagues took advantage of this circumstance to create a remarkable achievement that changed the course of public health administration in twentieth-century China.

Dr. Chen Zhiqian and His Education in Public Health

Born to a modest but scholarly family in Sichuan's provincial capital of Chengdu in 1903, until the age of ten Chen Zhiqian received at-home instruction in the Confucian classics from his grandfather. According to Chen's memoir, this education gave him the same conviction that inspired the entire May Fourth and New Culture generation of reformers: the belief that "scholars are a special class, but that, with this respected status, went the responsibility, as educated men, of working for the good of the common people."[5] His sense of medical responsibility began in his childhood, when six of his family members died of illness, including both of his siblings and his mother. He never knew his paternal grandparents, and his bustling childhood home of seven people became a lonely household of three. After all of these deaths, as well as his own illness from malaria, the specter of death visited his home once again when his stepmother contracted a severe case of pulmonary tuberculosis. Chen accompanied her to the French consulate in Chengdu, where she consulted a foreign physician as a last resort. Traumatized by the family deaths and greatly impressed with this foreign physician's diagnostic tools—a thermometer, a sphygmomanometer, and a stethoscope—the fourteen-year-old Chen reportedly decided in that very moment "to become a modern physician."[6]

To achieve this goal, Chen needed much more than knowledge of the Confucian classics. He received his most formative educational experience at the Rockefeller Foundation–funded Peking Union Medical College (PUMC) in Beijing (which he attended from 1921 to 1929), as well as during his master's degree in public health from the Harvard School of Public Health (1931), which catapulted him into the vanguard of China's medical professionals. This education in scientific biomedicine and public health further convinced him that "it was true . . . that poor health was in part responsible for China's weakness." Coupled with his early encounters with illness, it also left him with a lifelong belief in the superiority of scientific biomedicine when compared to Chinese medicine.[7] This combination of personal experience and education transformed Chen Zhiqian into an avid champion of an erstwhile foreign medicine, who ultimately worked to promote its indigenization in his home province in southwestern China.

As a man born in the last decade of Manchu rule, educated in the Confucian classics as well as in English and biomedicine, convinced both of the superiority of biomedicine and that his knowledge of it vested him with a profound responsibility to share it with the common people, Chen Zhiqian was a prototypical Chinese public health reformer of the early twentieth century. However, two things made him distinct from the average health professional with whom he worked. First, as a man of Sichuan, Chen hailed from a less developed part of China—indeed, his was the first health administration to exist in the province when it opened in 1939—which exposed him to more poverty and greater public need than health professionals from eastern cities such as Beijing, Tianjin, Nanjing, Shanghai, and Guangzhou typically witnessed.[8] Second, Dr. Chen's belief in scientific medicine was not a rhetorical commitment to modernity, but a heartfelt passion rooted in the personal experiences of his formative childhood years. His observation of ritual practices aimed at expelling demons and the healing methods of local physicians who failed to cure his loved ones compelled him to find more effective, life-saving methods. He developed an ardent determination to do everything in his power to alleviate the suffering of illness and untimely death, and he believed that "in a just society, medical care of good quality should be easily available to all the people."[9] In other words, throughout his career Chen Zhiqian remained staunchly committed to "serving the people" in a fashion often solely attributed to members of the Chinese Communist Party, yet he began his career under the Nationalist state. This suggests that a passion for public service does not belong to any single political ideology, and partially explains why he served both regimes so faithfully.

Already possessing a strong drive to serve his compatriots, at PUMC the young Chen met Dr. John B. Grant, director of the college's Public Health Department. Grant convinced this intelligent and passionate young man that a foreign medical system could only benefit Chinese people if adapted to local conditions and needs, and that establishing a private medical practice would benefit a few hundred people, whereas devoting oneself to public health would benefit thousands. These two aims—to use public health work to indigenize scientific biomedicine and adapt it to Chinese cultural practice for the benefit of the rural majority—formed Dr. Chen's lifelong career goals.[10]

Chen Zhiqian's disposition requires further explanation to place his service to the people in proper historical context. Many of his peers, armed with the same elite education at PUMC and its frequent companion of Rockefeller Foundation–funded graduate work abroad, used their credentials to advance their own careers with much more alacrity than they advanced health services to the rural poor. They did not necessarily believe that poor farmers in remote areas of the country would accept "modern medicine," and they rarely troubled themselves with questions of whether or not their impoverished countrymen and women deserved better health services. Many developed obscure medical specialties, established private practices, and served wealthy patients who could afford their high fees. Had he followed this path, Chen Zhiqian would have made much more money and lived a more comfortable life, particularly during the war when all government bureaus suffered from lack of funding and civil servants had to tighten their belts more each year.[11] The degree of personal sacrifice required for Chen to create a legacy of public health in wartime Sichuan deserves recognition.

For his part, John B. Grant occupied a specific position in a debate taking place in his own country—the United States—where, since the late eighteenth century, physicians and authorities had weighed the relative benefits of public sanitation and private medical practice. By the early twentieth century, this oft contentious discourse began to lean in favor of private practitioners and medical technology.[12] Grant expressed his continued belief in medicine as public service through his directorship of the Public Health Department at PUMC, from which position he educated young Chinese students in the importance of public health and advised the Nationalist government on the creation and staffing of its new public health bureau in 1928.[13]

Upon graduating from PUMC in 1929, Chen Zhiqian immediately seized the opportunity to put his goals into action; he spent a year directing the Xiaozhuang Rural Health Demonstration Program in a small town outside Nanjing. Chen described this year as the foundation of his later work in Dingxian.[14] After working in Dingxian for five and a half years, even the Japanese invasion and departure from his family did not deter Chen, who in 1939 moved to Sichuan, where he "organized a province-wide system of state medicine, based on the Dingxian model."[15] From his appointment in May 1939, Dr. Chen had a dual goal of directing the provincial capital's fledgling Provincial Health Administration in the city of Chengdu, and of organizing rural health services throughout the province. By 1945, the SPHA had established 131 county health centers in a province where not a single one had existed previously. This left a mere eight counties in the entire province without health services.[16] With this rate of activity, Sichuan alone accounted for nearly 19 percent of the wartime growth in CHCs (from 242 countrywide to 938). Additionally, under Chen's direction the SPHA "took up all the essential functions of a government health service," despite the fact that it was created principally to perform medical relief for air-raid victims.[17] This put 45 million Sichuan residents under its care, with directives from the provincial governor and funding from the National Health Administration (NHA).[18]

Each CHC in Sichuan employed one to two doctors, two nurses, and three midwives to reflect Chen's dedication to improving maternal and child health (MCH).[19] Remarkably even distribution throughout the province ensured that remote counties had some form of health services, although model counties received better-trained staff and more resources. As with the model county of Hebei, the cooperation of local leaders was of paramount importance, and Chen reported good relations with county leaders in almost all of Sichuan.[20] This was crucial because in a village setting, everything from purchasing or leasing a building in which to operate to obtaining the trust of the villagers rested on maintaining good relations with the local leadership.

In certain locations, village leaders included local practitioners of Chinese medicine who resented outsiders encroaching on their clientele. Chen understood the sensitivity of this issue and trained his staff to avoid "creating competitive pressure on traditional practitioners." However, he also had a strident preference for biomedicine that manifested in his exclusive use of biomedically trained staff in all county health centers. Indeed, he directed his entire career toward figuring out how to "best introduce modern scientific medicine into a predominantly rural population and make it take root there for the benefit of the entire country."[21]

Concomitant with his belief in biomedicine as a superior method for treating disease, within Chengdu Chen Zhiqian focused primarily on disease prevention. This emphasis included vaccination campaigns wherein some of the materials came from scientific laboratories, but also general public health work such as trash collection and latrine construction. However, conditions of war impeded sanitation work, particularly air raids and the prohibitive cost of construction supplies and labor in the wartime economy.[22] Chen also used his directorship of the administration to build the provincial capital's health services from scratch. By 1941, Chengdu had three MCH centers and five hospitals with a total of five hundred beds.[23] While actual need for medical and public health services far surpassed the supply during the war years, the SPHA launched a new era in central state commitment to providing such services in Sichuan.

A Comparative Analysis of Four County Health Centers

Each of the 131 county health centers sent frequent reports on its work to the SPHA headquarters, and all of the extant reports are held in the Sichuan Provincial Archives in Chengdu.[24] Rather than attempt a full analysis of all public health work throughout the province, this chapter highlights the health services developed in four counties in rural Sichuan—Bishan, Hechuan, Yibin, and Songpan—to demonstrate that, even as resources differed by locale, the distribution of health personnel and facilities during the war marked a key moment in China's medical history.

Women had the best chance of surviving childbirth and having healthy children in Bishan County, at the time a mere thirty kilometers west of the wartime capital of Chongqing (and now part of Chongqing municipality). Bishan had the most successful maternal and children's health program of all four counties discussed here, perhaps in all of Sichuan Province. Its CHC, established in October 1939 with Yu Wei as director and a monthly budget of 1,559 yuan, managed eight hospitals and twelve clinics, and became the Demonstration Health Center in 1940 through a special grant from the NHA.[25] By 1945, its budget exceeded that of any CHC in Sichuan, allowing it to run not only the center in the county seat but also six village health clinics in smaller locations throughout the county.[26] None of the other counties discussed here had any village health clinics, meaning that anyone who needed medical attention throughout these counties had first to travel to the county seat to receive the services offered at the CHC. The distance would have been prohibitive to many, especially those rendered weak from illness, and it is therefore safe to assume that many residents of small villages continued to use traditional medicine despite the presence of a government-funded county health center.

The singularity of Bishan's CHC highlights two distinctions between Chen Zhiqian's rural health work and the Barefoot Doctor program of the 1960s and '70s. First, the latter program successfully exploited cheap labor as a means of extending health services to the truly remote areas of rural China to a much greater degree than the SPHA managed to do. The Barefoot Doctors were often recruited from the same small villages that they served, and they had the authority to refer patients up the medical hierarchy to the county hospitals. Some doctors even accompanied their patients to these hospitals, administering medications along the way, providing the means of transportation, or helping the patient and his or her family negotiate with hospital staff. In a second, related difference between the two approaches, the Barefoot Doctor program departed from Dr. Chen's emphasis on elite individuals with advanced training, in that it formed its ranks primarily from young, unmarried rural residents from lower-class families with a middle school education and a few scant weeks of medical training.[27] If Dr. Chen had not transitioned into medical education in the late 1940s, he would have advised that the relatively uneducated rural doctors be given far fewer medical responsibilities and far less control over significant medical procedures.[28] These differences in approach demonstrate that the Barefoot Doctor program did indeed bring biomedicine to the greatest percentage of people, yet they do not belie the fact that Chen Zhiqian played a major role in shifting the focus of China's health administration from urban centers to the villages where the majority of the population lived.

In addition to receiving better funding, demonstration health centers tended to attract the best staff, and Bishan's CHC boasted more personnel than Chengdu and the other three counties combined; it also trained the greatest number of new colleagues.[29] Although the women's and children's health center (*fuying baojiansuo*) was not established until December 1943, the CHC trained new midwives, accepting only local women around twenty-five years of age, with the additional requirements that they be "healthy in body and pure in mind" (*sixiang chunzheng*), possess "gentle spirits" (*taidu wenrou*), and have had no previous experience in midwifery. These qualities presumably left the young women impressionable and ready to accept the training without questioning the ways in which its foundational principles differed from those of traditional village midwifery. The explicit goals of the two and a half months of training included instructing students to "understand the importance of 'new-style midwifery' (*xinfa jiesheng*) and decide to earnestly promote it," and "to learn to eat bitterness, endure hardship, and obey orders" (*xunlian chiku nailao fucong zhihui*).[30]

Despite the moralistic tone of the midwife training manuals, people working in maternal and child health in wartime China faced formidable foes. Health professionals and philanthropic organizations throughout the world spent much of the late nineteenth and early twentieth centuries combating the biggest killers of newborn infants and gestating women: infantile tetanus and puerperal fever.[31] In China, people with knowledge of germ theory and the importance of sterility believed that the practices of traditional midwives caused these deaths. Traditional midwives, usually older village women who had birthed several children themselves and successfully delivered as many as several hundred babies over the years, often severed a newborn child's umbilical cord with unsterilized knives and packed the cut with animal dung, dirt, or ash from the kitchen stove. While these materials were believed to contain ritualistic healing properties, they could also contain harmful bacteria, and frequently led to unnecessary deaths from infantile tetanus. The midwives' tendency to attend to a woman in childbirth without sterilizing their hands also alarmed the germ-conscious, in addition to sometimes causing unnecessary maternal deaths from childbed fever. The NHA estimated that 15 per 1,000 women and 200–250 per 1,000 infants died each year from these two diseases.[32] The Chongqing Bureau of Public Health, established in 1938, placed great emphasis on MCH services despite the hardships of war.[33] MCH staff in Bishan, part of a national movement in wartime China, brought this same level of attention to a more remote location.

Bishan's MCH programs also garnered success from the staff members' willingness to compromise. For example, MCH staff performed a far greater number of pre- and postnatal exams as well as births in women's homes than at the clinic, showing a willingness to honor people's preference for a familiar environment when submitting to a new medical practice.[34] Nevertheless, when patients did come into the clinic, staff took full advantage of their presence in the waiting room, delivering over one hundred public health talks to their captive audiences over a six-month period.[35] This practice built on the legacy of medical missionaries, who had subjected waiting patients to Christian sermons and teachings from the Bible. Health staff took advantage of this moment because their patients often resisted unsolicited advice. For example, mothers in Bishan showed reluctance to attend mothers' meetings where staff gave parental advice, with only four people appearing at the sole meeting in half a year in 1940, but they avidly participated in well-baby competitions, and also took greater advantage of the clinic's outpatient services than did men.[36] The staff eventually earned enough trust to overcome patient resistance. By 1945, CHC staff had made such an impression that over four hundred women attended mother's meetings, and well-baby meetings continued to draw large crowds.[37] Furthermore, staff in Bishan performed the greatest number of pre- and postnatal exams and delivered the most babies of any CHC, including that of Lu Zuofu's progressive city Beibei.[38]

Nevertheless, even at a successful county health center such as this, staff conducted far more general public health activities—such as hygiene lectures and scabies treatments at the county seat's bus terminal—than sophisticated medical services.[39] For example, the knowledgeable PUMC graduate Zhu Baotian (class of 1938) worked in Bishan, devoting several years to treating and preventing trachoma, one of the most common ailments among children in both urban and rural China during wartime.[40] This approach accorded with both the dominant model of rural health development at the time and with the needs of rural communities.[41] In the beginning stages of institutionalized health, reforms in basic sanitation and nutrition have been proven to make the greatest difference in public welfare.[42]

Health services in Hechuan County contrast slightly with those in Bishan. Beginning inside a missionary hospital, the Universal Love Hospital (Bo'ai yiyuan), the Hechuan CHC boasted a healthy number of medical staff and received adequate funding.[43] It also grew tremendously quickly; by 1946, Hechuan had five hospitals and twenty-four health clinics.[44] In the same year, the CHC reported 210 cases of dysentery and only one death, demonstrating admirable rapidity and effectiveness in treating this deadly disease that had afflicted millions of people during the war.[45] This marked a considerable improvement since 1939, when cholera vaccines were in such short supply throughout the country that the CHC was reduced to conducting compulsory health inspections with little treatment recourse in response to a local cholera epidemic. The CHC director appealed to the provincial governor and to Dr. Chen of the SPHA for more vaccine, but received a reply from the latter stating that cholera had been so rampant throughout the year that the entire province was out of vaccine, and that backup supplies had not yet arrived from the National Epidemic Prevention Bureau, which had recently relocated to Kunming.[46]

Slightly northwest and outside of Chongqing proper during the war (and now part of Chongqing municipality), Hechuan had been the scene of antiforeign riots in the late nineteenth century, though they were not "antiforeign" in the pure sense—no actual foreigners from Western countries ever died in these riots, but many Chinese Christians did.[47] There is no evidence that Hechuan residents felt more strongly antiforeign than did people in other regions of Sichuan during the war years, or were more reluctant to accept "foreign" scientific biomedicine. In fact, in 1946 the county had twenty-five doctors of biomedicine and thirty-two of Chinese medicine.[48] The balance between the two types of physicians in Hechuan County corroborates the fact that, by the early twentieth century, scientific biomedicine no longer seemed very foreign to most people in China.[49] Even rural Chinese decorated their walls with medicine advertisements from contemporary newspapers and magazines and kept abreast of new medical products. Moreover, Chinese entrepreneurs deliberately marketed locally produced drugs as foreign, complete with the endorsements of fictive Western doctors, in order to capitalize on the cultural cachet of foreign medicines, which were more likely to be accepted than rejected based on their supposed foreignness.[50]

Yibin County is equidistant from both major cities in Sichuan, 288 kilometers southwest of Chongqing and 286 kilometers southeast of Chengdu, marking a corner of an equilateral triangle in the heart of the province. Its CHC, established in July 1940 under the directorship of Qiu Zhengwen, received more funding than most.[51] Its general funding came from individual donations from people working in education, local government, and the military who pooled together their resources, illustrating that China's philanthropic tradition survived even the privations of war.[52]

Although the Yibin CHC reported to the SPHA infrequently, it was one of the most active county health centers in Sichuan, coordinating the work of four hospitals (with a staff of thirty-two doctors, thirty-two nurses, and six midwives) and fourteen health clinics (with a staff of fourteen doctors, three nurses, and three midwives).[53] As a promoter of scientific biomedicine, the Yibin CHC had a strong basis on which to build; American Baptist missionaries ran separate men's and women's hospitals in Yibin County (Ren'ai Men's Hospital and Mingde Women's Hospital), where Baptist medical missionary Dr. C. H. Finch began his work in 1892. Dr. Finch reported seeing twenty to thirty patients per day from the very beginning and recalled being "surprised at the confidence placed by the Chinese in the foreign doctor, willingly submitting to the knife or to the anesthetic, provided I would promise to cure."[54]

The CHC in Songpan County provides a stark contrast to the work achieved in the foregoing well-developed and centrally located counties. In this region of far northwest Sichuan bordering Gansu Province, Han Chinese lived as a minority among Tibetan, Hui, and Qiang Chinese. Songpan's CHC was situated in its county seat, 325 kilometers northwest of Chengdu. The county seat also housed the county's single hospital (the least of all locales discussed here) with three physicians, one pharmacist, two nurses, and one midwife, as well as a single health clinic (again, the least of all locales), with one doctor and two nurses on staff.[55] The sole hospital and health clinic could not have provided immediate succor to people living in the distant villages within Songpan County. However, geographical remove sometimes served one well; in 1944, neither remote Songpan nor relatively well-funded Chongqing had any cholera cases while most of Sichuan Province furiously battled the deadly disease.[56] Other diseases did plague the county, though, including kala-azar, leprosy, malaria, hookworm, schistosomiasis, and relapsing fever; nevertheless, in more than seven hundred reported cases of illness, not a single death occurred.[57]

The Songpan CHC reported to the SPHA even less often than did the CHC in Yibin, most likely because its paucity of staff made health work and compilation of statistics difficult and sporadic. Staff still performed general public health activities, including vaccination and cleanliness campaigns, well-baby contests, mothers' meetings, and hygiene demonstrations, as well as MCH work and treatments for venereal disease.[58] Perhaps due to its low number of staff, funding of the Songpan CHC paled in comparison to that of its sister organizations, though it is clear that the center performed an impressive amount of work considering these limitations.[59] For example, staff delivered one hundred babies in 1945, more than in Hechuan County and only slightly less than in Beibei, and vaccinated more people than did their colleagues in Hechuan that year and again the following year.[60] This level of activity indicates a high degree of trust between CHC staff and the local population in Songpan, and it belies a simple narrative of superior health services in urban centers and inferior services in the hinterland.

This brief examination of health work in 4 of Sichuan's 139 total counties illustrates shades and degrees of rurality. A woman and her infant in Songpan County might not survive a difficult childbirth, but both were highly likely to recover from the trauma—or escape it entirely—if the birth occurred in Bishan. Likewise, a person with a sudden case of dysentery could easily pass away before getting to the nearest health center in Songpan, while the same person might receive life-saving treatment in Hechuan. At the same time, public health staff in Bishan, trained in the country's best medical university, treated trachoma and delivered babies, while the sparse and poorly funded staff in remote Songpan outperformed their Hechuan colleagues working in the vicinity of the wartime capital.

Even a preliminary examination makes clear that the SPHA made such astonishing achievements during the trying war years due to the unflagging energy and heartfelt devotion of Dr. Chen Zhiqian, a man who never took the Rockefeller Foundation's generous support of his public health projects for granted, and who expressed profound humility in reflecting on his life's work.[61] Hundreds of others worked in the provincial health administration and, on a semivolunteer basis, in the CHCs, but they would never have had the opportunity to do so were it not for the unique personage of Dr. Chen, a man with one foot in the elite world of the American Rockefellers and the other in China's rural heartland.

Crafting New Bodies: A Coalescence of Desires in Wartime China

World War II created a unique moment in the histories of medicine and public health. Facing the imperative to fill battlefields and factories with healthy men and women, political leaders of countries around the world strove to keep their respective populations as healthy as possible. Scientists worked at a breakneck pace in laboratories to produce penicillin, pharmaceutical companies manufactured large quantities of sulfa drugs around the clock, and charitable organizations developed new methods of delivering medical aid to wounded soldiers and civilians.[62]

In China, astute health officials like Chen Zhiqian seized this opportunity to expand their work in a direction that Nationalist Party leaders associated with their political rivals, the Communists: public health services in the rural countryside. While similar projects came under closer scrutiny and were occasionally shut down in peacetime, health workers enjoyed greater autonomy during the war when more pressing issues distracted central government officials. This helps to explain how more than one hundred CHCs throughout Sichuan Province received financial and administrative support in a period of political and financial disarray. While never enough to cover actual needs, the financial contributions from outside a given county sometimes reached astonishing heights. For example, financial reports from the Yibin CHC demonstrate that financial assistance from the Executive Yuan (via the SPHA) and outside sources accounted for more than 86 percent of the operating budget.[63] Here again is another instance in which Chen Zhiqian's role as director of the SPHA was key. As a respected alumnus of the Peking Union Medical College, and one of John B. Grant's protégés, Chen received regular grants from the Rockefeller Foundation's China Medical Board to support the various county health centers as well as the public health work he directed in Chengdu. This funding included more than US$4,000 in the administration's inaugural year of 1939.[64] The SPHA also received large donations of materials from the American Red Cross. Dr. Chen made judicious use of his social connections to benefit the rural poor.

Even as he built the provincial capital's public health infrastructure from the ground up, Chen fought to uphold the primacy of rural public health in his organization's funding structure. He divided the funding the SPHA received from the NHA equally between the CHCs and SPHA headquarters in Chengdu.[65] Chen also used the outside monies he managed to recruit from US donors to further bolster the 131 CHCs. Rockefeller philanthropists gladly supported the SPHA because they had experienced dismay when the Japanese invasion curtailed rural health programs that they had funded previously.[66]

Besides helping to open up new opportunities for national government and international charity support, the threat of losing the country to an invading foreign army inspired compliance with government programs to remake the populace. The New Life Movement was the Nationalist government's attempt to instill Confucian-style morality as well as political obedience and bodily discipline in all citizens. Designed by middle- and upper-class Chinese for the supposed improvement of the lower classes, the New Life Movement embodied elite attitudes about the poor. First Lady Song Meiling gave voice to prevailing cultural attitudes about poverty and rural people when she wrote, in 1937, that the movement included "intensive course[s]" for rural Chinese "in public sanitation, rural economy, village industries, military discipline, and, most emphasized of all, methods of teaching the people to become self-respecting and worthwhile citizens."[67] Sean Hsiang-lin Lei concludes that the New Life Movement and related public health campaigns aimed to "habituate morality" and create "a new technology of the individual," according to which citizens related more readily to the nation-state than to their own families and willingly worked on behalf of the nation.[68]

Lei's analysis provides the proper context in which to understand Madame Song Meiling's use of the expression "worthwhile citizens." Without a doubt, rural Chinese were the most worthwhile and productive citizens in wartime China; not only did they feed soldiers and civilians alike through their agricultural work, they also served as soldiers themselves and, after migrating into the cities, performed a variety of manual labor that kept these cities functioning. Yet in the eyes of the New Life Movement's architects, rural Chinese would not become "worthwhile citizens" until they cast aside their values for those that government leaders deemed worthy. In the realm of public health, this required a repudiation of dirt and a hearty embrace of cleanliness. Therefore, teaching rural Chinese to give birth in a sterile environment and accept vaccination shots not only saved their lives—as public health workers wished to do—but, as state officials desired, enveloped them into the disciplined body of the nation.

228 ❧ NICOLE ELIZABETH BARNES

Notes

1. C. C. Chen, in collaboration with Frederica M. Bunge, *Medicine in Rural China: A Personal Account* (Berkeley: University of California Press, 1989), 57.

2. C. C. Chen, "A Statement of the Szechuan Provincial Health Administration," December 1, 1939, 1, folder 161, box 18, series 601, Record Group (RG) 1.1, Rockefeller Foundation Archives, Sleepy Hollow, New York [hereafter cited as RFA], Rockefeller Archive Center [hereafter cited as RAC].

3. Xiaoping Fang, *Barefoot Doctors and Western Medicine in China* (Rochester, NY: University of Rochester Press, 2012).

4. In its first year of operation (1929), the Ministry of Health received 0.11 percent of the national budget. The health budget grew to a still paltry 0.7 percent by 1936. Ka-che Yip, *Health and National Reconstruction in Nationalist China: The Development of Modern Health Services, 1928–1937* (Ann Arbor, MI: Association for Asian Studies, 1995), 63.

5. Chen, *Medicine in Rural China*, 2.

6. Ibid., 21–23. One thing that Dr. Chen fails to make clear in his memoir is that his stepmother also perished from this illness, even after visiting the French physician. Rather, he briefly mentions the death of his stepmother in a different context prior to relating the story of his first exposure to biomedical diagnostics (Ibid., 9).

7. Ibid., 1, 2, 25.

8. When he entered the Peking Union Medical College in 1921, Chen discovered that he was the only student from the entire southwestern region of China, and that "most of the others were from coastal cities, mainly Shanghai and Guangzhou." Ibid., 33.

9. Ibid., 209.

10. Ibid., 3, 25.

11. According to Chen, financial woes constituted his most difficult problem in retaining quality staff as well as the greatest reason for popular discontent with the Nationalist Party. See C. C. Chen to M. C. Balfour, November 6, 1940, folder 161, box 18, series 601, RG 1.1, RFA.

12. Paul Starr, *The Social Transformation of American Medicine: The Rise of a Sovereign Profession and the Making of a Vast Industry* (New York: Basic Books, 1982), 180–97.

13. Liping Bu, "John B. Grant: Public Health and State Medicine," in *Medical Transitions in Twentieth-Century China*, ed. Bridie Andrews and Mary Brown Bullock (Bloomington: Indiana University Press, 2014), 212–26; Yip, *Health and National Reconstruction*, 45–46, 50.

14. Chen, *Medicine in Rural China*, 66–69; Yip, *Health and National Reconstruction*, 18. On Chen's work in the model county in Hebei Province, see C. C. Chen, "Ting Hsien and the Public Health Movement in China," *Milbank Memorial Fund Quarterly* 15, no. 4 (October 1937): 380–90; and Jing Jun, *Dingxian shiyan: Shequ yixue yu huabei nongcun* [The Ding County experiment: Community medicine and rural North China] (Beijing: Qinghua University, Department of Sociology, 2004).

15. Chen, *Medicine in Rural China*, 106. Ka-che Yip, a scholar of Chinese medical history, has also stated that the health work Dr. Chen directed in Dingxian served as the model for other rural health programs in the Republican period. Yip, *Health and National Reconstruction*, 19.

16. C. C. Chen, "A Review of Government Health Services in Szechuan, China, for the period 1939–1945," 1–2, 1946, folder 2721, box 218, series 3, RG 5, International Health Board Archives, RCA.

17. "Report of Committee on Health and Medical Care," submitted to the Commission on Investigation and Planning of Relief and Rehabilitation of the Executive Yuan, July 1, 1944, Chongqing, 1, 3, folder 156, box 22, China Medical Board (CMB), RFA.

18. Chen, "Review of Government Health Services," 1.

19. Ibid., 2. On Dr. Chen's dedication to MCH, see Chen, Medicine in Rural China, 90–91.

20. Chen, "Review of Government Health Services," 3.

21. Chen, Medicine in Rural China, 25, 83; C. C. Chen, "Resume of Activities in January to August, 1940," 2, folder 161, box 18, series 601, RG 1.1, RFA.

22. "Report of Szechuan Provincial Health Administration for the Year of 1941," 10, folder 2719, box 218, series 3, RG 5.3, International Health Board Archives, RCA.

23. "Report of Szechuan Provincial Health Administration for the Year of 1941," 8, RFA; "Report of Committee on Health and Medical Care," 32, RFA; "Hospital Name Chart" [Yiyuan mingcheng yilanbiao], June 5, 1944, 113-1-1076, 8, Sichuan Provincial Archives [hereafter cited as SPA].

24. As of 2012, these CHC reports can be referenced in a paper index held in the SPA reading room; documents are in paper copy.

25. "Report on Health Improvements in This Province" [Bensheng tuijin weisheng baogao], 1940, 113-116, 10, SPA; Chen, "Resume of Activities in January to August, 1940," 2, RFA; "1945 Complete Statistical Health Report Compiled by the Sichuan Provincial Health Administration" [Sichuansheng weishengchu bianzhi 34 niandu weisheng tongji zong baogao], 1945, 113-1-118, 106–8, SPA.

26. Bishan's 1945 budget was over 1 million yuan (1,100,189 to be precise). Yibin's CHC budget followed very closely behind at 1,027,808 yuan. "1945 Complete Statistical Health Report," 15–21. For a thorough study of one of the village health clinics in Bishan County, see Isabel Brown Crook et al., Prosperity's Predicament: Identity, Reform, and Resistance in Rural Wartime China (Lanham, MD: Rowman and Littlefield, 2013).

27. Fang, Barefoot Doctors, 47–51, 136–37.

28. Chen noted that the Dingxian model included "a cardinal principle . . . that the health worker should never act, or be called on to act, as a physician . . . [that he or she] not commit serious errors," and emphasized the importance of a hierarchy in responsibility based on staff members' medical education and experience. See Chen, Medicine in Rural China, 83, 194; and Xiaoping Fang, "From Union Clinics to Barefoot Doctors: Healers, Medical Pluralism and State Medicine in Chinese Villages, 1950–1970," Journal of Modern Chinese History 2, no. 2 (December 2008): 233.

29. Bishan County reported seventy-two medical personnel, whereas Chengdu had twenty-three, Yibin County had nineteen, Hechuan County had thirteen, and Songpan County had eight, for a grand total of sixty-three. "1945 Complete Statistical Health Report," 105. Nonetheless, the exigencies and stressors of war made staff turnover incredibly high, and these numbers fluctuated wildly.

30. Bishan CHC Work Report, July 1944, 113-1-694, SPA; Bishan County Health Center Report on Personnel Training, February 1942, 96–100, SPA.

31. Tina Phillips-Johnson, *Childbirth in Republican China: Delivering Modernity* (Lanham, MD: Lexington Books, 2011), xxvi.

32. Yang Chongrui and Wang Shijin, *The Study of Maternal and Children's Health* [*Fuying weisheng xue*] (Chongqing: National Institute of Health, 1944), 3.

33. Nicole E. Barnes, "Disease in the Capital: Nationalist Health Services and the 'Sick (Wo)man of East Asia' in Wartime Chongqing," *European Journal of East Asian Studies* 11, no. 2 (December 2012): 292–94.

34. Bishan CHC Work Report, January–June 1940, 113-1-129, 84–85, SPA.

35. Ibid., n.p.

36. Ibid., n.p. Women constituted 61 percent of outpatients during the reporting period, an astonishingly high number given that in other counties and cities men regularly outnumbered women as recipients of hospital care.

37. "1945 Complete Statistical Health Report," 98–99.

38. Ibid., 90–92.

39. Bishan CHC Work Reports, March and April 1943, 113-1-926, 16, 22, SPA.

40. John R. Watt, *Saving Lives in Wartime China: How Medical Reformers Built Modern Healthcare Systems amid War and Epidemics, 1928–1945* (Leiden: Brill, 2014). A school health survey conducted in Chongqing in March 1945 found that nearly 65 percent of schoolchildren suffered from trachoma, the highest incidence of any one disease among over 5,000 children surveyed. Yong Zhou, ed., *Chongqing tongshi* [General history of Chongqing], vol. 3 of *A Comprehensive History of Chongqing* (Chongqing: Chongqing Press, 2002), 1145.

41. Yip, *Health and National Reconstruction*, 81.

42. Thomas McKeown first made this argument early in the scholarly debates on public health. See Thomas H. McKeown, *The Modern Rise of Population* (New York: Academic Press, 1976); Thomas H. McKeown, *The Role of Medicine: Dream, Mirage, or Nemesis?* (Princeton, NJ: Princeton University Press, 1980), 120.

43. "Hospital Name Chart," 8.

44. "1946 Complete Statistical Health Report Compiled by the Sichuan Provincial Health Administration" [*Sichuansheng weishengchu bianzhi 35 niandu weisheng tongji zong baogao*], 1946, 113-1-119, n.p., SPA.

45. Ibid.

46. Hechuan County Governor Xie Tianmin to Sichuan Provincial Governor Wang [*Hechuan xian xianzhang Xie Tianmin zhi Sichuan shengzhengfu zhuxi Wang*], 1939, 113-1-129, 44–46, SPA.

47. Judith Wyman, "The Ambiguities of Chinese Antiforeignism: Chongqing, 1870–1900," *Late Imperial China* 18, no. 2 (December 1998): 62.

48. "1946 Complete Statistical Health Report," n.p.

49. Bridie Andrews, *The Making of Modern Chinese Medicine, 1850–1960* (Vancouver: University of British Columbia Press, 2014), 51–68.

50. Sherman Cochran, *Chinese Medicine Men: Consumer Culture in China and Southeast Asia* (Cambridge, MA: Harvard University Press, 2006), 39–44, 71, 72, 160–61.

51. "Report on Health Improvements," 10. The Yibin CHC received 1,600 yuan in regular monthly funding and 600 yuan per month in additional assistance from the SPHA.

52. "Yibin County Donations to County Health Center," 1941, 113-1-867, 11–12, SPA.

53. "1945 Complete Statistical Health Report," 106–8.

54. "Medical Work," *West China Missionary News* 39, no. 9 (September 1937): 15.

55. "1945 Complete Statistical Health Report," 106–8.

56. Ibid., 34.

57. Ibid., 44–47.

58. Ibid., 28–30, 63–66, 98–99, 90–92.

59. Ibid., 15–21. The Songpan CHC received 310,162 yuan annually, while the Bishan and Yibin CHCs each received over 1 million yuan, and the Hechuan CHC received 779,848 yuan.

60. Ibid., 90–92; "1946 Complete Statistical Health Report," n.p.

61. Dr. Chen's many reports to the Rockefeller Foundation are all very long and full of detail, and every budget he submitted includes apologies for the degree to which inflation forced him to ask for additional funding, as well as immediate adjustments thereof when necessary. See files in box 18, series 601, RG 1.1, RFA. In his memoir, Dr. Chen reflected on his half century of service to public health by writing, "Most of us are apt to be surprised to realize how little we have accomplished in our lifetimes." Chen, *Medicine in Rural China*, 5.

62. John E. Lesch, *The First Miracle Drugs: How the Sulfa Drugs Transformed Medicine* (Oxford: Oxford University Press, 2007). See also the chapter by Mary Augusta Brazelton.

63. SPHA County Health Center Survey Reports, Yibin County, December, no year, 113-1-389, 7–12, SPA. While the CHC took in a monthly average of 400 yuan in patient fees, its monthly output was 2,880 yuan. Director Qiu Zhengwen's monthly salary alone was 200 yuan.

64. SPHA Grant Memo, November 1943, 43214, folder 161, box 18, series 601, RG 1.1, RFA.

65. Chen, "Resume of Activities in January to August, 1940," 2, RFA.

66. Paul B. Trescott, "H. D. Fong and the Study of Chinese Economic Development," *History of Political Economy* 34, no. 4 (2002): 800.

67. Song Meiling, *Madame Chiang Kai-shek on the New Life Movement* (Shanghai: China Weekly Review Press, 1937), 69.

68. Sean Hsiang-lin Lei, "Habituating Individuality: Framing Tuberculosis and Its Material Solutions in Republican China," *Bulletin for the History of Medicine* 84 (2010): 248–79.

Afterword

Western Medicine and Global Health

WILLIAM H. SCHNEIDER

A main goal of this volume has been to show how China-based developments in Western medicine incorporated China as an integral site in the creation of global biomedicine. Beginning in the nineteenth century, Western Europe developed an approach to medicine based on new scientific discoveries that had a global application by the beginning of the twentieth century. Gao Xi provides a case study of this development in her chapter on Patrick Manson and the medical missionaries in China beginning in the 1870s, but there are myriad examples of this from China and elsewhere. At the end of the century, Alexandre Yersin and Shibasaburo Kitasato made their dramatic discoveries of the cause of bubonic plague while working in Hong Kong; and before the outbreak of World War I, the Manchurian Plague Prevention Service hosted research by a team of international scholars. Other early global biomedical research included Ronald Ross's work on malaria in India, which won international notoriety (Nobel Prize in Physiology or Medicine 1902), as did the research of Alphonse Laveran in Algeria (Nobel Prize 1907). Algeria was also where Charles Nicolle made his discovery of the cause of typhus in 1912 (Nobel Prize 1928). In Brazil Oswaldo Cruz established an institute at the beginning of the twentieth century modeled on the Pasteur Institute, where he had trained.[1]

This afterword looks at the history of Western medicine in China from the perspective of today's global health concerns. Comparing contemporary efforts to improve health for all can help in understanding the growth of Western medicine in China, which typically has been studied as an arm of imperial domination or the inevitable growth of Western science. Likewise, this history of Western medicine in China can help to understand global health today if it is studied as a precursor or early example whose similarities and differences help clarify what is new and what is a continuation of earlier efforts.

Any examination of global health and the history of medicine in China begins with the question of what is meant by global health. The problem is that the concept is not very well defined, nor is there much common agreement.[2] One phrase commonly found in definitions is the goal of "access to healthcare" by those most in need. For example, J. P. Koplan et al. define global health as "an area for study, research, and practice that places a priority on improving health and achieving health equity for all people worldwide."[3] Similarly, S. B. Macfarlane and colleagues describe global health as being the "worldwide improvement of health, reduction of disparities, and protection against global threats that disregard national borders."[4] I. Kickbush places even greater emphasis on this transnational element: "those health issues that transcend national boundaries and governments and call for actions on the global forces that determine the health of people."[5] Condensing these, Robert Beaglehole and Ruth Bonita define global health as "collaborative trans-national research and action for promoting health for all."[6]

These are very present-minded definitions, and most authors ignore the fact that such concepts as world or international health or tropical medicine were used as far back as the end of the nineteenth century to describe cross-border efforts—first to identify and treat disease, then later to justify organizations whose purpose was to improve health for populations worldwide. Historians Theodore M. Brown et al. have identified the use of the phrase "global health" as early as the 1970s, but in the current sense only as recently as 2000.[7] Their conclusion is that tropical medicine and international health at the end of the nineteenth and beginning of the twentieth centuries were concerned primarily with identification, monitoring, and prevention of epidemics of infectious diseases. The establishment of a League of Nations Health Organization and more importantly the World Health Organization (WHO) after 1945 created intergovernmental bodies of international health to coordinate national efforts not only to prevent epidemics but also to improve access to new and more effective medical care using Western scientific medicine.

These international efforts had historical roots in colonial medical services; by the 1920s in Africa (depending on the colony), there was annual reporting of the main diseases, as well as monitoring of periodic epidemics such as smallpox and sleeping sickness.[8] In addition to this work and the newly established and more highly publicized campaigns that toured the countryside to combat these diseases,[9] most time and resources went into the establishment and operation of hospitals and clinics, at first in capitals and European enclaves, but also increasingly in more remote districts. The "health for all" goal was enunciated at the WHO Alma Ata Conference of 1978 and reflected a new emphasis on this "horizontal" as opposed to "vertical" access to health care, even as the international organization was completing its most successful disease campaign that culminated in the eradication of smallpox.[10] The new concept of global health arose, according to

Brown et al., not only from the growth of these activities, but also from the work of numerous new nongovernmental organizations that were becoming involved in cross-border health and the inability of WHO to control or coordinate them.[11]

What follows is an examination of some key features of global health as they apply to the history of Western medicine in China to 1950. This will take into account the breadth of the definition as well as the geographical regions of greatest activity. It will identify the focus of efforts, specifically the question of the priority of disease control versus health for all (vertical versus horizontal), as well as the donor-recipient relationship implicit in much of global health. Crucial to the latter is the role of local national government, especially as viewed by outside donors.

One problem with applying the concept of global health to historical circumstances (or even contemporary practices) is the broad and pervasive scope of cross-national efforts to improve the health of all. Assuming that all governments favor the improvement of everyone's health, then whenever they utilize outside assistance or collaboration, their efforts could be considered as part of global health. Hence the term risks being so broad as to be of little use. Nevertheless, in comparing the specific circumstances that have varied considerably over time and in different places in the world, even the broad concept of global health can help to identify the relative importance of key elements, such as ability to protect heath, willingness and ability to obtain outside assistance, and interest of outsiders to provide it.

For example, the place today most associated with work in global health is sub-Saharan Africa, and whether intended or not, many of the efforts at improving health in that region have fostered perceptions that are similar to those about China during the nineteenth century and first half of the twentieth century. The high death rate from infectious diseases, the lack of access to effective and adequate health care, periodic famines and epidemics, problems of warfare, and corrupt and ineffective government—these are just some of the problems seen in sub-Saharan Africa today that were once observed and described in similar terms concerning China.[12] The corresponding health concerns both historically in China and today in Africa have elicited responses within the countries affected, as well as significant assistance from outside to improve the situation. Indeed, one need look no further than the similar interest in health of the dominant foundation in the first half of the twentieth century (Rockefeller) and the largest one today (Gates) to find that their greatest expenditures have been on health in China (Rockefeller) and Africa (Gates).

Another feature of global health is the disagreement about priorities that has emerged between those concerned with infectious disease and those concerned with access to general health care.[13] Today all countries are involved in monitoring infectious diseases, especially new emerging ones.

The WHO still plays the most important coordinating role, although one offshoot of this part of global health—prevention and eradication of disease—has also involved a number of other agencies, nongovernmental organizations, foundations, and bilateral agreements not always well coordinated by the WHO.[14] Although the efforts to combat the AIDS epidemic in Africa (and more recently SARS and Ebola) have received the most attention, historically the eradication of smallpox has inspired similar campaigns against polio and childhood diseases, plus renewed campaigns against malaria and tuberculosis.[15] Earlier, China, along with India, were identified by Westerners as the locations of the greatest epidemics in the nineteenth and first half of the twentieth century. In fact, contagious disease was a paramount concern both to the Chinese and to foreigners who came to visit, trade, and live in China, and this was among the main reasons for the outside interest in medical assistance. Although eradication was not a viable option, the periodic epidemics and efforts to introduce preventive measures were comparable to much contemporary global health work in Africa.[16]

Those concerned with health for all and access to care have sometimes been at odds with the disease campaigns, particularly as far as resource priorities are concerned. In fact, some scholars have charged that philanthropic donors have deliberately backed disease-specific campaigns instead of primary health care because the campaigns were less expensive than the higher cost of developing the health infrastructure. For example, the Gates Foundation has been criticized in this regard.[17] Providing basic infrastructure, such as adequate hospitals or training for doctors, nurses, and other health workers requires extensive and ongoing commitment of resources. Another noteworthy consequence of building infrastructure as shown by the history of Western medicine in China is that the process of securing extensive resources to build costly or complicated infrastructure is much more likely to introduce a long-term donor-recipient relationship of dependency. Based on the experience in China to 1950 and in sub-Saharan Africa to the present day, whereas disease campaigns usually take a much shorter time and are less costly, the transfer of resources and knowledge from the richer countries to build the infrastructure (e.g., hospitals and medical schools) to make more effective health care available to the population takes longer and is much more expensive.

One problem that often arises in the donor-recipient relationship is the tendency of the donor to blame problems on the weakness of the local (recipient) government. This is a common complaint about most contemporary African governments, and it was also the case with China from 1800 to 1950.[18] In this matter, the history of Western medicine in China might at first glance resemble more the history of medicine in India or the Islamic world rather than Africa, because China, India, and the Middle East were highly populated regions with histories of strong central government and widely used, indigenous medical traditions that were challenged in the nineteenth and twentieth centuries by Western powers militarily and politically. The result was weakened political rule at the same time that more promising new medical treatments also appeared.[19] When combined with Western racism, the confidence of outsiders in local government was greatly reduced, both in Islamic lands as well as the Indian subcontinent and China as well as Africa. One crucial difference, however, was that formal colonial rule was not established in China. As a result, China was presented with a greater variety of outside influences in areas such as medicine and education, because there was no single colonial administration attempting to control and limit such assistance to Chinese institutions. In fact, colonial medical officers were sometimes wary of health and other assistance from organizations in their home country such as missionaries and universities. They feared such efforts might overshadow the benefits of colonial rule that the outside power wished to demonstrate to its subjects through such amenities as providing health care and education.[20]

In one sense the weak and divided Chinese government of the Republican period, like African governments today, was less able to resist and more likely to take advantage of multiple outside offers of assistance, both because of lack of resources to take advantage of them as well as the inability to overcome internal criticism if it were to turn down much-needed assistance. Ironically, this same weakness was criticized by outsiders in both circumstances as hindering the development of health facilities. In any case, the similarities of poor health status, weak or ineffective local governments, and interest of outsiders in providing assistance historically to China from 1800 to 1950, and today in sub-Saharan Africa, make the comparison of these two situations useful in understanding each. Of course, Africa has lacked some important features that China, South Asia, and Islamic states had, such as a strong tradition of literate physicians and a unified rule under a strong government. This explains in part some of the more deeply seated reasons why health in Africa is a greater problem than in other regions.

Evidence of the important role of government can most visibly be seen in the development of health infrastructure. Hospitals and medical schools are the two most important institutional reflections of Western medicine, and both colonial Africa and China before 1950 saw the establishment of hundreds of hospitals. There were more missionary hospitals in China than in Africa, reflecting the greater activity of missionaries there, but colonial governments added significantly to the numbers in Africa, reflecting the strategy after the 1920s and especially after 1945 of providing additional medical services to demonstrate concretely the benefits of colonial rule.[21] But investment in medical schools was a different story because they quickly became much more expensive and took longer in terms of payoff. Excluding South Africa, there were only a handful of medical schools established in sub-Saharan Africa by the time of independence, most notably in Kampala, Uganda, and Ibadan, Nigeria, and both of those only began to be phased in after 1945.[22] In contrast, China saw the creation of dozens of medical schools starting in the nineteenth century. Some were short lived, but a 1931 report by the League of Nations found thirteen such schools in existence.[23] This was a small number in comparison to need, but a reflection in part of the existence of an independent government that supported or encouraged their creation.[24]

The fact that missionaries in China relied on "union" schools (e.g., Chengdu, Shandong, and Beijing) was in part a response to the increasing costs of Western medical education by the beginning of the twentieth century, thanks to new discoveries and technology that were at the core of laboratory-based scientific biomedicine.[25] These new schools typically required the resources of a government or the Rockefeller Foundation to sustain them. Other evidence of the crucial role of government is the fact that in Africa it was not until shortly after independence that the number of hospitals dramatically increased, especially in districts outside the capitals and big cities. In almost every African country, at least one medical school was soon established.[26]

Paradoxically, governments whose weakness attracts outside assistance have often been criticized by those offering it for being weak, ineffective, and corrupt. In other words, the very weakness that makes governments themselves unable to afford investments in health—and that is among the main reasons that outside institutions and governments offer assistance in health care—also test the patience and confidence of outside donors as to what they expect local governments to produce. The expectation most commonly disappointed is that the recipient government would make some matching financial contribution. For example, the policy of the Rockefeller Foundation worldwide, especially in funding infrastructure, was to expect that a share of costs would be paid by the local government. Yet in the case of PUMC, by far the single biggest project investment of the foundation in the first half of the twentieth century, its officers were almost always disappointed.[27]

Criticism of African governments by the European and US press for ineffectiveness at the least, and corruption or dictatorial brutality at the worst, is widespread.[28] Neoliberal development experts have characterized this differently, arguing since the 1980s for "structural adjustment," by which they meant less government involvement in the economy in favor of open markets.[29] As a result, governments cut back on support of health infrastructure. Critics of this strategy have concluded that rather than the expected demand for health care stimulating the private sector to respond, that need has been met instead by international health assistance, or global health. In a 2010 cross-national study entitled "Public Financing of Health in Developing Countries," Lu et al. found that in all developing countries government financing of health nearly doubled from 1995 to 2006. At the national and regional levels, however, they found that "while shares of government expenditures to health increased in many regions, they decreased in many sub-Saharan African countries. The statistical analysis showed that DAH [development assistance for health] to government had a negative and significant effect on domestic government spending on health such that for every dollar of DAH to government, government health expenditures from domestic resources were reduced by $0.43 (p = 0) to $1.14 (p = 0)."[30]

This broad comparison risks raising more questions than it answers, but hopefully it demonstrates the need for further work. One should not expect neat and simple lessons when comparing such complex developments as the history of Western medicine in China and the activities of global health today. Nevertheless, looking at China's historical experience in a global context has two important values. It guards against the tendency to isolate China and see its history and conditions as so peculiar as to be unique. At the same time, it is a warning against present-mindedness by contemporary health practitioners who are caught up so intently in meeting immediate needs that they ignore potentially useful lessons from the past.

Notes

1. Anne-Marie Moulin, "Patriarchal Science: The Network of the Overseas Pasteur Institutes," in Patrick Petitjean, Catherine Jami, and A. M. Moulin, eds., *Science and Empires: Historical Studies about Scientific Development and European Expansion* (New York: Springer, 1992), 307–22. There is a large and growing body of scholarship on this concept of global biomedicine. In addition to other contributions in *Science and Empires*, see a recent provocative work by David Baronov, *The African Transformation of Western Medicine and the Dynamics of Global Cultural Exchange* (Philadelphia: Temple University Press, 2008). For broader reconsiderations of "Western" science, including medicine, see Roy MacLeod, "Introduction," in *Nature and Empire: Science and the Colonial Enterprise*, vol. 15 of *Osiris*, 2nd ser. (2000): 1–13; and Marwa Elshakry, "When Science Became Western: Historiographical Reflections," *Isis* 101 (2010): 98–109.

2. Oliver-James Dyer and Ayesha de Costa, "What Is Global Health?" *Journal of Global Health* 1, no. 1 (Spring 2011): 31–32.

3. J. P. Koplan et al., "Towards a Common Definition of Global Health," *Lancet* 373 (2009): 1993–95.

4. S. B. Macfarlane, M. Jacobs, and E. E. Kaaya, "In the Name of Global Health: Trends in Academic Institutions," *Journal of Public Health Policy* 29 (2008): 383–401.

5. I. Kickbush, "The Need for a European Strategy on Global Health," *Scandinavian Journal of Public Health* 34 (2006): 561–65.

6. Robert Beaglehole and Ruth Bonita, "What Is Global Health?" *Global Health Action* 3, no. 5142 (2010), https://www.ncbi.nlm.nih.gov/pmc/articles/PMC2852240/.

7. Theodore M. Brown, Marcos Cueto, and Elizabeth Fee, "'International' to 'Global' Public Health," *American Journal of Public Health* 96 (2006): 62–72. Brown, Cueto, and Fee cite, for example, James E. Banta, "From International to Global Health," *Journal of Community Health* 26 (2001): 73–76; Supinda Bunyavanich and Ruth B. Walkup, "US Public Health Leaders Shift Toward a New Paradigm of Global Health," *American Journal of Public Health* 91 (2001): 1556–58; Derek Yach and Douglas Bettcher, "The Globalization of Public Health, I: Threats and Opportunities," *American Journal of Public Health* 88 (1998): 735–38; and "The Globalization of Public Health, II: The Convergence of Self-Interest and Altruism," *American Journal of Public Health* 88 (1998): 738–41.

8. William H. Schneider, "Smallpox in Africa during colonial Rule," *Medical History* 53 (2009): 193–228.

9. For examples in addition to Schneider, "Smallpox in Africa," see Maryinez Lyons, *The Colonial Disease: A Social History of Sleeping Sickness in Northern Zaire, 1900–1940* (Cambridge: Cambridge University Press, 1992); and Jean-Paul Bado, *Eugène Jamot, 1879–1937: Le médecin de la maladie du sommeil ou trypanosomiase* (Paris: Karthala, 2011).

10. Frank Fenner, *Smallpox and Its Eradication* (Geneva: World Health Organization, 1988).

11. Brown, Jacobs, and Kaaya, "'International' to 'Global,'" 62; James Webb and Tamara Giles-Vernick, "Introduction," in *Global Health in Africa: Historical Perspectives on Disease Control* (Athens: Ohio University Press, 2013), 10–11.

12. Although frequently mentioned by Westerners in residence in China at the time, the perception of health and disease has not often been the focus of scholarly study. More general examinations of how China was perceived can be found in Harold Isaacs, *Scratches on Our Minds: American Images of China and India* (New York: John Day, 1958); David Martin Jones, *The Image of China in Western Social and Political Thought* (New York: Palgrave Macmillan, 2001); T. Christopher Jesperson, *American Images of China, 1931–1949* (Stanford, CA: Stanford University Press, 1996); and Jonathan D. Spence, *The Chan's Great Continent: China in Western Minds* (New York: Norton, 1990).

13. Webb and Giles-Vernick, "Introduction," 8–10.

14. Devi Sridhar, Lawrence O. Gostin, and Derek Yach, "Healthy Governance: How the WHO Can Regain Its Relevance," *Foreign Affairs*, May 24, 2012, http://www.foreignaffairs.com/articles/137662/by-devi-sridhar-lawrence-o-gostin-and-derek-yach/healthy-governance.

15. See, for example, Joel G. Breman, Ciro A. de Quadros, and Paulo Gadelha, "Smallpox Eradication after 30 Years: Lessons, Legacies and Innovations," Proceedings of a Symposium held at the Oswaldo Cruz Foundation, special issue of *Vaccine* 29, Supplement no. 4 (December 30, 2011): D1–D164.

16. In addition to the contribution by Gao Xi in the present volume, see the recent book by Marta Hanson, *Speaking of Epidemics in Chinese Medicine: Disease and the Geographic Imagination in Late Imperial China* (New York: Routledge, 2011).

17. Anne-Emmanuelle Birn, "Gates's Grandest Challenge: Transcending Technology as Public Health Ideology," *Lancet* 366 (2005): 514–19. More generally, see Marcos Cueto, "The Origins of Primary Health Care and Selective Primary Care," *American Journal of Public Health* 94, no. 11 (2004): 1868–70; and Webb and Giles-Vernick, "Introduction," 5–7.

18. For China, see references in note 12 above. Much recent scholarship on weak states in Africa is concerned with terror—for example, Stewart M. Patrick, *Weak Links: Fragile States, Global Threats, and International Security* (New York: Oxford University Press, 2011). Nonetheless, weak health infrastructure is commonly associated with poor health in Africa. See "African Governments Still Underfunding Health, Warns UN watchdog," *Guardian*, July 24, 2013, http://www.theguardian.com/global-development/2013/jul/24/african-governments-funding-world-health-organisation.

19. For a comparison between Egyptian and Chinese reactions to "Western" science beginning in the nineteenth century, see Elshakry, "When Science Became Western," 98–109.

20. See, for example, Osaak Olumwullah, *Dis-ease in the Colonial State: Medicine, Society, and Social Change among the AbaNyole of Western Kenya* (Westport, CT: Greenwood Press, 2002), 182; and, more recently Anna Greenwood, ed., *Beyond the State: The Colonial Medical Service in British Africa* (Manchester: University of Manchester Press, 2016).

21. Knud Faber, *Report on Medical Schools in China* (Geneva: League of Nations Health Organization, 1931), 9, reports that in 1931 half of the Western hospitals in China were missionary hospitals. Colonial officials in Africa kept close watch on missionary hospitals, whose numbers varied from colony to colony but by the 1930s rarely accounted for more than one-third of hospitals. After World War II, there was a significant increase in government funding for hospitals. See William Schneider, *History of Blood Transfusion in Sub-Saharan Africa* (Athens: Ohio University Press, 2013), 28–29.

22. The *Sub-Saharan African Medical Schools Study* (2011), funded by the Gates Foundation and led by George Washington University and the University of Pretoria, is the first comprehensive study of medical education. https://www.k4health.org/sites/default/files/Sub-Saharan%20African%20Medical%20School%20Study.pdf.

23. Faber, *Report on Medical Schools*, 10–18.

24. See chapter 3 by Daniel Asen and David Luesink in the present volume.

25. The same process resulted in consolidation of medical education in the United States at this time, accelerated by the Flexner Report of 1910. For a recent biography, see Thomas Neville Bonner, *Iconoclast: Abraham Flexner and a Life of Learning* (Baltimore: Johns Hopkins University Press, 2002).

26. See Schneider, *History of Blood Transfusion*, 18, 30–31, 70, 82–83. For more detailed studies of specific regions of Africa, see John Iliffe, *East African Doctors: A History of the Modern Profession* (Cambridge: Cambridge University Press, 1998); André Prost, *Services de santé en pays africain: Leur place dans des structures socio-économiques en voie de développement* (Paris: Masson, 1970); and J. J. André, J. Burke, J. Vuylsteke, and H. van Balen, "Evolution of Health Services," in P. G. Janssens, M. Kivits, and J. Vuylsteke, eds., *Health in Central Africa* (Brussels: King Baudouin Foundation, 1997), 89–158.

27. Raymond Fosdick, *The Story of the Rockefeller Foundation* (New York: Harper & Brothers, 1952), 89. For problems between the foundation and PUMC, see, inter alia, Mary Brown Bullock, *An American Transplant: The Rockefeller Foundation and Peking Union Medical College* (Berkeley: University of California Press, 1980), 48–77.

28. For examples, see Ian Birrell, "Our Image of Africa is Hopelessly Obsolete," *Guardian*, August 25, 2012, http://www.theguardian.com/commentisfree/2012/

aug/26/ian-birrell-emergence-new-africa; or Paul Stoller, "Media Myopia and the Image of Africa," *Huffington Post,* January 12, 2014, http://www.huffingtonpost.com/paul-stoller/media-myopia-and-the-imag_b_3704865.html.

29. There is a huge literature on structural adjustment. The bedrock study is World Bank, *Accelerated Development in Sub-Saharan Africa: An Agenda for Action* (Washington, DC: World Bank, 1981). For a later assessment, see Robert H. Bates, *When Things Fell Apart: State Failure in Late-Century Africa* (Cambridge: Cambridge University Press, 2008).

30. Lu Chunling et al., "Public Financing of Health in Developing Countries: A Cross-National Systematic analysis," *Lancet* 375 (2010): 1375–87.

Chinese and Japanese
Terms and Names

Terms

Aiyou xuehui 艾酉學會
ai ye 艾葉
Beijing yixue zhuanmen xuexiao 北京醫學專門學校
Beiping yikan 北平醫刊
Bishan 璧山
Bo'ai yiyuan 博愛醫院
chanpo 产婆
Chi shizi hui 赤十字会
Dade 大德
Dingxian 定县
feng 风
fenghan 风寒
fuying baojiansuo 婦嬰保健所
guixie 鬼邪
Guoli Beijing yike daxue 國立北京醫科大學
han 寒
Hechuan xian 合川縣
Hechuan 合川
honghuaping 红花瓶
houdan 喉痹
houyong 喉癰
igaku senmon gakkō 醫學專門學校
ika daigaku 醫科大學
jibing 急病
jiwen 祭文
jugong li 鞠躬禮
Kanritsu igaku senmon gakkō kitei 官立醫學專門學校規程
kōtō gakkō 高等學校

lao 癆
laobing 老病
midwives *zuchanshi* 助产士
muxiao 母校
nao sangzi 闹嗓子
Guoqing jinian ri 國慶紀念日
nüeji 疟疾
ri 热
sangu liupo 三姑六婆
zuchan jiangxisuo 助產講習所
Seijō gakkō 成城學校
Shanghai nuzi zhuanmen yixuexiao 上海女子專門醫學校
shanghan 傷寒
shi 湿
shi 食
shuoming yuan 說明員
Sichuan sheng weishengchu 四川省衛生處
sixiang chunzheng 思想純正
Songpan xian 松潘縣
Songpan 松潘
taidu wenrou 態度溫柔
tan 痰
Tongde 同德
Tongsu yishi yuekan 通俗醫事月刊
Tongyi jinian ri 統一紀念日
wenpo 稳婆
xian weishengyuan 縣衛生院
xinfa jiesheng 新法接生
Xiyuanlu 洗冤錄
xue peng jing 血盆经
xunlian chiku nailao fucong zhihui 訓練吃苦耐勞服從指揮
yaopo 药婆
yaozi 疟子
yi 疫
Yibin xian 宜賓縣
Yibin 宜賓
yike daxue 醫科大學
yixue guan 醫學館
yizhe luanbao 醫者亂暴
you 酉
Yu Wei 郁維
Zhongde 中德
zuchanpo 助产婆

Names

Chen Yongsheng 陈泳声
Chen Zhiqian 陈志潜
Fan Yuanlian 范源濂
Ikegami Keiichi 池上馨一
Ishikawa Yoshinao 石川喜直
Jin Baoshan 金宝善
Jin Yamei 金雅妹
Li Jinghan 李景汉
Li Rulin 李入林
Lin Qiaozhi 林巧稚
Liu Ruiheng 刘瑞恒
Murakami Shōta 村上庄太
Nakano Chūtarō 中野鑄太郎
Ni Baochun 倪葆春
Ni Fengsheng 倪逢生
Qian Baohua 钱宝华
Qiu Zhengwen 邱正文
Shi Meiyu 石美玉
Tang Erhe 湯爾和
Yan Yangchu 晏阳初
Yang Chongrui 杨崇瑞
Yao Xunyuan 姚寻源
Zhang Jingxia 张静霞
Zhang Xiangwen 张湘纹
Zhang Zhujun 张竹君
Zhu Baotian 朱寶鈿

Selected Bibliography

Primary Sources

Aside from the vast corpus of periodicals published in China in Chinese and English, sources include the Beijing Municipal Archives; Peking University Health Science Center Archives; Sichuan Provincial Archives; Chongqing Municipal Archives; Yunnan Provincial Archives; Hunan Provincial Archives; Central South University Archives, Changsha; Institute of Modern History Archives, Academia Sinica, Taipei; ABMAC Records, Columbia University; Archives of the League of Nations; Rockefeller Foundation Archives; Cambridge University Archives; and Manuscripts and Archives, Yale University Library. Some of the primary sources cited in the individual chapters of this volume are available at "The History of Western Medicine in China Resources Portal," http://ulib.iupui.edu/wmicproject/project, cosponsored by Indiana University and the Peking University Health Science Center. This project has received support from the Rockefeller Archive Center and a generous grant from the Henry Luce Foundation. It includes a wide collection of information—archive guides, primary sources, digitized materials—selected to assist laypeople and undergraduate students, as well as established scholars and graduate students. Most sources to date focus on the period from the beginning of the nineteenth century to the formation of the People's Republic of China.

Secondary Sources

Anderson, Warwick. *Colonial Pathologies: American Tropical Medicine, Race and Hygiene in the Philippines.* Durham, NC: Duke University Press, 2006.

Andrews, Bridie. *The Making of Modern Chinese Medicine, 1850–1960.* Vancouver: University of British Columbia Press, 2014.

Annals of Shanghai Women Editorial Committee. *Shanghai funv zhi* [Annals of Shanghai women]. Shanghai: Shanghai Academy of Social Sciences Press, 2000.

Arkush, R. David, and Leo O. Lee. "Excerpts from 'Observations on a Trip to America' by Liang Qichao." In *Chinese Civilization: A Sourcebook.* New York: Patricia B. Ebrey, 1993.

Arnold, David. *Colonizing the Body: State Medicine and Epidemic Disease in Nineteenth-Century India*. Berkeley: University of California Press, 1993.

Asen, Daniel. *Death in Beijing: Murder and Forensic Science in Republican China*. Cambridge: Cambridge University Press, 2016.

"Bainian yaolan tianshi qugao wanren tideng renjian nuanhe: Jinian Xiangya huli jiaoyu 100 zhounian" [In memory of the 100th anniversary of Hunan-Yale-in-China nursing education]. *Zhongnan daxue xuebao* [Journal of the Central South University] 21, no. 1 (2011): 1.

Balme, Harold. *China and Modern Medicine: A Study in Medical Missionary Development*. London: United Council for Missionary Education, 1921.

Barry, John M. *Great Influenza: The Story of the Deadliest Pandemic in History*. New York: Penguin Books, 2005.

Bartholemew, James. *The Formation of Science in Japan: Building a Research Tradition*. New Haven, CT: Yale University Press, 1993.

Basalla, George. "The Spread of Western Science." *Science*, n.s., vol. 156, no. 3775 (1967): 611–22.

Bates, Robert H. *When Things Fell Apart: State Failure in Late-Century Africa*. Cambridge: Cambridge University Press, 2008.

Beaglehole, Robert, and Ruth Bonita. "What Is Global Health?" *Global Health Action* 3, no. 5142 (2010). https://www.ncbi.nlm.nih.gov/pmc/articles/PMC2852240/.

Bello, David A. "To Go Where No Han Could Go for Long: Malaria and the Qing Construction of Ethnic Administrative Space in Frontier Yunnan." *Modern China* 31, no. 3 (July 2005): 283–317.

Benedict, Carol. *Bubonic Plague in Nineteenth-Century China*. Stanford, CA: Stanford University Press, 1996.

Birn, Anne-Emmanuelle. "Gates's Grandest Challenge: Transcending Technology as Public Health Ideology." *Lancet* 366 (2005): 514–19.

Bonner, Thomas Neville. *Becoming a Physician: Medical Education in Britain, France, Germany, and the United States, 1750–1945*. New York: Oxford University Press, 1995.

———. *Iconoclast: Abraham Flexner and a Life of Learning*. Baltimore: Johns Hopkins University Press, 2002.

Borowy, Iris, ed. *Uneasy Encounters: The Politics of Medicine and Health in China, 1900–1937*. Frankfurt: Peter Lang, 2009.

Bowers, John Z. *Medical Education in Japan: From Chinese Medicine to Western Medicine*. New York: Hoeber Medical Division, Harper & Row, 1965.

———. *Western Medicine in a Chinese Palace: Peking Union Medical College, 1917–1951*. Philadelphia: Josiah Macy Jr. Foundation, 1972.

Breman, Joel G., Ciro A. de Quadros, and Paulo Gadelha. "Smallpox Eradication after 30 Years: Lessons, Legacies and Innovations." Proceedings of a Symposium held at the Oswaldo Cruz Foundation. Special issue of *Vaccine* 29, Supplement no. 4 (December 30, 2011): D1–D164.

Brook, Timothy, and Bob Wakabayashi. *Opium Regimes: China, Britain and Japan, 1839–1952*. Berkeley: University of California Press, 2000.

Brown, E. Richard. *Rockefeller Medicine Men: Medicine and Capitalism in America*. Berkeley: University of California Press, 1979.

Brown, Theodore M., Marcos Cueto, and Elizabeth Fee. "'International' to 'Global' Public Health." *American Journal of Public Health* 96 (2006): 62–72.

Brunero, Donna. *Britain's Imperial Cornerstone in China: The Chinese Maritime Customs Service, 1854–1949.* New York: Routledge, 2006.

Bu, Liping, and Darwin Stapleton. *Science, Public Health and the State in Modern Asia.* New York: Routledge, 2012.

Buck, Peter. *American Science and Modern China, 1876–1936.* Cambridge, MA: Harvard University Press, 1980.

Bud, Robert. *Penicillin: Triumph and Tragedy.* Oxford: Oxford University Press, 2007.

Bullock, Mary Brown. *An American Transplant: The Rockefeller Foundation and Peking Union Medical College.* Berkeley: University of California Press, 1980.

———. *The Oil Prince's Legacy: Rockefeller Philanthropy in China.* Washington, DC, and Stanford, CA: Woodrow Wilson Center Press and Stanford University Press, 2011.

Bunyavanich, Supinda, and Ruth B. Walkup. "US Public Health Leaders Shift toward a New Paradigm of Global Health." *American Journal of Public Health* 91 (2001): 1556–58.

Butler, Thomas. *Plague and Other Yersina Infections.* New York: Plenum Medical Book Company, 1983.

Cao Xuetao. "Immunology in China: The Past, Present, and Future." *Nature Immunology* 9, no. 4 (April 2008): 329–43.

Chakrabarti, Pratik. *Medicine and Empire.* London: Palgrave Macmillan, 2014.

Chan, Alan K. L., Gregory K. Clancey, and Hui-Chieh Loy, eds. *Historical Perspectives on East Asian Science, Technology, and Medicine.* Singapore: Singapore University Press: World Scientific, 2001.

Chapman, Nancy E., and Jessica C. Plumb. *The Yale-China Association: A Centennial History.* Hong Kong: Chinese University Press, 2001.

Chen, Bangxian. *Zhongguo yixue shi* [Chinese medical history]. Beijing: Tuanjie Publishing, 2005.

Chen, C. C., with Frederica M. Bunge. *Medicine in Rural China: A Personal Account.* Berkeley: University of California Press, 1989.

Chen, Kaiyi. "Quality versus Quantity: The Rockefeller Foundation and Nurses' Training in China." *Journal of American–East Asian Relations* 5, no. 1 (2003): 77–104.

———. *Seeds from the West: St. John's Medical School, Shanghai, 1880–1952.* Chicago: Imprint Publications, 2001.

Chen Mingyuan. *The Intellectuals' Economic Life.* Shanghai: Wenhui Press, 2007.

Cheng, Guangsheng, Ming Li, and George F. Gao. "Recollection: 'A Friend to Man,' Dr. Feifang Tang: A Story of Causative Agent of Trachoma, from 'Tang's Virus' to Chlamydia Trachomatis, to 'Phylum Chlamydiae.'" *Protein Cell* 2, no. 5 (2011): 349–50.

Cheung, Yuet-Wah. *Missionary Medicine in China.* Lanham, MD: University Press of America, 1988.

Chiang, Howard, ed. *Historical Epistemology and the Making of Modern Chinese Medicine.* Manchester: University of Manchester Press, 2015.

Chieko Nakajima. "Medicine, Philanthropy, and Imperialism: The Dōjinkai in China, 1902–1945." *Sino-Japanese Studies* 17 (2010): 46–84.

Choa, Gerald H. *"Heal the Sick" Was Their Motto: The Protestant Medical Missionaries in China.* Hong Kong: Hong Kong University Press, 1990.

Cochran, Sherman. *Chinese Medicine Men: Consumer Culture in China and Southeast Asia.* Cambridge, MA: Harvard University Press, 2006.

Croizier, Ralph. *Traditional Medicine in Modern China: Science, Nationalism, and the Tensions of Cultural Change.* Cambridge, MA: Harvard University Press, 1968.

Crook, Isabel Brown, and Christina Kelley Gilmartin, with Yu Xiji. *Prosperity's Predicament: Identity, Reform, and Resistance in Rural Wartime China.* Lanham, MD: Rowman and Littlefield, 2013.

Crosby, Alfred. *Ecological Imperialism: The Biological Expansion of Europe, 900–1900.* Cambridge: Cambridge University Press, 1986.

Cueto, Marcos. "The Origins of Primary Health Care and Selective Primary Care." *American Journal of Public Health* 94, no. 11 (2004): 1868–70.

Davis, Paxton. *A Boy's War.* Winston-Salem, NC: J. F. Blair, 1990.

Ding, Weiliang (W. A. P. Martin), Shen Hong, Yun Wenjie, and Hao Tianhu, trans. *Huajia jiyi—yiwei Meiguo chuanjiaoshi yanzhong de wan Qing diguo* [Recollections from 60 years on: The late Qing Empire from the perspective of an American missionary]. 1896. Reprint, Guangxi: Normal University Press, 2004.

Dirlik, Arif. "Reversals, Ironies, Hegemonies: Notes on the Contemporary Historiography of Modern China." *Modern China* 22, no. 3 (July 1996): 243–84.

Dyer, Oliver-James, and Ayesha de Costa. "What Is Global Health?" *Journal of Global Health* 1, no. 1 (Spring 2011): 31–32.

Edgerton-Tarplay, Kathryn. *Tears from Iron: Cultural Responses to Famine in Nineteenth-Century China.* Berkeley: University of California Press, 2008.

Ehrlich, Paul. "Die Wertbemessung des Diphterie serums und deren theoretische Grundlagen" [The value assessment of diphtheria serums and their theoretical foundations]. *Klinische Jahrbuch* [Clinical yearbook] 6 (1897): 299–326.

Elshakry, Marwa. "When Science Became Western: Historiographical Reflections." *Isis* 101 (2010): 98–109.

Eyler, John M. *Victorian Social Medicine: The Ideas and Methods of William Farr.* Baltimore: Johns Hopkins University Press, 1979.

Fairbank, John K. *Trade and Diplomacy on the China Coast: The Opening of the Treaty Ports, 1842–1854.* Stanford, CA: Stanford University Press, 1953.

Fan, Fa-ti. *British Naturalists in Qing China: Science, Empire and Cultural Encounter.* Cambridge, MA: Harvard University Press, 2004.

Fang, Xiaoping. *Barefoot Doctors and Western Medicine in China.* Rochester, NY: University of Rochester Press, 2012.

———. "From Union Clinics to Barefoot Doctors: Healers, Medical Pluralism and State Medicine in Chinese Villages, 1950–1970." *Journal of Modern Chinese History* 2, no. 2 (December 2008): 221–37.

Fenner, Frank. *Smallpox and Its Eradication.* Geneva: World Health Organization, 1988.

Ferguson, Mary E. *China Medical Board and Peking Union Medical College: A Chronicle of Fruitful Collaboration, 1914–1951.* New York: China Medical Board of New York, 1970.

Finnane, Antonia. *Changing Clothes in China: Fashion, History, Nation.* New York: Columbia University Press, 2008.

Fitzgerald, John. *Awakening China: Politics, Culture, and Class in the Nationalist Revolution*. Stanford, CA: Stanford University Press, 1996.

Fosdick, Raymond. *The Story of the Rockefeller Foundation*. New York: Harper & Brothers, 1952.

Frank, Andre Gunder. *On Capitalist Underdevelopment*. Oxford: Oxford University Press, 1976.

Frank, Andre Gunder, Sing C. Chew, and Robert Allen Denemark. *The Development of Underdevelopment: Essays in Honor of Andre Gunder Frank*. Armonk, NY: Sage Publications, 1999.

Fu Hui and Deng Zongyu. "The Struggle between the German-Japanese Group and the Anglo-American Group." In Wenshi ziliao xuanji bianjibu, *Wenshi Ziliao Xuanji*, vol. 119, 64–74. Bejing: Zhongguo Wenshi Chubanshe, 1989.

Furth, Charlotte. *A Flourishing Yin: Gender in China's Medical History, 960–1665*. Berkeley: University of California Press, 1999.

Fuyi, Luo, Ruth Rogaski, and Xiang Lei, trans. *Weisheng de xiandai xing: Zhongguo tongshang kou'an weisheng yu jibing de hanyi* [The modernization of hygiene: The meaning of hygiene and disease in China's treaty ports]. Nanjing: Jiangsu People's Press, 2007.

Gamsa, Mark. "The Epidemic of Pneumonic Plague in Manchuria, 1910–1911." *Past and Present* 190 (2006): 147–83.

Gao, Xi. *Dezhen zhuan: Yige Yingguo chuanjiaoshi yu wan Qing yixue jindai hua* [A biography of John Dudgeon: An English missionary and the modernization of late Qing medicine]. Shanghai: Fudan University Press, 2009.

Glosser, Susan. *Chinese Visions of Family and State, 1915–1953*. Berkeley: University of California Press, 2003.

Gong Chun. "Woguo jinbainian lai de yixue jiaoyu" [The last hundred years of Western medical education in China]. *Zhonghua yishi zazhi* 12, no. 4 (1982): 209.

Goodman, Bryna, and David Goodman, eds. *Twentieth-Century Colonialism and China: Localities, the Everyday, and the World*. New York: Routledge, 2012.

Grypma, Sonya. *Healing Henan: Canadian Nurses at the North China Mission, 1888–1947*. Vancouver: University of British Columbia Press, 2008.

Hamashita, Takeshi. *Trade and Finance in Late Imperial China: Maritime Customs and Open Port Market Zones*. Singapore: Singapore University Press, 1989.

Hamlin, Christopher. *The Cholera Stigma and the Challenge of Interdisciplinary Epistemology: From Bengal to Haiti*. London: Routledge, 2010.

Hanson, Marta. *Speaking of Epidemics in Chinese Medicine: Disease and the Geographic Imagination in Late Imperial China*. New York: Routledge, 2011.

Harrell, Paula. *Sowing the Seeds of Change: Chinese Students, Japanese Teachers, 1895–1905*. Stanford, CA: Stanford University Press, 1992.

Harrison, Henrietta. "Rethinking Missionaries and Medicine in China: The Miracles of Assunta Pallotta, 1905–2005." *Journal of Asian Studies* 71 (2012): 127–48.

Harrison, Mark. *Contagion: How Commerce Has Spread Disease*. New Haven, CT: Yale University Press, 2012.

Hayhoe, Ruth. *China's Education and the Industrialized World: Studies in Cultural Transfer*. Shanghai: Shanghai People's Publishing House, 1990.

Haynes, Douglas M. *Imperial Medicine: Patrick Manson and the Conquest of Tropical Disease*. Philadelphia: University of Pennsylvania Press, 2001.

He Xiaolian. "The Social Status of Western Medical Doctors in Modern Shanghai." *Social Science* (Shanghai) 8 (August 2009): 137.

———. *Xiyi dongjian yu wenhua tiaoshi* [Western medicine's eastern advance and cultural accommodation]. Shanghai: Shanghai Guji Chubanshe, 2006.

Hershatter, Gail. *The Gender of Memory: Rural Women and China's Collective Past.* Berkeley: University of California Press, 2014.

Hevia, James. *English Lessons: The Pedagogy of Imperialism in Nineteenth-Century China.* Durham, NC: Duke University Press, 2003.

Hinrich, Larissa. *The Afterlife of Images: Translating the Pathological Body between China and the West.* Durham, NC: Duke University Press, 2008.

Hu Cheng. *Yiliao, weisheng yu shijie zhi zhongguo: Kua guohe kua wenhua shiyu zhi xia de lishi yanjiu* [Medicine, hygiene and China in the world: A transnational and transcultural history study]. Beijing: Kexue Publishing, 2013.

Hu, Guotai. *Yu Huo Chong Sheng: Kangzhan Shiqi de Gaodeng Jiaoyu* [Reborn of fire: Higher education during the Second Sino-Japanese War]. Taipei: Daoxiang Press, 2004.

Huang, Shanqi. *Xiangya lao gushi* [Old stories of Yale-in-China]. Changsha: Central South University Press, 2012.

Iliffe, John. *East African Doctors: A History of the Modern Profession.* Cambridge: Cambridge University Press, 1998.

Isaacs, Harold. *Scratches on Our Minds: American Images of China and India.* New York: John Day, 1958.

Isao, Sugimoto, ed. *History of Science in Japan.* Translated by Zheng Pengnian. Beijing: Commercial Press, 1999.

Israel, John. *Lianda: A Chinese University in War and Revolution.* Stanford, CA: Stanford University Press, 1998.

Janssens, P. G., M. Kivits, and J. Vuylsteke, eds. *Health in Central Africa.* Brussels: King Baudouin Foundation, 1997.

Jensen, Kimberly. *Mobilizing Minerva: American Women in the First World War.* Urbana: University of Illinois Press, 2008.

Jesperson, T. Christopher. *American Images of China, 1931–1949.* Stanford, CA: Stanford University Press, 1996.

Jing Jun. *Dingxian shiyan: Shequ yixue yu huabei nongcun* [The Ding County experiment: Community medicine and rural North China]. Beijing: Qinghua University Department of Sociology, 2004.

Jones, David Martin. *The Image of China in Western Social and Political Thought.* New York: Palgrave Macmillan, 2001.

Kao Tien and Ha Hongchien. "Taiwan jiepou ji kao" [Anatomy cadaver ceremonies in Taiwan]. *Zhonghua yishi zazhi* 29, no. 3 (1999): 175–77.

Keishuu, Sanetou. *History of Chinese Students in Japan.* Translated by Lin Qiyan and Tan Ruqian. Beijing: SDX Joint Publishing Company, 1983.

Kickbush, I. "The Need for a European Strategy on Global Health." *Scandivanian Journal of Public Health* 34 (2006): 561–65.

Kim, Hoi-eun. *Doctors of Empire: Medical and Cultural Encounters between Imperial Germany and Meiji Japan.* Toronto: University of Toronto Press, 2014.

Kirby, William. *Germany and Republican China.* Stanford, CA: Stanford University Press, 1984.

Ko, Dorothy. *Cinderella's Sisters: A Revisionist History of Footbinding.* Berkeley: University of California Press, 2005.

Koplan, J. P., T. C. Bond, M. H. Merson, K. S. Reddy, M. H. Rodriguez, N. K. Sewankambo, J. N. Wasserheit, for the Consortium of Universities for Global Health Executive Board. "Towards a Common Definition of Global Health." *Lancet* 373 (2009): 1993–95.

Kusama, Yoshio. "Medical Education in Japan." *Journal of Medical Education* 31, no. 6 (June 1956): 393–98.

Ladurie, Emmanuel Le Roy. *The Mind and Method of the Historian.* Chicago: University of Chicago Press, 1984.

Lary, Diana. *The Chinese People at War: Human Suffering and Social Transformation, 1937–1945.* Cambridge: Cambridge University Press, 2010.

Lei, Sean Hsiang-lin. "From Changshan to a New Anti-Malarial Drug: Re-Networking Chinese Drugs and Excluding Chinese Doctors." *Social Studies of Science* 29, no. 3 (1999): 323–58.

———. "Habituating Individuality: Framing Tuberculosis and Its Material Solutions in Republican China." *Bulletin for the History of Medicine* 84 (2010): 248–79.

———. *Neither Donkey nor Horse: Medicine in the Struggle over China's Modernity.* Chicago: University of Chicago Press, 2014.

Lesch, John E. *The First Miracle Drugs: How the Sulfa Drugs Transformed Medicine.* Oxford: Oxford University Press, 2007.

Leung, Angela Ki Che. *Leprosy in China: A History.* New York: Columbia University Press, 2009.

———. "Organized Medicine in Ming-Qing China: State and Private Medical Institutions in the Lower Yangzi Region." *Late Imperial China* 8, no. 1 (1987): 134–66.

———. "Yiliao shi yu zhongguo xiandai xing wenti" [The history of medicine and the problem of modernity in contemporary China]. *Zhongguo shehui lishi pinglun* [Chinese social history review], vol. 8. Tianjin: Tianjin guiji chubanshe, 2007.

Leung, Angela Ki Che, and Charlotte Furth, eds. *Health and Hygiene in Chinese East Asia: Policies and Publics in the Long Twentieth Century.* Durham, NC: Duke University Press, 2010.

Li Chuanbin. Tiaoyue tequan zhidu *xia de yiliao shiye: Jidujiao zai hua yiliao shiye yanjiu (1835–1937)* [Healing activities under the unequal treaties: Research on Christian healing activities in China, 1835–1937]. Changsha: Hunan Renmin Chubanshe, 2010.

Li, Hongshan. *U.S.-China Educational Exchange: State, Society, and Intercultural Relations, 1905–1950.* New Brunswick, NJ: Rutgers University Press, 2008.

Li Shenglan. "Refashioning Care: Nursing, Intimacy, and Citizenship in Wartime China, 1930–1950." PhD diss., Binghampton University, 2017.

Li Wenhai, ed. *The Corpus of the Republican Social Survey.* Fuzhou: Fujian Education Press, 2005.

Liu, Lydia. *The Clash of Empires: The Invention of China in Modern World Making.* Cambridge, MA: Harvard University Press, 2004.

Liu, Michael Shiyung. *Prescribing Colonialization: The Role of Medical Practices and Policies in Japan-Ruled Taiwan, 1895–1945.* Ann Arbor, MI: Association of Asian Studies, 2009.

———. "The Ripples of Rivalry: The Spread of Modern Medicine from Japan to Its Colonies." *East Asian Science, Technology and Society* 2 (2008): 47–71.

Livingston, Julie. *Improvising Medicine: An African Oncology Ward in an Emerging Cancer Epidemic.* Durham, NC: Duke University Press, 2012.

Lo, Ming-cheng M. *Doctors within Borders: Profession, Ethnicity, and Modernity in Colonial Taiwan.* Berkeley: University of California Press, 2002.

Lorber, Judith. *Women Physicians: Careers, Status, and Power.* London: Tavistock Publications, 1984.

Lu Chunling, Matthew T. Schneider, Paul Gubbins, Katherine Leach-Kemon, Dean Jamison, and Christopher J. L. Murray. "Public Financing of Health in Developing Countries: A Cross-National Systematic Analysis." *Lancet* 375 (2010), 1375–87.

Lucas, AnElissa. *Chinese Medical Modernization: Comparative Policy Continuities, 1930–1980s.* Westport, CT: Praeger Publishers, 1982.

Luesink, David Nanson. "Dissecting Modernity: Anatomy and Power in the Language of Science in China." PhD diss., University of British Columbia–Vancouver, 2012.

Lutz, Jessie. *China and the Christian Colleges, 1850–1950.* Ithaca, NY: Cornell University Press, 1971.

Lyons, Maryinez. *The Colonial Disease: A Social History of Sleeping Sickness in Northern Zaire, 1900–1940.* Cambridge: Cambridge University Press, 1992.

Lyons, Thomas P. *China Maritime Customs and China's Trade Statistics, 1859–1948.* Trumansburg, NY: Willow Creek of Trumansburg, 2003.

Macfarlane, S. B., M. Jacobs, and E. E. Kaaya. "In the Name of Global Health: Trends in Academic Institutions." *Journal of Public Health Policy* 29 (2008): 383–401.

McKeown, Thomas H. *The Role of Medicine: Dream, Mirage, or Nemesis?* Princeton, NJ: Princeton University Press, 1980.

———. *The Modern Rise of Population.* New York: Academic Press, 1976.

Minden, Karen. *Bamboo Stone: The Evolution of a Chinese Medical Elite.* Toronto: University of Toronto Press, 1994.

Mu Jingjiang. *Minguo xiyi gaodeng jiaoyu (1912–1949)* [Advanced medical education in Republican China, 1912–1949]. Hangzhou: Zhejiang Gongshang University Press, 2012.

Murdock, Michael. *Disarming the Allies of Imperialism: Agitation, Manipulation, and the State during China's Nationalist Revolution, 1922–1929.* Ithaca, NY: Cornell University Press, 2006.

Osterhammel, Jürgen. "'Technical Co-operation' between the League of Nations and China." *Modern Asian Studies* 13, no. 4 (1979): 661–80.

Ou, Ge. *Xieheyishi* [Medical Affairs at Peking Union Medical College]. Beijing: Sanlian Book Co., 2007.

Patrick, Stewart M. *Weak Links: Fragile States, Global Threats, and International Security.* New York: Oxford University Press, 2011.

Peckham, Robert, and David M. Pomfret. *Imperial Contagions: Medicine, Hygiene, and Cultures of Planning in Asia.* Hong Kong: Hong Kong University Press, 2013.

Petitjean, Patrick, Catherine Jami, and A. M. Moulin, eds. *Science and Empires: Historical Studies about Scientific Development and European Expansion.* New York: Springer, 1992.

Phillips-Johnson, Tina. *Childbirth in Republican China: Delivering Modernity.* Lanham, MD: Lexington Books, 2011.

Pomeranz, Kenneth. *The Making of a Hinterland: State, Society, and Economy in Inland North China, 1853–1937.* Berkeley: University of California Press, 1993.

Porter, Roy, ed. *The Cambridge Illustrated History of Medicine.* Cambridge: Cambridge University Press, 1996.

———. *The Greatest Benefit to Mankind: A Medical History of Humanity from Antiquity to the Present.* New York: Norton, 1997.

Prost, André. *Services de santé en pays africain: Leur place dans des structures socio-économiques en voie de développement.* Paris: Masson, 1970.

Qiusha, Ma. *To Change China: The Rockefeller Foundation's Century-Long Journey in China.* Guilin: Guangxi Normal University Press, 2013.

Quataert, Jean. "Gendered Medical Services in Red Cross Field Hospitals during the First Balkan War and World War I." In *Peace, War and Gender from Antiquity to the Present: Cross-Cultural Perspectives,* ed. Jost Dulffer and Robert Frank, 219–33. Essen: Klartext Verlag, 2009.

Renshaw, Michelle. *Accommodating the Chinese: The American Hospital in China, 1880–1920.* New York: Routledge, 2005.

Reynolds, Douglas. *China, 1898–1912: The Xinzheng Revolution and Japan.* Cambridge, MA: Council on East Asian Studies, Harvard University, 1993.

Rogaski, Ruth. *Hygienic Modernity: Meanings of Health and Disease in Treaty-Port China.* Berkeley: University of California Press, 2004.

Ruiting, Huang. *Fayi qingtian: Lin Ji fayi shengya lu* [A righteous medico-legal expert: A record of the career of the medico-legal expert Lin Ji]. Beijing: Shijie tushu chuban gongsi, 1995.

Sanetō, Keishū. *Zhongguo ren liuxue riben shi* [History of Chinese students in Japan]. Translated by Lin Qiyan and Tan Ruqian. Beijing: Beijing University Press, 2012.

Scheid, Volker. *Currents of Tradition in Chinese Medicine: 1626–2006.* Seattle: Eastland Press, 2007.

Schneider, Laurence. *Biology and Revolution in Twentieth-Century China.* New York: Rowman and Littlefield, 2005.

Schneider, William. *History of Blood Transfusion in Sub-Saharan Africa.* Athens: Ohio University Press, 2013.

———. "Smallpox in Africa during Colonial Rule." *Medical History* 53 (2009): 193–228.

Schoppa, Keith. *In a Sea of Bitterness: Refugees during the Sino-Japanese War.* Cambridge, MA: Harvard University Press, 2011.

Shemo, Connie. *The Chinese Medical Ministries of Kang Cheng and Shi Meiyu, 1872–1937.* Lehigh, PA: Lehigh University Press, 2011.

Shu, Yang. "Plans for Studying in Japan." In *Resources for the History of Chinese Modern Education,* ed. Chen Xueyun, vol. 1. Beijing: People's Education Press, 1987.

Silverstein, Arthur. *History of Immunology.* London: Elsevier, 1989.

———. "History of Immunology: Cellular versus Humoral Immunity; Determinants and Consequences of an Epic 19th-Century Battle." *Cellular Immunology* 48 (1979): 208–21.

Sivin, Nathan, ed. *Science and Technology in East Asia.* New York: Science History Publications, 1977.

———, ed. *Traditional Medicine in Contemporary China*. Ann Arbor: University of Michigan Center for Chinese Studies, 1987.

Spence, Jonathan D. *To Change China: Western Advisers in China*. New York: Penguin, 1980.

———. *The Chan's Great Continent: China in Western Minds*. New York: Norton, 1990.

Starr, Paul. *The Social Transformation of American Medicine: The Rise of a Sovereign Profession and the Making of a Vast Industry*. New York: Basic Books, 1982.

Summers, William C. *The Great Manchurian Plague of 1910–1911: The Geopolitics of an Epidemic Disease*. New Haven, CT: Yale University Press, 2012.

Sun Daixing and Wu Baozhang, eds. *Yunnan kangri zhanzheng shi: A History of Anti-Japanese War in Yunnan*. Kunming, China: Yunnan daxue chubanshe, 2005.

Takahashi, Aya. *The Development of the Japanese Nursing Profession: Adopting and Adapting Western Influences*. London: Routledge Curzon, 2004.

Taylor, Kim. *Chinese Medicine in Early Communist China, 1945–63: A Medicine of Revolution*. London: Routledge Curzon, 2005.

Thomas, Lewis. *The Youngest Science: Notes of a Medicine-Watcher*. New York: Viking, 1983.

Trescott, Paul B. "H. D. Fong and the Study of Chinese Economic Development." *History of Political Economy* 34, no. 4 (2002): 789–809.

Unschuld, Paul. *Medicine in China: A History of Ideas*. 1985. Reprint, Berkeley: University of California Press, 2010.

Vuic, Kara Dixon. *Officer, Nurse, Women: The Army Nurse Corps in the Vietnam War*. Baltimore: Johns Hopkins University Press, 2010.

Waley-Cohen, Joanna. "China and Western Technology in the Late Eighteenth Century." *American Historical Review* 98, no. 5 (1993): 1525–44.

Wang Hsiu-yun. "Refusing Male Physicians: The Gender and Body Politics of Missionary Medicine in China, 1870s–1920s." *Bulletin of the Institute of Modern History, Academia Sinica* 59 (2008): 29–67.

Wang Yi Chu. *Chinese Intellectuals and the West, 1872–1949*. Chapel Hill: University of North Carolina Press, 1966.

Wang Zheng. *Women in the Chinese Enlightenment: Oral and Textual Histories*. Berkeley: University of California Press, 1999.

Watt, John R. *A Friend in Deed: ABMAC and the Republic of China, 1937–1987*. New York: American Bureau of Medical Aid to China, 1992.

———. "Public Medicine in Wartime China: Biomedicine, State Medicine, and the Rise of China's National Medical Colleges, 1931–1945." Rosenberg Institute Occasional Paper No. 1, 70–71. Boston: Rosenberg Institute for East Asian Studies, Suffolk University, 2012.

———. *Saving Lives in Wartime China: How Medical Reformers Built Modern Healthcare Systems amid War and Epidemics, 1928–1945*. Leiden: Brill, 2014.

Webb, James, and Tamara Giles-Vernick. *Global Health in Africa: Historical Perspectives on Disease Control*. Athens: Ohio University Press, 2013.

Wendland, Claire. *A Heart for the Work: Journeys through an African Medical School*. Chicago: University of Chicago Press, 2010.

Weston, Timothy B. *The Power of Position: Beijing University, Intellectuals, and Chinese Political Culture, 1898–1929*. Berkeley: University of California Press, 2004.

Wong, K. Chi-min, and Wu Lien-teh. *History of Chinese Medicine*. Shanghai: National Quarantine Service, 1936.

World Bank. *Accelerated Development in Sub-Saharan Africa: An Agenda for Action.* Washington, DC: World Bank, 1981.

Wu, Yi-Li. *Reproducing Women: Medicine, Metaphor, and Childbirth in Late Imperial China.* Berkeley: University of California Press, 2010.

Wu Songdi. "Cognition and Utilization of Chinese Traditional Maritime Customs Trade Return." *Journal of Historical Science,* no. 7 (2007): 33.

———. "An Essay on the Publications of the Chinese Imperial Maritime Customs." *Journal of Historical Science,* no. 12 (2011): 54–63.

Wyman, Judith. "The Ambiguities of Chinese Antiforeignism: Chongqing, 1870–1900." *Late Imperial China* 18, no. 2 (December 1998): 86–122.

Xiaoli Tian. "Rumor and Secret Space: Organ-Snatching Tales and Medical Missions in Nineteenth-Century China." *Modern China* (March 2014): 1–40.

Xu, Xiaoqun. *Chinese Professionals and the Republican State: The Rise of Professional Associations in Shanghai, 1912–1937.* Cambridge: Cambridge University Press, 2001.

Xu Youchun, *Minguo renwu da cidian* [Biographical dictionary of Republican China]. Shijiazhuang: Hebei renmin chubanshe, 1991.

Yach, Derek, and Douglas Bettcher. "The Globalization of Public Health, I: Threats and Opportunities." *American Journal of Public Health* 88 (1998): 735–38.

———. "The Globalization of Public Health, II: The Convergence of Self-Interest and Altruism." *American Journal of Public Health* 88 (1998): 738–41.

Yang Nianqun. *Zaizao "Bingren": Zhongxi yi chongtu xia de kongjian zhengzhi* [Remaking "Patients": Spatial politics in the conflict between Chinese and Western medicine]. Beijing: China Renmin University Press, 2006.

Ye Weili. *Seeking Modernity in China's Name.* Stanford, CA: Stanford University Press, 2001.

Yeh, Wen-Hsin. *The Alienated Academy: Culture and Politics in Republican China, 1919–1937.* Cambridge, MA: Harvard University Press, 1990.

Yip, Ka-che. *Disease, Colonialism and the State: Malaria in Modern East Asian History.* Hong Kong: Hong Kong University Press, 2009.

———. "Health and Nationalist Reconstruction: Rural Health in Nationalist China, 1928–1937." *Modern Asian Studies* 26, no. 2 (May 1992): 395–415.

———. *Health and National Reconstruction in Nationalist China: The Development of Modern Health Services, 1928–1937.* Ann Arbor, MI: Association for Asian Studies, 1995.

Young, Theron Kue-Hing. "A Conflict of Professions: The Medical Missionary in China, 1835–1890." *Bulletin of the History of Medicine* 47 (1973): 250–72.

Yu Xinzhong. "Guanzhu shengming—Haixia liang an xinqqi jibing yiliao shehui shi yanjiu" [Saving lives—the rise of historical research into disease and medicine on both sides of the Taiwan Strait]. *Zhongguo shehui jingji shi yanjiu* [Journal of Chinese social and economic history] 3 (2002): 94–98.

———. "Hewei weisheng: Zhongguo jinshi weisheng shi yanjiu chuyi" [What is hygiene? My humble opinion on the historiography of hygiene in China]. *Research on the Theory of History* 4 (2011): 133–41.

———. *Qingdai Jiangnan de wenyi yu shehui: Yi xiang yiliao shehui she de yanjiu* [Epidemics and society in Qing Jiangnan]. Beijing: Beijing Normal University, 2014.

———. *Qingdai weisheng fangyi jizhi jiqi jindai yanbian* [Qing-era hygienic prevention mechanisms and their modern transformation]. Beijing: Beijing shifan daxue chubanshe, 2016.

————. "Writing about a Different Kind of Medical History: A Critical Review of *Zaizao "Bingren"* by Yang Nianqun." Translated by Li Yi. *Journal of Modern Chinese History* 1, no. 2 (2007): 239–48.

Zhang Daqing. *Zhongguo jindai jibing shehui shi* [A social history of diseases in modern China]. Jinan: Shandong Jiaoyu chubanshe, 2006.

Zhang Mingdao, ed. *Shanghai weisheng zhi* [Annals of Shanghai public health]. Shanghai: Shanghai Academy of Social Sciences Press, 1998.

Zhao, Hongjun. *History of the Modern Controversies over Chinese vs. Western Medicine.* Hefei: Anhui kexu Jishu chubanshe, 1989.

Zhou, Yong, ed. *Chongqing tongshi* [General history of Chongqing]. Vol. 3 of *A Comprehensive History of Chongqing.* Chongeqing: Chongqing Press, 2002.

Contributors

DANIEL ASEN is assistant professor of history at Rutgers University–Newark.

NICOLE ELIZABETH BARNES is assistant professor of history at Duke University.

MARY AUGUSTA BRAZELTON is university lecturer in global studies of science, technology, and medicine in the Department of History and Philosophy of Science at the University of Cambridge.

GAO XI is professor of history at Fudan University in Shanghai.

HE XIAOLIAN is an independent scholar based in Ithaca, NY.

LI SHENGLAN is assistant professor of history at Wheaton College in Massachusetts.

DAVID LUESINK is assistant professor of history at Sacred Heart University in Connecticut.

WILLIAM H. SCHNEIDER is professor emeritus of history and medical humanities at Indiana University Purdue University Indianapolis.

SHI YAN is senior editor at the People's Education Press in Beijing.

YU XINZHONG is professor of history at Nankai University in Tianjin.

ZHANG DAQING is professor and director, Institute of Medical Humanities at Peking University in Beijing.

Index

CCP and, 208n31; Chen Zhiqian and, 215–21, 223, 225–27, 231n61; education and training, 128n48, 160, 191; exhibition, 71; facilities, 56; groups, 206; history of, 18, 37; imperialism, 6; Janus-faced nature of, 17; Japanese influence, 103n10; magazine, 212; McKeown, Thomas, and scholarly debates, 230n42; nursing and, 165, 173–75; personnel, 22; politicization of, 18; research, 184; stations, 200; systems, 37, 40, 42–46; teams, 201; vital statistics and, 58, 69

Qilu University Medical College. *See* Cheeloo University
Qing Dynasty (government, state), 2–3, 7–12, 17, 24, 63, 72, 86, 115, 134, 170, 190; court dress, 71; Ministry of Education, 102n5; Qing-era forensic handbook, 99; Qing-era hygiene, 37–40, 43–44, 46
quarantine, 38, 42, 45; laissez-faire approach, 10

rabies, 192, 200, 202
racism, 236
Red Cross: American, 197, 227; Chinese, 149, 170, 185, 189, 197; International, 216; Japanese, 165
reform and opening up, 40
refugees, 14, 22, 160, 162, 164–65, 175, 186, 190
relapsing fever, 190, 225
Renji Hospital, 139–40
Republic of China (ROC), 8, 14, 81, 86, 151
rights, 43; collective, 23; equal, 135, 148; individual, 46–47; marriage, 11; of medical practitioners, 125n7; nurses, 172; women's, 150, 152
rituals, collective, 93–94
Rockefeller Foundation, 1, 12, 16, 20, 24–25, 88, 110, 113, 116–17, 121, 161, 184, 201, 205, 217–18, 237; Archives, 247; Chen Zhiqian and, 231

Rogaski, Ruth, 17, 160
Ross, Ronald, 232
rumors, 8, 150, 163
Russia, 2, 45, *55*; Boxer Indemnity, 128; Russo-Japanese War (1904–5), 112

sanitation, 220, 223; history of sanitization, 40, 42–44; public, 219, 227; urban, 174
SARS, 17, 235
"saving the nation," 81, 147
schistosomiasis, 225
science, 11, 90, 116, 232; education, 115; medical, 1–3, 25, 31n76, 42–43, 45–46, 52–53, 67, 81–82, 91, 113, 117, 184, 190, 197; scientism, 152; technology and, 71; wartime, 205; Western, 232, 238n1, 240n19
scientization (*kexuehua*), 15
Second Sino-Japanese War. *See* war
semicolonial condition, 2, 6, 15, 20, 37, 84, 132
sera, 22–23, 183, 185, 189, 197, 200, 205–6
Shanghai, 9, 12–13, 17, 21, 38, 53–54, *55*, *58*, 69, 70, 73n23, 97, 107n62, 113, 131–33, 136–42, 144, 149–50, 152, 154n20, 186–87, 203–4, 218, 228n8; British and American settlements, 62; Customs Station, 50; Health Bureau, 140, 154n10; Municipal Council, 69, 77n85; Physicians Guild, 125n7; Police Bureau, 140
Shanghai Women's (Technical) Medical School (*Shanghai nuzi zhuanmen yixuexiao*), 89, *98*, 138
shanghan
Shi Meiyu (Mary Stone), 9, 133, 135, 142, 144, 245
Sichuan, 101, 162, 171, 215–16, 218–21, 224–26
Sichuan Provincial Health Administration (SPHA, *Sichuan sheng weishengchu*), 23, 215, 244
Sick Man of East Asia, 10, 40, 82
Simmons, Duane B., 54, 66–67, 69

Printed in the United States
By Bookmasters